Happy
Hours

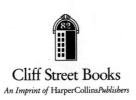

Cliff Street Books

An Imprint of HarperCollins*Publishers*

Happy Hours

Alcohol in a Woman's Life

DEVON JERSILD

The names of women in recovery have been changed to protect their privacy. In some cases, other identifying details have also been altered.

HarperCollins books may be purchased for educational, business, or sales promotional use. For information please write: Special Markets Department, HarperCollins Publishers Inc., 10 East 53rd Street, New York, NY 10022.

FIRST EDITION

DESIGNED BY DEBORAH KERNER

Printed on acid-free paper

Library of Congress Cataloging-in-Publication Data

Jersild, Devon.
    Happy Hours : alcohol in a woman's life / by Devon Jersild.
        p.   cm.
    Includes bibliographical references.
    ISBN 0-06-019268-2
    1. Women alcoholics.   2. Women—Alcohol use.   3. Alcoholism—
Treatment.   I. Title.

HV5137 .J47 2000
362.292'082—dc21   00–035880

00   01   02   03   04   RRD   10   9   8   7   6   5   4   3   2   1

*To the memory of
my mother,
and to my father
and Dee*

Contents

Acknowledgments

I AM DEEPLY GRATEFUL TO THE WOMEN IN RECOVERY WHO shared their stories with me. I learned far more than I expected to learn, and not just about problems with alcohol. These women taught me to look at my own life in a new way. Their stories, whether or not they appear in these pages, are close to my heart.

I am indebted to the many clinicians, researchers, scientists, and psychologists who took time to talk with me and, in many cases, sent me copies of their research. Among these, I owe particular thanks to Sharon Wilsnack, who was endlessly gracious; to Claudia Bepko, Diane Byington, Rita Teusch, Elizabeth Zelvin, Sylvia Staub, George Lewis, and Leslie Ann Sparks, who shared their clinical experience; to John Searles and Henri Begleiter, for clarifications of scientific material; and to Sheila Blume, who answered questions and challenged me in helpful ways. Whatever errors appear are my own.

My agent, Geri Thoma, supported me from this project's inception and guided me wisely throughout. I relied on her good spirits, energy, and insight. My editor, Diane Reverand, communicated her confidence in the book, and this sustained me at crucial moments. I am grateful to Diane and Janet Dery for editorial direction. Early on, Tricia Welsch told me to scrap my impossible outline and write about what interested me; for listening deeply, I thank her. Michael Lowenthal, Pamela Erens, Yonna McShane, Linda Meyers, Audrey Galex, and Joyce Henderson read drafts of the manuscript at different stages and gave me essential feedback. Shauna Hill, Christina Norris-Watts, and Eric Munson were resourceful, reliable, and patient research assistants. At the copyediting stage, Susan Gamer's astute and sensitive work improved the book significantly.

I appreciate the generosity of family members and friends who gave me lodging and comfort on research trips and writing retreats, especially Tom and Kathleen Strombeck, Lola Van Wagenen and George Burrill, Mary Kelley and Phil Pochoda. Thanks also to the Bishop Booth Episcopal Retreat Center.

My father, Harold, was a loving background presence throughout this project, as he has been all of my life. My stepmother, Dee, has for years supported me more than she knows, with her enthusiasm and her unfailing interest.

Thanks to my husband, Jay Parini, for his loving attention, for giving me time and space, for offering counsel when I needed it, and for caring, always. Nothing was too big for him to help me with, and nothing was too small. For coping cheerfully with my absences, more thanks to Jay and to our children—Leo, who missed me; and Will and Oliver, who swear they didn't. I am glad for their ebullient presence and even their interruptions.

Without Polly Young-Eisendrath, I could not have carried this book through, or even imagined writing it. I am grateful beyond words.

During the three years I worked on this book, I became aware of how much I am supported by dear friends, some close at hand, some very far away. I have relied on our shared meals, walks, and conversations. Their encouragement and love have made me feel very much blessed.

Special thanks to my sister, Carri, for her generous spirit, her loyalty, and her willingness to share her story, which is so much a part of mine.

Foreword

IN *HAPPY HOURS*, DEVON JERSILD'S ELOQUENT RENDER-
ing of the stories of women and their alcohol problems is supported by
her research in the field of alcohol studies. She has captured this huge
literature in an engaging and scientifically objective manner, and she
has woven the information into an enlightening, moving, and em-
pathic book.

   Her subject is important to all of us, whether or not we ourselves
drink. The women in *Happy Hours* are our friends and neighbors, the
driver of the car next to us on the highway, the patient being taken to
the hospital in the ambulance for whom we pull over to the side of the
road, the surgeon who will operate on that patient, and the nurse who
will monitor her vital signs. *Happy Hours* is about the teachers and
coaches and school bus drivers to whom we entrust our children. Devon
Jersild introduces us to these women and to alcohol.

   When we contemplate how deeply alcohol is embedded in American culture, it is easy to conclude that nearly all Americans drink. But
that isn't so. As of 1990, over 40 percent of American women and
nearly 30 percent of men reported that they did not use alcohol, so the
guest next to you at the party may very well be drinking club soda or
ginger ale. There are many reasons that people choose not to drink.

Some abstain for religious reasons, but most do so for reasons of health. Alcoholism is a disease that runs in families. Both those who suffer from the disease and those at high genetic risk because of alcoholism in the family are safest if they do not drink. Others may wish to abstain to avoid "empty calories," the dangers of drinking during pregnancy, or the interaction of alcohol and medications. Finally, there are the millions of men and women who have had problems related to alcohol and have chosen to give up drinking, sometimes easily but often in an intense and ongoing struggle—a life-and-death conflict.

Many of these men and women (especially women) have been my patients during the thirty-eight years of my career in addiction medicine. Like the women you will meet in *Happy Hours*, they have come from all walks of life and developed their alcohol problems at varying ages, from childhood to postretirement. What they share is an all-consuming love-hate relationship with their drug of choice, and the increasing knowledge that the substance that has been their best friend will kill them if they don't stop using it.

Like most physicians, I learned almost nothing about alcoholism during my medical education. As an honors graduate of Harvard Medical School in the late 1950s, I began my career without a working knowledge of addiction. Not that we didn't treat alcoholics at Harvard. We learned most of our medicine and surgery treating alcoholic patients for the complications of their alcoholism, everything from trauma to infertility, and we learned about the effects of ethyl alcohol on organs and tissues. But we never learned why alcoholics drink or how to help them stop.

I recall vividly the first patient I saw as a third-year student in the neurology clinic. He was a seaman in his forties, with tattoos on both forearms. He came to the clinic after having had a seizure, and it was my job to discover why. After a history and physical examination, I made a diagnosis of rum fits (alcohol withdrawal seizures) and presented the case to my professor. I was praised for the thoroughness and accuracy of my work, although neither my professor nor I seemed to think it was part of our duty to intervene in the man's alcoholism, and we made no referral for that purpose. In fact, at that time standard medical histories often began, "This thirty-eight-year-old alcoholic male comes to the hospital complaining of abdominal pain . . ." or "This fifty-eight-year-old alcoholic woman with a history of multiple abdominal surgery . . ." The word "alcoholic" was merely a descriptor, like "French," or "Presbyterian." It carried no implication that we were responsible for treating it.

With this educational background and an internship in pediatrics I began a residency training in psychiatry on September 9, 1962, and also began my lifelong fascination with alcoholism in women. I arrived on that day at Central Islip State Hospital, a 10,000-bed facility on Long Island in New York. My assignment was the women's admission service. Unfortunately, my slender background in psychiatry at Harvard had been limited to an introduction to psychoanalytic concepts, and I found little application to the group of twenty-five desperately ill women who were put in my care. I had been taught that I should regularly spend a "fifty-minute hour" with each patient, but this was not possible. I selected the patient who seemed to be the most sick and the one who seemed least sick, and I spent as much time as possible with them, to learn. For the others, I did as my colleagues did, prescribing the few medications available to us, giving advice, and charting their progress.

The woman I had chosen as least sick was an elementary school teacher who suffered from alcoholism. Like many of the women in *Happy Hours*, she was desperate to stop drinking, but neither she nor I knew how she could do so. As I struggled to understand her problem, I learned that the hospital had little to offer her other than our sessions together. There was no medication that would help her quest for sobriety, and the environment designed for psychotic patients was absolutely boring for her. After several weeks, I did what any good student would do. I made an appointment to see the chief of service and asked for help. His two-word answer set me on my lifelong career. He said, "Why bother?"

This attitude toward alcoholics was not unusual in the 1960s. By "why bother?" he meant two things: that I should spend my energies on a truly worthy person rather than a drunk, and that you can't help those people anyway. Alcoholism was seen as hopeless. I didn't see it that way. I left vowing that I would help her get well. I went to the library and read the little there was about alcoholism in the textbooks. I was lucky that the hospital had a book by a layperson, *Marty Mann's New Primer on Alcoholism*. Marty Mann was the first woman to recover in Alcoholics Anonymous and had later founded the National Council on Alcoholism. Her book made sense of my patient's symptoms, and she considered alcoholism a treatable disease. Shortly afterward, I started a group for alcoholic women in the hospital, unaware that it was probably the first program for alcoholic women in the state system. I discovered that there was an AA meeting in our hospital (on the men's unit, for men only). With great effort, I was able to open it to the members of my group. I'm glad to report that the first patient eventually got well, as did others in the group, though unfortunately not all of them. I learned that overcoming alcoholism is a lifelong task, but a rewarding one that is well worth the effort.

Later, I was given the job of running a newly opened alcoholism rehabilitation unit at the hospital (for men, as I learned most alcoholism programs were), but I took the job only on the condition that we develop one for women. In 1968, we opened that first women's unit, and I ran both of them until they merged in the 1970s. In 1979, I was appointed a state commissioner, director of the New York State Division of Alcohol Abuse and Alcoholism, a recently created agency. In that position I had the opportunity to influence the development of services throughout the state and to promote public policy initiatives that would benefit alcoholic women. After retiring from state service, I ran addiction programs in the private sector, again concentrating on developing responses to the needs of women and teaching this knowledge and skill to others. I felt that the wheel had turned full circle when the National Council on Alcoholism and Drug Dependence awarded me its Marty Mann Founder's Award in October 1999 for my work in advocacy for addicted women.

Throughout my year in the field, I felt that there was a need for a popular book on women and alcohol that portrayed women's drinking problems in all their complexity. *Happy Hours* is such a book. In it, Devon Jersild presents both the scientific facts and the human faces of drinking and alcoholism in women. The book reads true to me. I recommend it to you in the hope that it helps generate the understanding and help that these women so desperately need.

—SHEILA B. BLUME, M.D.

Happy
Hours

Introduction

TWO YEARS AGO, AS I WAS STARTING THIS BOOK, MY OLDER sister called me from a hospital where she had gone to dry out for the weekend. In a monotone of resignation and despair, she told me her blood alcohol level—0.36. (A friend had once told me that his blood alcohol was 0.29 after a dozen beers and several shots of tequila, so I could imagine what it took to pump hers up to 0.36.) She told me that withdrawal was agony; her mind and body were on fire. It felt like death. "If I had a dollar," she said, "I'd walk out and buy a beer. But I don't have any money."

When I hung up, I tried to get my bearings, but a part of me, as always, was stumbling in the dark with Carri. She was in grave danger—of accidents (there have been many), alcohol poisoning, organ damage, abuse by men, an early death. For a long time she had resisted the notion that she was alcoholic, but she was beyond that now. She drank, she said, because she couldn't stand the tension of being sober. During her last treatment (she's been treated three times), the doctors were unable to find an antidepressant that didn't give her panic attacks; they sent her back to her usual psychiatrist, who also had no luck. Sure enough, when depression came down on her three months later, she picked up the bottle again.

As a girl, she was full of spunk and grit. She organized neighborhood carnivals and collected large sums of money. In the summer,
when it got dark, she'd round us all up for games of Cops and Robbers.
She swam on a team. As a horsewoman, she entered jumping competi-
tions—the foul-mouthed trainer made the other girls cry, but Carri
grinned and shrugged it off. She loved the camera and jumped in front
of it at any opportunity. With her beauty, we all thought, she might
one day be a movie star. When company came, she'd play her guitar
and belt out songs from Peter, Paul, and Mary. My brother remembers
her making up dance routines to the Rolling Stones, crying "Hey, you!
Get off of my cloud!" She had a raucous, unladylike laugh, and a smart
answer to every question. She got good grades without studying. She
read fat books like *Gone with the Wind* with tears streaming down her
face.

Then came the storm of Carri's adolescence, which blew through
our family and very nearly tore us apart. She picked fights with my
brothers and me and knew just what to say to make us cry in fury. She
felt excluded by her girlfriends, and she wept over boys until the rest of
us wanted to wring her neck. She became obsessed with weight and
dieting. Moping about the house and staring into the mirror, she never
entered into any of the family fun. My mother, trying to counsel and
encourage her, was strained beyond endurance.

In *Reviving Ophelia,* Mary Pipher describes how common this loss
of resilience and optimism is among adolescent girls. "Just as planes
and ships disappear mysteriously into the Bermuda Triangle," she
writes, "so do the selves of girls go down in droves. They crash and
burn in a social and developmental Bermuda Triangle." Carri might
have crashed and burned in the best of circumstances, but in my family, she became a kind of scapegoat. I personally blamed her for all our
problems, especially the guilt that wore my parents down.

As the rest of us struggled to make sense of Carri's problems, we
didn't worry about her occasional alcohol binges—these were common
among high school students. Later, we were distracted from her drinking by more obvious chaos: marriage and divorce at age eighteen, col-

lege started and abandoned, jobs she didn't keep. In our minds, the problem was Carri, and her drinking was just another sign of her lack of self-discipline. In those days, there was less awareness of alcoholism. The word "alcoholic" conjured up a wino lying in the gutter—it certainly didn't apply to anyone we knew. Not, that is, until Carri was thirty and getting smashed every day.

Why did a child of such promise turn to food stamps and empty beer bottles? For twenty-some years, my family has struggled with this question. Was it low self-esteem that led Carri to the bottle, or did her addiction damage her sense of who she was? Which came first, the problem drinking, or the tumultuous relationship that ended in an early marriage and divorce? Did my sister's difficult relationship with my mother lead her to the bottle, or did the bottle turn her into an addict with an addict's personality, including the tendency to find excuses to explain her addiction in order to justify another drink? At the age of twenty, she had some frightening hallucinations. Were these the result of a mental disorder, or were they alcohol-induced? Was her drinking an attempt to medicate herself to relieve herself of depression, or did the depression grow out of the addiction?

Like most families of alcoholics, we had different "answers" at different times. I have seen similar swings of feelings and perceptions in the families of other women alcoholics. One day our sister or mother or child or wife is, through no fault of her own, the victim of a terrible disease; the next day it's her stubborn selfishness that got her where she is. Then all her problems can be traced to her sexual appetite. She is loving and generous, in spite of everything; she's hard-hearted and unnatural, intent on her own destruction; she is mentally ill and needs to be cared for like a child. Feelings swing from hostility to pity, from fear to love and compassion, from a desire to protect the drinker from herself and public scrutiny to a wish that she would walk into a snowbank and end it there.

In part, these perceptions and feelings vary wildly because the behavior of an alcoholic is changeable and confusing. But often our attitudes arise from our own assumptions. For instance:

How a woman ought to behave. When a drinking man gets boisterous, he's still acting like a man. He can get drunk and still be macho—maybe even more macho. But a drinking woman who gets loud or rude, who slurs her words or forgets to keep her knees together—well, is she really a *lady?* Because our expectations about femininity are still strong, people are often disgusted by a woman under the influence of alcohol—especially if her appearance becomes sloppy or she is openly sexual.

Our view of alcoholic women as sexually available. There is an ancient and persistent misconception that alcohol heightens sexual responsiveness in women. Though alcohol may help a drinker lose her inhibitions, it interferes with physiological sexual arousal, and women alcoholics are likely to lose interest in sex. If an alcoholic woman does engage in indiscriminate sex, she is scorned by society and even by her family. Her actions are dangerous and self-destructive, but instead of hearing a cry for help, or seeing her behavior as an expression of self-loathing, we shame and condemn her further. When she most needs help, she slips outside the range of our compassion. All alcoholic women are hurt by the stereotype of the fallen woman, which is summed up in the saying, "A man who drinks is a drunk, but a woman who drinks is a slut." Worse, alcoholic women are seen as fair targets for sexual aggression.

What we need—or want—from a woman. If a man stumbles home drunk when his children are asleep, he is likely to evoke disapproval. If a woman does the same thing, she's likely to evoke outrage and disbelief. We still think of women as the glue holding families together. We also depend on women to nurture us, and we become enraged when they fail to deliver.

What we think it means to be alcoholic. Until recently, alcoholism was considered a man's disease, and clinical studies about alcohol-related disorders were conducted almost entirely on men—in spite of the fact that at least 25 percent of alcoholics are women, and in spite of the fact that, physiologically, alcohol affects women differently from men. In the last few decades, we've made great progress in our knowledge about women's problem drinking, but we have a great deal more to learn. We need a better idea of why women use alcohol; what the risk factors are for problem drinking; how symptoms of abuse are exhibited; what the medical, social, and personal consequences are; what motivates women to seek treatment; and what their needs are in recovery.

As I researched this book, many people mentioned women alcoholics among their friends and relatives whose story they believed was unique. "My daughter is alcoholic, but you won't want to interview her," one woman told me. "She's not your typical case." This woman had been told that alcoholism has nothing to do with personality problems or life events. She believed her daughter's drinking, on the other hand, was completely intertwined with relationship problems, and with an effort to battle depression. Another woman said that her lesbian lover was an alcoholic, but not a "real" one—alcoholics, this woman had been told, are not physiologically capable of controlling their drinking, but her lover had no problem drinking moderately for over twenty years. Her abusive drinking began when her alcoholic mother came to visit, and memories of her traumatic past rose up and overwhelmed her. For years, I also imagined the complexity of my sister's case to be unique, but in my research and interviews for this book, I have discovered that thousands of women and their families have similar stories to tell.

Why does each woman's story seem to be an exception? Perhaps this is partly because when we think of an alcoholic, we still conjure up a man. He may be a businessman at a three-martini lunch, or a romantic drunken writer, or that wino in the gutter. If we are familiar with Alcoholics Anonymous, we may think of a man describing his experience, telling a classic story of drinking and recovery—though this is now a story women also tell. Often, the alcoholic starts off economically stable and productive; he is emotionally stable; his problem is physiological, without compounding psychological vulnerability or a hostile environment. He hits an identifiable bottom, and then he wants to get sober. He once had fellowship, family and friends, employment, dignity, and respect. Through AA, and by admitting his powerlessness over alcohol, he is capable of getting all this back. This tale of addiction and recovery has enormous value; thousands of people around the world have gotten sober when they took it to heart.

Many of the women I interviewed for this book tell their own version of this story in deeply moving detail. It is a story that offers hope and companionship. When it fits, it consoles the alcoholic by revealing that her problems are not, in fact, unique. Like many other people, she has a particular vulnerability to alcohol, which she cannot control. Other people have been in thrall to alcohol and have done the same crazy, humiliating things. They have suffered, but they have come through. The behavior they regret—whatever it may be—can be forgiven, and life can be rebuilt on sturdier ground, as long as they keep fresh in their minds how low they can sink if they take alcohol. This story has an archetypal shape, as well it might, since AA began as a Christian fellowship, and its twelve steps draw on the procedures of the evangelical Oxford Group—giving in to God, listening to God's direction, checking guidance, making restitution, and sharing. Within this framework, a life that was confused and chaotic takes on a human shape. At AA, when a woman tells her story and communicates it to others, she gives meaning to her life, and she can begin to heal.

Yet this particular story reflects many assumptions that do not apply equally to everyone struggling with addiction—not surprisingly, since Bill Wilson, the cofounder of AA, based the all-important Big Book on the experiences of a hundred white, Protestant, mostly upper-middle-class men and one woman. Unlike these people, there are women (and men) who walk into the halls of AA without ever having known a life they would like to recover. The AA approach, which confronts the false pride of the alcoholic, may not be helpful to a woman who needs to build her self-esteem from the ground up. Many alcoholic women have histories of childhood trauma that AA is not meant to address. New research has established that sexual problems are frequently interwoven with women's alcohol problems—they usually begin before the addiction and continue after it—but AA is not the place to bring these up. Many alcoholic women are dependent on men, and many start drinking in response to depression. Taking responsibility for their lives may require them to look at how they have been socialized to relinquish their power to men, and to recognize the role that alcohol has played in these dynamics. AA discourages discussion of social and political factors contributing to alcoholism. A single, needy woman may also meet with male "assistance" that amounts to sexual harassment (what's known as "thirteenth stepping").

In many places, AA is adapting to women and minorities—particularly in cities, there are same-sex groups that avoid some of these problems—and women currently make up 40 percent of its membership. Some have made good use of AA by remembering the slogan "Take what you need and leave the rest." But where is a woman to turn for help with issues that AA cannot address? In today's climate of managed care, substance abuse treatment is likely to be brief. There is often no time to address the life issues bound up with a woman's drinking, and in any case, these require ongoing support. My point here is that the dominant images of alcoholism and recovery are based on men's experience. For women—and many men—the reality is often quite different. We need to know more about this group of people who do not fit the mold, and we must acknowledge and act on information we already have about specific aspects of women's alcohol problems.

Happy Hours explores the world of women whose drinking has led to dependence. It is aimed at any woman who has ever wondered whether she drinks too heavily or too often, and at anyone who has a sister, mother, grandmother, child, or friend whose drinking has caused concern. I come to the subject as a layperson, with no scientific expertise or firsthand experience—only a strong connection to my sister, and a wish to understand how alcohol takes over a woman's life. I interviewed many treatment providers, researchers, alcohol counselors, psychologists, and scientists, but I focus on stories gathered from interviews with forty recovering women, to whom I owe an enormous debt of gratitude. These women came from a range of racial backgrounds. They were teenagers and over-sixties, heterosexuals and lesbians, well-

to-do professionals and working poor. Daphne was a housewife who hid
her drinking from her husband for many years; by the time she sought
treatment, her life was in ruins. Alice shocked her colleagues at a high-
powered law firm when, after a year of stellar performance, she
announced she needed treatment for alcoholism. Samantha and Rachel,
Native Americans of the Ojibwa tribe, grew up on reservations where
drinking problems were epidemic. No one drank much at all in Lindsey's family. Eighteen at the time of our interviews, she grew up in
rural Vermont, where her family was forced out of their farmhouse
when it was quarantined by the state. Her drinking picked up when
her father was sent to jail. Nell, also eighteen, grew up in Manhattan,
where she drank Stoli martinis and snorted cocaine among the rich and
famous. Marianne, a doctor's wife and mother of four, didn't touch
alcohol until she was in her forties. Sophie, a dancer, remembered gulp-
ing down the half-glass of sherry her mother allowed her when they
dressed up and went out to have tea "with the ladies."

A few of these women were still struggling with relapses when I
interviewed them. Others had been sober for more than twenty years.
They spoke with the hope that some woman, somewhere, would read
their story and recognize the warning signs earlier than they did, that
women trapped in an alcoholic nightmare might discover that they are
not alone, that their individual voices help dispel the stereotypes that
have shamed many women and deterred them from seeking treatment,
and that families might better understand. When I questioned my sister, Carri, about whether she was comfortable with my divulging some
details of her life, she answered, "If one woman is helped by my story, it
will be worth it."

In telling these women's stories, I have tried to stay away from the
language of cause and effect. I have come to feel strongly that as much
as we want to find a single answer (as groups with specific orientations
often do), alcoholism cannot be reduced to any single precipitating factor—not a cluster of genes, or psychopathology, or a difficult family
background, or a bad peer group, or poverty or economics, or a culture
of addiction. These factors may all come together to influence alcoholic

drinking, yet none by itself is sufficient. Some patterns may be typical, but the variables depend on the person. Perhaps more than any other disease, alcoholism challenges simplistic equations. It is both cause *and* effect. It is shaped by a personal and social context, and it shapes that context in turn. The process is circular, and trying to fix a beginning is pointless.

Today, there is a good deal of excitement about research into the physiological aspects of addiction. In one avenue of exploration, scientists are learning how addictive substances enter into the "reward pathways" of the brain and cause changes in dopamine functioning. Normally, the brain releases a certain amount of dopamine with everyday kinds of pleasure—a good meal, an accomplishment, sex. Drugs (including alcohol) short-circuit this process, triggering a flood of dopamine that results in instant euphoria. Over time, the brain is tricked into thinking it can't get pleasure any other way. Instead of seeking out ordinary satisfactions, the addict goes to the drug. The drug eventually stops providing this initial high, but the addict now needs the drug just to function. Her life may be falling apart, but she will, if she needs to, lie, cheat, and steal to get her drug, because her brain has been tricked into thinking she can't survive without it.

In recovery, long after the last withdrawal symptoms, powerful emotional memories, in which the drug is associated with survival, may come back to overwhelm the recovering addict. She will surely relapse if she has not developed strategies to cope with her persistent craving. This is an important point, because it highlights the fact that although drugs can take over a portion of the brain, recovering addicts can be engaged. They can reeducate the brain. They can deliberately remind themselves of the negative consequences of alcohol and learn new ways of achieving satisfaction. Some people are also helped by new medications that turn down the volume of the craving, so to speak, and put it in a manageable range.

The explosion of research on human and animal genetics promises to help us better understand what is inherited in the predisposition to alcoholism, and who is at risk. If we can identify people who are at risk

but do not develop the syndrome, we may learn more about environmental factors that protect vulnerable people. A better understanding
of the specific mechanisms of risk may also help us develop more
focused programs of treatment and prevention.

Although alcohol impairs the brain, this does not mean that
addiction is entirely a "brain disease." We have a tendency to talk
about the brain as if it existed in a vacuum, influenced by nothing but
itself. We know, however, that environmental influences are crucial to
alcoholism—rates of alcoholism in a population will vary even with the
price of alcohol. It is tremendously difficult to measure environmental
influences; the precision of a scientist's laboratory is a far cry from the
messy business of a person's whole life, not to mention the world in
which the person lives. Still, there have been some significant findings.
In one study of alcoholic women who have an identical twin—with,
obviously, the same genetic structure—30 percent of the co-twins were
also alcoholic, 70 percent were not. This points to the powerful influence of both genetic and environmental factors.

The potential environmental factors are enormously diverse. The
strong association between childhood trauma and alcoholism is now
well-established. Cultural norms—attitudes about whether, how
much, and when a person should drink—can influence individual
drinking. An Asian-American woman living in an ethnic community
is likely to drink little, if at all. A young woman living in a sorority
house may find that she can drink nine beers in a row without causing
anyone to think she is out of line. On the familial level, parental support, good communication, and close monitoring discourage alcohol
abuse in teenagers, even when a parent drinks abusively. George Vaillant, reporting on a thirty-three-year longitudinal study, found that an
early unstable family environment was a more potent predictor of later
alcohol problems than the number of alcoholic relatives. Psychologists
now know that there is no definable "alcoholic personality," though
alcoholics and nonalcoholics may differ somewhat on certain personality scores, such as "behavioral undercontrol" and "negative emotional-
ity," or a tendency to feel distressed. Our expectations with regard to

alcohol (such as the beliefs we hold about its effects) figure prominently in current cognitive research, especially since the surprising results of a study published in 1973. This study found that when alcoholics and social drinkers believed they were drinking vodka and tonic, they consumed more ounces, even if, in reality, they were drinking only tonic. They consumed less when they were told the drink was tonic water, even when it actually contained one part vodka to five parts tonic. In other words, in this experiment, what the men believed was in the glass had more influence on their drinking than the alcohol itself.

With alcoholism—as with so much else—to think in terms of nature versus nurture is to misunderstand the profound interdependence of the mind and the environment. With our penchant for quick fixes, and with scientists dependent on millions of research dollars from pharmaceutical companies, we have a tendency to see all our problem behaviors and states of mind as stemming from biological abnormalities: biology is the cause, behavior is the effect, a drug is the cure. Biochemical expressions of disorders are presented—by drug companies, by health practitioners, and sometimes by scientists themselves—as if they were proven causes of suffering, rather than correlates. Many people are told that their depression is biochemical, caused by high cortisol; they are often not told that cortisol levels are themselves affected by environmental stress. A researcher finds differences in the way a group of adults with symptoms of hyperactivity metabolize glucose in the brain, compared with a control group, and assumes that hyperactivity is caused by a brain abnormality. Other research into cerebral glucose metabolism suggests that it is also affected by the environment. In a group of people diagnosed with obsessive-compulsive disorder, behavior therapy gave rise to a change in cerebral glucose metabolism and a reduction of symptoms, in the same way Prozac did.

In addiction, as in many disorders, biological, psychological, and sociocultural factors interact and influence each other. Genetic vulnerability increases the risk of addiction, and the environment—especially traumatic events—also has an impact on an individual's biology, perhaps even altering gene-regulating hormones. Experiences early in life can alter the way the brain works in the future. Indeed, the brain itself is built in interactions between genes and the environment. In recent years, some researchers have begun to develop conceptual models that allow them to explore this complex interplay as it relates to alcohol—specifically, to the way drinking behavior develops gradually over time—but there is still a strong tendency to pit biological and nonbiological factors against each other.

Given this context, it's not surprising that many people, hearing about my work on this book, asked me, "But isn't alcoholism genetic?" They had the impression that alcoholism is predetermined, passed on from parent to child like cystic fibrosis or flat feet. Dr. Henri Begleiter, professor of psychiatry and neuroscience at State University of New York College of Medicine at Brooklyn, is head of the Collaborative Study on the Genetics of Alcoholism (COGA), a national and international study that is among the most promising and carefully designed research projects in the area of alcoholism and genetics. He clarifies certain points that commonly cause confusion:

- There is no gene or set of genes that causes alcoholism.
- There may be a group of genes that predispose a person to addiction.
- You do not have to be genetically predisposed to addiction to become alcoholic. According to Begleiter, a conservative estimate is that 50 to 60 percent of people who develop alcoholism have genes that would predispose them to addiction.
- We do not know the rate of transmission of this predisposition. Health professionals sometimes tell recovering alcoholics what the chances are, statistically, that their children will be alcoholic; this is irresponsible. Not only—to repeat—do we not know the rate of transmission of this predisposition; we do not even know how frequently the predisposition actually leads to alcoholism. Other statistical evaluations of risk that are based on population samples vary, depending on who is sampled.
- The important thing, says Begleiter, is that "with alcoholism, genes are not destiny." In Mendelian disorders—those involving a single

gene, such as Huntington's disease—if you inherit the gene, you are in trouble. This is not true of the predisposition to alcoholism.

In the words of a report to the U.S. Congress from the Secretary of Health and Human Services, "No gene exists with the primary function to make its possessor drink chronically and abusively."

THE GENETICS OF ALCOHOLISM

TO DATE, the clearest association between genetics and alcohol consumption is a trait that *protects* certain populations from becoming alcoholic. Alcohol is first broken down in the body by the enzyme alcohol dehydrogenase (ADH), and this process creates a toxic metabolite called acetaldehyde. Normally, blood levels of acetaldehyde are low, because it is quickly broken down by another enzyme, called aldehyde dehydrogenase (ALDH). Studies of Asian men and women (Japanese, Chinese, and Korean) have found that about 10 percent of Asians inherit a form of ALDH that is biologically inactive, and another 40 percent inherit a partially inactive form. As a result, when these people drink alcohol, more acetaldehyde circulates in the blood, causing an increased heart rate, skin flushing, and sometimes nausea and vomiting. Not surprisingly, Asians with one of these variations of ALDH are considerably less likely to drink to the point of alcohol dependence. They make up about half of the Asian population, but they are less than 10 percent of the alcoholics in these countries.

Though this may change in the next few years, research into genetic factors that *predispose* a person to alcoholism is less definitive. One promising avenue of research involves studying individuals who have a low level of response to alcohol. In a study of 450 sons of alcoholics and controls, Dr. Marc Schuckit at the department of psychiatry, University of California, San Diego School of Medicine, found that the sons of alcoholics were more likely to exhibit a low level of response to alcohol in their late teens or early twenties: they needed to drink more than the controls to achieve the same effect. These young men were also more likely to develop alcohol-related problems by the time of the eight-year follow-up. The implications for women are not clear. Schuckit is engaged in a newer, unpublished study, which is obtaining similar results with women; but another large-scale investigation of sensitivity to alcohol and inheritance of a risk of alcoholism, this one published in 1999 by Andrew Heath and colleagues, found no relationship between a low level of response to alcohol and alcohol dependence in women. Attempts to locate genes which might influence alcohol sensitivity are mostly at initial stages. Research is focused largely on genes related to brain serotonin and other neurochemical receptors.

Another (somewhat contradictory) prominent model proposes that sons of alcoholics are hypersensitive to the pleasant effects of alcohol, and less responsive to the unpleasant ones.

If you look at the studies of enzymes and the studies of responses to alcohol together, a certain commonsense logic emerges. If, when you drink alcohol, it makes you feel terrible, you're not likely to drink much or often. If, on the other hand, you have to drink twice as much as everybody else to get a buzz, you might be likely to drink more, and you therefore become susceptible to addiction. Similarly, if drinking makes you feel especially good, and you don't suffer much from hangovers, you have more incentive to drink. Negative physiological responses can be overridden, however. In a study of Japanese-Americans living in Los Angeles, 53.7 percent of a sample of the college students who experienced a fast flushing response reported having drunk heavily, compared with only 14.5 percent of the sample from the general community. For the college students, cultural influences were more powerful than their bodies' response to alcohol.

The genetic research of Dr. Henri Begleiter's group is focused on a less specific relationship between genes and alcohol. They are looking at abnormal brain wave patterns (especially variations in the P300 brain wave) that might predispose a person to a range of disorders, including addictions of all kinds. According to Begleiter's research, people who are predisposed to alcoholism exhibit hyperexcitability of the central nervous system. The best "cure" for this hyperexcitability is alcohol—which is why alcohol looks so attractive. Begleiter believes, however, that alcoholism is one of many possible outcomes of the same genetic material. "There is no specificity," he told me. "One is predisposed to any behavior which implies a lack of normal homeostatic inhibition." In other words, the brain lacks control over behavior, and this leads to impulsivity. The same excitability could lead to a range of cognitive and mood disorders, including attention deficit and hyperactivity disorder; conduct disorder; anxiety and depression; and addictions to caffeine, cocaine, or any other addictive substance, including alcohol. Dr. Begleiter believes that the COGA study could isolate the first (of many) genes that influence the P300 brain wave within a year. "And the first is the hardest to isolate," he noted.

In all the models above, genes exert an indirect influence on drinking behavior. When alcoholism does develop in a genetically susceptible individual, this is because alcohol plays a unique role in that person's life. The pathway to addiction involves many biochemical, physiologic, and psychological steps. In every step, genes interact with the environment. Furthermore, the individual traits that predispose a person to alcoholism are determined independently of one another—in other words, they are not passed on as an indivisible set. This confirms that alcoholism is very much a heterogeneous disease. Its biological underpinnings may vary from person to person.

For a while, the explosion of research into biological mechanisms of addiction created the hope of a miracle drug that would cure alcoholism. However, while new medications can be helpful to many people, none of them is a magic bullet. To complement the continuing genetic research, the National Institute on Drug Abuse has promoted a multidimensional research agenda. Investigators are encouraged to explore how neurobiological, psychological, social, and cultural factors interact at different stages of involvement in drugs, and how these factors change over time. Such research is expensive, difficult, and time-consuming, but complex models are crucial to understanding such a complex disease as alcohol and drug addiction.

• • •

When I use the term "disease" in this book, I use it in a very broad sense, with the understanding that alcoholism has a complex etiology that includes personal, social, and cultural factors, and the belief that, ultimately, the alcoholic must assume responsibility for her own life. Alcoholism is a medical problem, a compulsive behavior, a family problem, a spiritual problem, and a reflection of our culture. If I have lingered here on the topic of the powerful interconnection between mind and body, it is to counter the strong tendency today to pull alcoholism out of its social and psychological context and to redefine it as a biological illness that needs strictly medical attention.

Such a narrow interpretation trivializes the lives of alcoholics. Take Amy, a painter whose story appears in Chapter 8. She drank moderately until she was nearly sixty years old, and then, when her beloved grandson moved away, she fell into a deep depression and drank a pint of whiskey every day. Was this strictly due to a brain disease? Or consider Ruth, whom you'll meet in Chapter 11. Her godfather sexually abused her from the age of five and gave her alcohol at each of their meetings. She got drunk every day from age six until age forty-one. Is this a brain disease, pure and simple?

Alcoholism is certainly a disease in that it has destructive effects on tissues and body functioning; it is more common among those with a genetic vulnerability; it requires skilled medical and pharmacological care during acute withdrawal; it leads to secondary health problems that also require medical attention; its victims need medical coverage, sick leave, and access to emergency rooms. For these reasons and more, most professionals agree that alcoholism is a disease. To those who say it is more of a bad habit, they may respond that many diseases are linked to bad habits. Diabetes and heart disease, for instance, may arise from dietary factors and obesity in combination with genetic vulnerability.

What's more, the disease concept of alcoholism has been very useful in moving public opinion from seeing alcoholism as a moral failing (the alcoholic as a sinner) to seeing it as an illness of which the sufferer and his or her family need not be ashamed. Critics of the disease concept have feared that it strips the alcoholic of responsibility for recovery, but most clinicians find that when alcoholics understand the physiological processes of addiction, it frees them from shame. Only when that has happened can they effectively take responsibility for managing their lives in the context of an addiction that would otherwise kill them.

Yet I fear that when the disease concept of alcoholism is narrowly interpreted—as it so often is—this strategy backfires, because people know that they are not merely victims of their biology, just as they are not mere victims of circumstance, no matter how hard their lives have been. There is more to it than that. Some people conclude that they or their loved ones are not "real alcoholics" because the reality of their problems is more complex than what they hear described. Others continue to struggle with the disease concept and have trouble reconciling their conflicting attitudes, which they often hide, because in many circles it is considered retrograde to question this concept. I have seen alcoholics and their families speak the language of brain disease for years, only suddenly to confess with anger that they don't believe it, and to start all over with the blame—of the alcoholic, of the family, of the culture.

Everyone agrees that letting go of blame is crucial to recovery. If we were more honest about alcoholism and its many facets—the pull of the body and the pull of the mind, the broad context in which it develops—perhaps we could accomplish this more fully.

In *Happy Hours*, I begin with the assumption that a woman may be genetically vulnerable to becoming alcoholic. Whether she begins to drink and whether she continues depend on a host of other factors. It is not my intent to unravel these. Rather, my aim has been to present women's own stories—their histories, their current context, their challenges in recovery. Most often, alcohol has been woven into the fabric of their lives, so that stories about women and alcohol are also dramas about women's relationships, their needs, their work, their feelings about their bodies, sexual abuse and other trauma, human loss, and spiritual development.

Part One, "The Impact of Alcohol," includes medical information and a history of perceptions about women and alcohol.

Part Two, "On the Job and in Families," deals with the relationship between women's alcohol problems and their social roles, in the family, among peers, and at work.

Part Three, "Take Two at Bedtime: Drinking as Self-Medication," examines some common conditions that accompany women's alcoholism. Chapter 7, "Love Hunger," tells the stories of women whose drinking was tied up with their romantic relationships. Depression is the psychiatric disorder most commonly diagnosed among alcoholic women, and it came up in varying degrees in a majority of my interviews. Even when depression was crucial to the women's stories, however, they did not present it to me as something they could disentangle from the circumstances of their lives. I have followed their lead, not devoting a separate chapter to depression but rather weaving it in wherever it comes up. I do address various ways of thinking about alcoholism and depression in Chapter 8, "Springs of Sorrow: Drinking at Times of Loss." Chapter 9 explores the place of alcohol in the lives of sexually abused women, who may be three times more likely than other women to become dependent on alcohol.

Finally, in Part Four, I turn to "Women's Paths in Recovery." The problem of treating a woman's alcohol problems begins at home, where her drinking is more likely than a man's to be missed or covered up. In the doctor's or therapist's office, a woman's alcoholism is not likely to be diagnosed, as described in Chapter 10, "Doctors Still Don't Get It." She is fortunate if her treatment includes specialized programs for women; we still know much more about treating men. Owing largely to child care issues and a lack of "wraparound care," especially important to women, she may not complete the course. In Chapter 11, "Working with Difference," I show how treatment that honors differences has affected the lives of some Native American and African-American women. In Chapter 12, "Recovery: Only Connect," I explore how women have adapted to the programs that are available.

During the very first interview for this book, I frantically scribbled in my notebook (my tape recorder broke) as a woman opposite me—Meredith, pregnant with her third child—talked about her near-death experience in a hospital ward, where she pinched shut the feeding tube going into her nose to avoid consuming calories, but desperately drank the beer sneaked in by her friends. I listened in shock, sadness, and dismay as she described her hunger, her refusal to eat, her loneliness, and her punishing drive to be perfect: thin and attractive, cheerful and smart, a model student, popular at parties. She always thought she was a failure, except when she was drinking. At the end of the interview, she said, "You know, addicts are not like other people, and we can always recognize each other."

I thought about that statement a lot, and from time to time I heard it from other people. It warned me not to assume too much or to make easy leaps of identification. I have not experienced the physical hold of addiction. I have not had a seizure or a blackout. I have not left a detox ward with no money in my pocket, looking for a beer. Alcoholics describe the canny ways of their disease, how it sneaks into nooks and crannies of their lives, looking for a foothold. That's why recovering alcoholics are best at counseling one another. They know about cravings; they know the kind of thinking that means danger is at hand.

Yet the more I listened to these women's stories, the less I was able to imagine that they were "not like me." I recognized their defenses. I admired them. I have experienced many of the pressures they described. I was fighting for the same kind of spiritual breakthroughs. The cultural forces that influence a woman's drinking—those connected to trauma, sexuality, and relationships—are common to many of us. Whether or not we have a problem with drinking, all of us are likely to have experienced something of the frustration, the self-doubt, the bouts of depression, and the sense of powerlessness that plague the alcoholic.

Among the women whose stories I tell here—and others whose stories don't appear but who helped me understand—some are still suffering in some way, and a few have relapsed. I hope they will be inspired by women who have fought their way out of a pit as black and deep as theirs. It's hard to imagine the courage it takes for a woman to acknowledge the devastation alcohol has wrought in herself and her family, and then to remake her life. I am moved by the determination and grace of those who have come through, and I am sometimes astonished by the sheer joy of their new lives. Meredith, after describing four miserable years of addiction, said, "I wouldn't trade those years for anything. If they hadn't been so bad, I could be out there still searching for a way to fill up my emptiness." Instead, she treasures her husband and children, takes pleasure in daily miracles and daily work, and looks for opportunities to reach out to others who suffer as she once did. Such women have transformed pain into gratitude and compassion, and they have something to offer us all.

Part One

The Impact
of Alcohol

1

Why Men Can
Outdrink Women

MYTHS ABOUT WOMEN AND ALCOHOL HAVE ALWAYS
abounded, and only in the mid-1970s, when clinical studies of alcohol-related disorders began to include women, did we begin to get real information. Although we still know far more about men's drinking than women's, researchers have begun to fill in some of the gaps in our understanding of women and alcohol.

There is mixed news for women who like to drink. The Harvard Nurses' Health Study found a U-shaped curve: light to moderate drinkers lived longer than women who were abstinent or heavy drinkers. It isn't clear whether these results are due to the benefits of alcohol or to the generally healthy habits of light drinkers, who may also be more likely to exercise and eat well. The U.S. Department of Health has defined moderate and acceptable alcohol intake for women as one drink a day—five ounces of wine, twelve ounces of beer, or one and a half ounces of eighty-proof distilled spirits (each of these contains 0.5 ounce of pure alcohol). (For men, it's two drinks a day.) Light drinking for women is defined as up to three drinks a week, moderate drinking as four to thirteen, and heavy drinking as fourteen or more. A woman who has two glasses of wine each evening is thus categorized as a "heavy drinker."

While ongoing research is likely to refine the picture, it now seems clear that in certain ways, women are more vulnerable than men to the immediate and long-term consequences of alcohol.

Women metabolize alcohol differently from men. Their bodies have a higher proportion of body fat, which carries little water. This means that alcohol is more concentrated in their body fluids. Women also have less of an enzyme that metabolizes alcohol in their stomach lining, so that for each ounce taken, a higher percentage of alcohol enters the bloodstream and liver (an effect that is enhanced by fasting). Fluctuations in hormonal levels during the menstrual cycle can slow the rate of alcohol metabolism, and oral contraceptives also slow it. All these factors probably contribute to the higher blood alcohol concentration in women, which increases the health risks of women who drink.

Take a couple—let's call them Pete and Laurie. Both are thirty-two years old, and both weigh 140 pounds. They drink the same amount. Every night, they have a glass of wine together as they make dinner and chat about their day at work. At the table, they polish off the bottle and open another. By the end of the evening, each has finished four glasses of wine.

What is the medical outlook for Pete and Laurie?

If their drinking remains constant over many years, both Pete and Laurie may suffer a variety of long-term effects. For Laurie, however, the picture may be worse. Her four glasses of wine will get her drunk faster and keep her drunk longer. She runs a significant risk of liver injury such as fatty liver (which is reversible when drinking stops) and more serious disorders such as hepatitis and cirrhosis (for women the risk of cirrhosis of the liver becomes significant at two drinks a day; for men, at six drinks a day). Sooner than Pete, she may develop digestive and nutritional problems such as anemia, peptic ulcers, and folic acid deficiency, which leads to severe diarrhea. A four-year study of 58,000 nurses demonstrated that in women, the risk of developing high blood pressure begins at about two to three drinks per day and increases with each drink. While light drinking may actually help counteract osteoporosis (because it raises estrogen levels), even small amounts of alcohol cause the body to excrete calcium at twice its normal rate. More research is needed to understand the overall effect of alcohol on women's bones.

Laurie's endocrine system may be impaired by alcohol, leading to menstrual irregularities, which increase with a woman's level of drinking. These can lead to infertility and early menopause. If Laurie becomes pregnant and continues to drink heavily, her risk of spontaneous abortion increases, and she also increases her risk of having a baby with some abnormality, including fetal alcohol effects. (Fullblown fetal alcohol syndrome may result from even heavier drinking.) While the infant death rate is 8.6 per 1,000 among women who do not drink during pregnancy, it is 23.5 per 1,000 births among those who have an average of two or more drinks per day.

Laurie is a little nervous about the link between alcohol and breast cancer—some studies suggest that women who drink alcohol may increase their risk of breast cancer by as much as 40 percent—but she was relieved by the 1999 report from the Framingham Heart Study, which followed the drinking habits of 2,800 women for more than forty years, and found that the incidence of breast cancer was roughly the same for all women, even those who had two or more drinks per day. This study, reasonably enough, eased the minds of many doctors and women who drink moderately. Yet the researchers cautioned that they could not draw conclusions about breast cancer among heavy drinkers, because their sample did not include enough women in this category. Earlier studies suggest strongly an increased risk at four to six drinks a day or more, perhaps related to the fact that alcohol raises estrogen levels.

Listening to the radio on her way home from work, Laurie was also pleased to hear about a study conducted by the American Cancer Society, which corroborated other studies that found moderate consumption of alcohol may protect men and women from heart disease. Her local food co-op sent out a flyer drawing on that study, touting the benefits of red wine (which it now sells).

Laurie, then, feels reassured about her drinking habits. But she has been misled. When a woman's production of estrogen decreases at menopause, her risk of heart attack increases; moderate consumption of alcohol may partly counteract this risk by significantly raising levels of estradiol (the most potent natural estrogen). Alcohol also reduces the likelihood of blood clots and raises the blood levels of the protective HDL cholesterol. At age thirty-two, however, Laurie is not among the postmenopausal women for whom alcohol has a protective effect. More important, "moderate drinking," in this study, is defined as one to two drinks a day. Above one drink per day, the overall death rate began to increase. Among women and men thirty to fifty-nine years old who were at low risk for cardiovascular disease, those who consumed four or more drinks daily had the highest rate of death from all causes. Indeed, though research is inconclusive, Laurie's twenty-eight drinks a week may put her more at risk even for cardiovascular disorders (as well as the cancers and cirrhosis that the mortality study cites). One study found that women who consumed six or more drinks a day were eight times more likely to develop cardiomyopathy, a degenerative disease of the heart muscle. Although in general men die of heart disease at a rate twice as high as women, an analysis of over 8,000 cardiovascular deaths demonstrated that women who drink heavily die young of these diseases at a rate equal to that of heavy-drinking men.

Because alcohol depresses the immune system, both Pete and Laurie will be predisposed to infectious diseases such as respiratory infections and pneumonia. Because they consume more than twenty-one drinks per week, they have almost a tenfold higher risk of esophageal cancer, compared with people who have fewer than seven drinks a week.

If both Pete and Laurie develop alcoholism, and both suffer damage to the liver, heart, nerve fibers, muscle tissue, and brain, all this damage will be likely to visit Laurie somewhat sooner than Pete. Should both members of the couple become sober, it will take Laurie's tissues longer to repair themselves. Should both persist in drinking, Laurie will be at graver risk for suicide and alcohol-related accidents. In the general population, women attempt suicide more frequently than men but are less likely to die in this way. Among alcoholics, however, women's rate of completed suicide appears to exceed even that of alcoholic men. In fact, if Laurie becomes alcohol-dependent, she will be five times more likely to commit suicide than women her age who don't drink; and in any given year, she will be twice as likely to die as Pete. This is especially grave when you consider that Pete will be three times as likely to die as men of his age who don't drink.

How Much Is Too Much?

PEOPLE OFTEN WANT to know how much alcohol constitutes a problem, but alcohol abuse and dependence are defined not by the quantity consumed but rather by the consequences of drinking. The term "alcohol abuse" (what is often referred to as "problem drinking") applies when there is a pattern of drinking that creates difficulty in one or more areas of life, for instance, being unable to meet the demands of school, work, or parenthood; driving while intoxicated; or getting into fights. "Alcohol dependence" (or "alcoholism") is more severe. According to criteria defined by the American Psychiatric Association, it is diagnosed by a cluster of symptoms, some of which last at least a year. These include increasing tolerance of alcohol (meaning that it takes more to feel high), difficulty cutting back, preoccupation with alcohol, and continued drinking despite problems with health, work, or relationships. In short, says one doctor, "alcohol abuse is too much, too often, and alcohol dependence is the inability to quit."

An individual's pattern of drinking also influences health risk in ways that are not fully understood. Three days of binge drinking followed by a period of abstinence will have effects on a woman's body that are different from those of the same amount of alcohol consumed in heavy daily doses over the course of a week. For example, in binge drinking alternating with abstinence, the liver has a chance to repair itself. On the other hand, binge drinking creates a graver risk of accidents and vulnerability to violence.

Women aged twenty-one to thirty-four have the highest rates of problem drinking. At age thirty-two, consuming four glasses of wine a day, Laurie is certainly a heavy drinker, and she is risking her health. She may or may not be headed for alcohol dependence. She is at high risk if there are alcoholics in her family, if she has a history of sexual or physical abuse, or if she suffers from depression. There is also the question of why she drinks. Her drinking is already problematic if its purpose is to relieve anxiety or otherwise regulate her mood, if she feels empty inside and drinks to fill herself up, if getting high with Pete smooths over problems in their relationship. It's already a problem if it interferes with her sleep (alcohol depresses the central nervous system, but there's a rebound effect when it wears off), or makes it hard for her to get to work in the morning or get through an evening during which there is no alcohol. It's also a problem if she's trying to get pregnant.

Alcohol is the leading single drug of abuse among American women. About 10 to 15 percent report some type of drinking-related problem, and about 4 percent meet diagnostic criteria for alcohol abuse or dependence. Most women who drink, however, are not clinically dependent, and in 1990 the Institute of Medicine stated that most alcohol problems—accidents, fights, and medical complications—are created not by "alcoholics" but by people with a broad range of problem drinking. A woman may abuse alcohol without ever drinking heavily and may, at different stages in her life, move in and out of "problem drinking" without ever having a diagnosable disorder. In a follow-up analysis of women's drinking habits over ten years, one study found that of the women who were problem drinkers to begin with, one-third got worse, one-third stayed the same, and one-third moved out of problem drinking altogether. Typically, both young women and young men are more likely to be heavier drinkers, though among African Americans and Hispanic Americans, heavy drinking more often peaks at a later age. In the general population, women under age forty drink more than older women. After age fifty, women's heavy drinking drops precipitously.

Women's physiology—their lower average body weight, their

greater sensitivity to alcohol, and their special risks during pregnancy—makes them more susceptible to alcohol problems if, like Laurie, they match a male partner's heavy drinking. But physiology is only
the beginning. Alcohol problems express themselves in a person's
whole life: in work and relationships and psychological well-being. It
is not surprising, then, that in certain ways, women and men experience alcohol problems differently. Women enter addiction on different
paths, with different histories. The triggers that set off drinking in
women may vary from those for men. Women may have different motivations for entering treatment, and their needs in recovery may also be
distinct.

Here are some facts that cry out for our attention.

- The alcoholic beverage industry is aggressively marketing to
  women, with ads linking drinking with glamour, independence,
  and liberation.
- Women in treatment for alcoholism are four times more likely than
  other women to have been abused by a partner. For a woman, being
  a victim of violence is both a risk factor for alcohol abuse and a
  potential consequence of it. A study of spousal abuse among alcoholic and nonalcoholic women found that alcoholic women were
  nine times more likely to be slapped by their husbands, five times
  more likely to be kicked or hit, five times more likely to be beaten,
  and four times more likely to have their lives threatened.
- Women who need treatment face particular barriers, including lack
  of special programming to meet their needs, exclusion of pregnant
  women from treatment, personal and family denial, lack of child
  care, and inadequate insurance coverage. Although insurance problems affect both men and women—some policies cover only hospital detoxification, for instance—women, particularly minorities, are
  more likely than men to be underemployed and underinsured.
- Alcoholic women frequently wind up with a cross-addiction to over-
  the-counter or prescription drugs. Overlooking or mistaking the
  markers of alcohol use, women's doctors often diagnose anxiety or

depression (which may also be present) and prescribe tranquilizers, which can be habit-forming and are dangerous to mix with alcohol.

- Tolerance for alcohol and prescription drugs decreases with age, and alcohol magnifies the effects of sedatives and tranquilizers and accelerates dependence on these drugs. Women—especially those over fifty-nine—are more likely than men to abuse these drugs together; this can cause confusion, delirium, heavy sedation, and such accidents as falls. White, higher-income women are the heaviest older drinkers.

- Oral contraceptives reduce a woman's ability to metabolize alcohol.

- Women in treatment for alcohol abuse report high rates of sexual problems, for example, lack of desire and difficulty achieving orgasm. These problems usually preceded their heavy drinking. When women use alcohol to "treat" this problem, they find themselves in a vicious circle. In a five-year follow-up of women showing signs of problem drinking in 1981, sexual dysfunction was the single strongest predictor of continued problem drinking in 1986.

- Women problem drinkers often use alcohol as a form of self-treatment. More often than men, they cite a traumatic event as precipitating abusive drinking, whether divorce or abandonment, a death in the family, a miscarriage, or a health problem.

- From 1977 to 1994, the number of male drivers involved in alcohol-related fatal traffic crashes decreased 25 percent; for females there was a 12 percent increase. Laboratory studies of the effects of alcohol on responding to visual cues suggest that there may be gender differences in how alcohol affects driving performance.

- Alcoholic women are more likely than alcoholic men to have a mental health disorder—especially depression, anxiety, or an eating disorder. (Among men, antisocial personality disorder—linked to aggression and criminality—comes first and is followed by additional substance abuse.) Although depression in men tends to follow alcohol abuse, depression in women more often comes first, and this means that it's less likely to go away when drinking stops.

- Women in treatment for alcoholism report childhood sexual abuse twice as often as women without alcohol problems. Their reports are corroborated by a study of women and men whose childhood sexual or physical abuse was substantiated by court records. For men, no relationship was found between alcohol problems and childhood victimization. For women, however, the relationship was significant, even after the researchers controlled for a family history of alcohol or drug problems, poverty, race, and age. Girls who are sexually or physically abused become problem drinkers in disproportionate numbers.

- Lesbian and bisexual women have been thought to be at particular risk for addiction, but the studies showing high rates of alcoholism among sexual minorities are not reliable, because they found their samples at least partly through gay bars, where heavy drinkers gather. Newer studies find no significant differences in the drinking habits of lesbian and heterosexual women, though more lesbian women report recovering from alcoholism.

- Though the number of women who drink has increased sharply, the ratio of alcohol *dependence* among men and women has stayed level at about three men to every woman. But this is changing among the young. Among men and women ages eighteen to twenty-nine, the ratio is 2.2 to 1, and in today's secondary schools as many girls drink as boys. If this trend persists, alcoholism among women will surely increase in years to come.

- In a study of 572 women in treatment for alcohol or drug addiction, or both, 79 percent of older women usually or always used only alcohol or only a single drug, compared with 47 percent of younger women. Women under age thirty-five were more likely to use several drugs, while women thirty-five and older more often used one or two, such as alcohol and a painkiller.

- Most men leave their alcoholic wives; most women stay with their alcoholic husbands. Women in treatment centers frequently report that their families have discouraged them from getting help for their drinking problems.

- Women who are not married but are living with a partner are 50 percent more likely to drink heavily than married women.

- The increased threats of prosecution and of losing child custody may frighten many pregnant alcoholic women away from seeking treatment.

- African-American women who drink heavily are 6.7 times more likely to have a child with fetal alcohol syndrome than white women who drink the same amount at the same frequency.

- Although the rate of alcohol dependence is lower for African-American women than for white women, mortality from cirrhosis is 83 percent higher among black females, and black alcoholic women suffer death rates that are nearly double those of white alcoholic women.

- Statistically, a woman is somewhat more at risk if she is childless, and less at risk if she is married and employed full-time. Women in their late thirties and forties are most at risk when they are divorced and unemployed and have no children living at home. (Drinking may have contributed to these losses.) Among women in their fifties and sixties, the risk is higher if they are not employed and have no children at home. Widows also have a higher risk. Like their male counterparts, white women are most likely to report problem drinking, followed by Hispanic women; African-American women are least likely. The more acculturated a minority woman is—that is, the more she has acquired mainstream attitudes and values—the more likely she is to drink heavily.

The health risk factors of women *in general* are different from those of men *in general*, but not all women are alike. The risks and benefits of drinking are influenced by a woman's age and overall health. A woman of sixty, for instance, is more susceptible to alcohol's effects than she was before menopause; but if she has high blood cholesterol and a family history of heart disease, with no special risk of cancer, and she is taking no other medications that might interact with alcohol, she may want to talk to her doctor about the protective effect of light drinking. A woman whose mother and sister died of breast cancer, and whose family tree is studded with alcoholics, may consider it wisest to abstain from drinking altogether.

The evidence for a genetic influence on addiction in women is somewhat mixed. Early twin studies indicated that environmental factors are more important both in the development of women's alcohol problems and in protecting women from the disease. Some recent research has had contrasting results; these studies suggest that about 50 to 60 percent of the liability to alcoholism is inherited, for women and for men. It may be that for women, genes have more influence over alcohol dependence than they do over alcohol abuse. In truth, however, most research along these lines is still focused on men, and the results of current work on women are often contradictory. We need to wait to see how research develops, but a woman with a family history of alcoholism should certainly consider herself at risk. Both her environment and her genes could be working against her.

In my own conversations with women, I have been struck by how many women who are not and never have been dependent on alcohol still find that there is a level of drinking, well below dependence, that impairs their health and relationships. One woman, an editor at a New York publishing company, said her two nightly drinks kept her from coming to grips with her teenage daughter's rebelliousness. Another woman found that one drink became two, and two became three, and several years passed before she faced the facts of her life: her husband was shutting her out, and the business she had started was not going to survive. For a period of time in these women's lives, the release they found in their evening cocktail ritual seemed like a godsend. Only gradually did they realize that this pleasant habit was not serving them well. The alcohol kept them from experiencing the frustration that might have impelled them to confront the sources of pain in their lives and find creative solutions.

One young woman who'd just come out of treatment told me a saying she'd heard, "If you care more about alcohol than you do about broccoli, you have a problem." I suspect that this definition, comical on its face, is meant to jolt people out of their certainty that they do not have a problem, that their story wouldn't belong in a book like *Happy Hours*.

And perhaps it wouldn't. Yet I suspect that any woman who has ever worried about her drinking, or had a few quick beers to be sociable, or to get in the mood for sex, or—like Sophie, whose story I tell in Chapter 7—to be "funnier, prettier, warmer," will find something familiar in these stories. There's a way of thinking that goes along with alcohol problems but is not unique to alcoholics. It has to do with looking for solutions outside yourself. It has to do with finding yourself unacceptable, trying to make yourself right, and having your efforts backfire. Those of us who never become dependent on alcohol can muddle through life without ever confronting this way of thinking and being. Alcoholics who want to stay sober do not have this option. For them, clarity about the choices they make and the way they live is a matter of life and death. They have to figure out what really matters and who is responsible for their lives.

2

Women and Drinking:
A Long Story in Brief

My own self let me more have pity on,
To my own sad self, hereafter, kind.
—GERARD MANLEY HOPKINS

AN EXTRA DOSE OF SHAME

SHAME IS THE FEELING OF BEING WORTHLESS. WHEN WE feel ashamed, we don't sense that we have made a mistake; we sense that we *are* a mistake. We have disgraced ourselves and our families. We're worse than nothing, and we deserve to be cast out. Alcoholism is referred to as a "shame-based disorder" because very often a drinking habit develops in part to drown out feelings of shame. Once addicted, the drinker has more to be ashamed of, and another drink helps dull the feeling of despair. The cycle takes another turn.

In women, shame is deepened by negative stereotypes about their sexuality. People mistakenly believe that alcohol is sexually arousing, and alcoholic women are presumed to be promiscuous. In fact, alcohol reduces physiological sexual responsiveness in both men and women. As Dr. Marc Schuckit has written, "The popular image of the scarlet woman is a fiction—promiscuity is appropriate to only 5 percent of all women drinkers. Most of the other 95 percent complain of diminished interest in sex." In a survey of the general population, women reported drinking deliberately when they planned to have sex, in order to lose their inhibitions, but only 8 percent of respondents said that they had ever become less particular in their choice of a sexual partner when they had been drinking. On the other hand, 60 percent said that someone else who was drinking had become sexually aggressive toward them. Here, the double standard becomes egregious. Women who drink are seen as fair targets for physical and sexual victimization. A psychologist's study using college students and rape scenarios found that a man is considered less responsible for raping a woman if he was drunk when he did it. But if the woman he raped was drunk, she is considered more to blame. Alcoholic women who internalize society's attitudes may be crippled by their shame.

Of course, some alcoholic women do have numerous sexual partners. Often, the sex they have is the result of not being sober or confident enough to manage a situation, especially when a man is emboldened by the belief that alcoholic women are fair game. Others are frantically casting about for some kind of human connection. Convinced they are unworthy, they believe they have only their bodies to offer. Many are economically dependent on men. They feel they need to comply with the man who is buying them drinks. In all of these cases, the woman's sexual behavior is a symptom of her belief that she is powerless. The shame heaped on her by society only confirms her in her self-loathing, which she drowns out with another drink.

Men are not spared the shame of alcoholism. In spite of massive education efforts, alcoholism is still associated with moral weakness and still felt as a sign of failure. Both women and men who are dependent on alcohol are likely to be deeply dissatisfied with themselves. They frequently describe themselves as awkwardly self-conscious and somehow "different" from other people. Many believe they are unworthy of affection, and though they may be very successful, they often play down their accomplishments; they fear that one day the truth will come out and they'll be seen as frauds.

Yet studies repeatedly find that alcoholic women suffer even worse anxiety, guilt, and depression than alcoholic men, have lower self-esteem, and, as we have seen, commit suicide more often.

For women, compared with men, alcohol problems have a greater impact on all areas of their lives. Among people who have had an alcohol-related accident, for instance, a woman is twenty-five times more likely than a man to report "failures" in her social roles and general demeanor, and these failures are significantly more closely linked to health problems. When a woman has alcohol problems, says Kaye Middleton Fillmore, a leading researcher in the field, "Everything tends to go wrong at once." Women's paralyzing sense of worthlessness can prevent them from reaching out for help. Typically, by the time they enter treatment, their alcoholism is further advanced, and their health more compromised, than men's. With any step toward health and wholeness, the old belief that they don't deserve it may reassert itself. "A man may come in for treatment with a puffed-up, false sense of masculinity," says Barry Carr, director of the Bournewood Substance Abuse Treatment Center in Bournewood, Massachussetts, "but a woman who comes in is typically in far worse shape. She's lost all her defenses. She's tremendously stigmatized by alcoholism."

WHY NO ONE WANTS A WOMAN TO DRINK LIKE A MAN

ONE CAN SEE the tenacity of negative stereotypes of drinking women by looking at early Roman society, in which a man had the power of life and death over his wife and children. Since a woman was her husband's property, women's gravest crime was adultery, and it was assumed that a woman who drank would wind up in another man's bed. "When she is drunk, what matters to the Goddess of Love?" wrote Juvenal. "She cannot tell her groin from her head." And so each day a wife was forced to kiss her husband and all her male relatives. If there was wine on her breath, the men gathered to decide whether to exercise their legal right to kill her on the spot.

Women in our society drink freely, but if a woman develops alcohol problems, gender roles and the imbalance of power still shape her relationship to alcohol: her reasons for drinking, her risks when she does, the forces that maintain her drinking, and her hope of getting help.

A taboo against drunkenness in women has persisted for centuries, as has a tendency to stigmatize and punish women for hard drinking. In her book *Women: The Invisible Alcoholics*, Marian Sandmaier recounts the history of women and alcohol in the Western world, pointing out that there has always been a special stigma attached to an alcoholic woman. This attitude has its roots in the perception that drinking takes a woman outside of a man's control and thus threatens the sexual status quo. "The real issue has never been drunkenness per se," writes Sandmaier, "but rather man's fear that the alcohol abusing woman will abandon her role and careen out of his control. Wherever drinking among women has been limited in history, it has been linked to promiscuity and neglect of home and hearth; it has always sparked a terrifying vision of what she might say, do, or be once freed by alcohol."

Sandmaier's interpretation may be bolstered by studies of cultures around the globe, suggesting that whenever gender roles are most clearly polarized, so too are women's and men's drinking patterns. Ethnographers point out that men drink in part to demonstrate their masculinity—they drink to show stamina, self-control, independence, and willingness to take risks. Men also drink to bond with one another despite social differences, and to escape control by others. There's no real parallel for women, no way in which drinking confirms them in their roles—quite the opposite. Because of the fear that alcohol will interfere with women's responsibilities, their drinking has often been restricted.

Whether restrained by society or choice, women have always drunk less than men and had fewer alcohol problems, and this remains true today. In every society that has been studied—primarily North Atlantic societies, but also across Africa, Asia and the Pacific, and Latin America—for all age groups and measures, men have higher rates of alcohol use and abuse. Even in cultures where women are equally likely to drink, they drink less than men and are more likely to abstain as they get older, and so as a group they have fewer alcohol problems.

To a degree, biological factors may explain these gender differences. Some researchers propose that women drink less than men because physiologically, as we have seen, it takes less alcohol to get the same results. Across cultures, as women age, the quantity of their drinking stabilizes more consistently than men's, and they are more likely to become abstainers over time. This could be in part because childbirth gives women a greater incentive to curtail their drinking. Women's social role as child rearers would also play a part.

It isn't clear why relatively small differences in metabolism become such large differences in drinking behavior, or why the differences between women's and men's drinking habits vary so much from one culture to the next. In 1998 a cross-cultural study that provided comparative data on women's and men's drinking in thirteen countries pointed out that female drinkers in the Netherlands drank on an average of ten occasions per month, but those in Finland drank on only about three occasions. Women in Prague drank more frequently than any other women in the study but did not have high rates of heavy drinking or intoxication. Swedish women drank heavily most often but had the lowest rate of adverse consequences. Czech men drank heavily more often than Czech women, but Czech women drank heavily as often as Israeli men.

The authors of this study propose that though biological differences explain why there are gender differences in drinking, cultural differences explain the great variation. In essence, each group begins with the fact of an observable biological difference and uses this as a basis for creating rules for social behavior and relationships that then magnify the difference, in varying degrees and ways. Perceptions of women and men become dichotomized until differences of degree become absolute divisions of roles and behavior. Differences in women's and men's responses to alcohol become a basis for decrees about what is appropriate drinking behavior for each.

This perspective makes sense of the ethnographic descriptions of drinking behavior, which report that women's drinking is most restrained where women are clearly subordinate to their husbands, con-

fined in the domestic sphere, while the husbands move freely in the
public realm and take on economic and political roles denied to
women. In Nigeria, for instance, where women's role is clearly circum-
scribed, the rare woman who abuses alcohol is subject to severe stigma
and insult; she falls "from a glorious Olympian height to the level of
the gutter." Another intriguing study looked at the lifetime prevalence
of drinking problems among native Korean men and women living in
two places: Kangwha, Korea; and Yanbian, China. In Kanghwa, the
ratio of men to women with alcohol problems was 17.5 to 1; but in
Yanbian, where traditional social values are more powerful, the ratio
was 115 to 1. In contrast, where gender roles are changing, and where
women are gaining access to education and employment, women seem
to be drinking more, even in cities in Nigeria. Researchers have noted
that even when the data suggest *stable* drinking patterns, public concern about women's alcohol consumption heightens during times when
women's rights and independence are most visibly expanding. In many
cultures, as Sandmaier suggests, a drunken woman is not considered
merely irresponsible, as a man would be. She is a metaphor for potential social disruption.

The disinhibiting effects of alcohol may cause any drinker, male
or female, to talk more loudly, become boisterous, or act on sexual or
aggressive impulses more typically suppressed. Drinkers may become
more expansive, more willing to take risks, even as the faculty of judgment is dulled. These alcohol-induced changes in personality may be in
keeping with traditional masculinity. A drinking man may feel *more*
masculine, bolder, and more powerful. The people around him, though
they may not be impressed, are likely to see his behavior as in keeping
with traditional norms. If a drinking woman gets loud and garrulous,
if she swears or gets crude or boisterous or angry, her behavior flies in
the face of traditional femininity. She is not just bad or immoral. She is
acting like a man—in a sense, unsexed. People are apt to respond with
disgust. Their disgust, say Sandmaier and others, punishes the woman
for stepping outside her feminine constraints, and reminds other
women what will happen to them if they step out of their place.

• • •

In the West, women's drinking has always been subject to more controls than men's, but the response to it has varied across the centuries and in different social climates. By the second century B.C.E., even Roman women were permitted to drink, and like Greek women, they performed rites of worship to the god of wine. In general, some degree of drinking by women has been permitted whenever they were given a degree of freedom in society, and when alcohol was seen more as a medicine or a symbol of hospitality than as a threat to sacred moral values. In medieval Europe, alcohol was widely available. Englishwomen drank at home but not in taverns. Ale and wine were drunk in monasteries and convents, and monastic rules noted, "It shall be the concern of the holy abbess to provide such wine as shall soothe those who are ill or who were raised more delicately." Social class has played a role. In Germany, for instance, beginning in the third century and for several hundred years, noble women were a strong social presence, and it was common for them to drink with men. During the Renaissance, when traditional views were being challenged on many fronts, highborn ladies again drank fairly openly. Today in America class continues to exert an influence on drinking habits: a female lawyer in San Francisco may drink freely in public or at home; a housewife in rural Georgia may well be in a different situation.

For centuries women were involved in brewing as part of their household duties, and in some countries in Europe and Africa it became an exclusively female trade. In colonial America, women brewed beer and fermented cider and were free to drink in public—especially upper-class women, who, in the mid-1700s particularly, enjoyed a more relaxed social code and were also free to play cards and shoot dice. On the pioneers' dance floors, whiskey bottles were passed briskly from mouth to mouth, regardless of the dancer's age or sex.

Alcohol has also been an essential ingredient in many medicinal remedies throughout the centuries, for everything from "foulness of breath" to deafness, swollen tonsils, indigestion, and "breeding sickness" in colonial America, where recipes were passed among women.

Eventually, such formulas evolved into the popular patented medicines of the nineteenth and early twentieth centuries such as "Lydia Pinkham's Pink Pills for Pale People," medicines aimed at "women's troubles," which contained up to 50 percent opiates or alcohol. Opium, mercury, morphine, and coca (from which cocaine is produced) were legal during this period and were often used to treat women's "nervous weakness." The excessive and often inappropriate medication of women by doctors and pharmacists, along with women's own self-medication, is a persistent theme in the history of women's addictions. Traditionally, drugs and alcohol have been condoned for women as long as they were used officially for medicinal purposes—and, most likely, taken in solitude, so that the woman's reputation would not be tarnished. Today's stereotypical image of a housewife hiding alcohol bottles in a closet has its basis in this history, and studies still show that, compared with men and younger women, older women are more likely to drink alone.

Although moderate use of alcohol was accepted in colonial America, the Puritans inveighed against drunkenness along with gambling, fighting, and adultery. Laws prohibited drinking more than half a pint per half-hour. Both men and women could be punished for infractions, though there are few accounts of drunkenness among women.

Perhaps the most extreme example of the scapegoating of women alcoholics occurred in England in the early eighteenth century, during the "gin epidemic." When Parliament lifted regulations on the production of domestic gin in the hope of creating revenues, cheap, often adulterated gin flooded the market. In the slums of London, where industrialization had created desperate poverty, women and men turned to the cheap gin available in every grocery shop for temporary escape from their intolerable lives. Though there were no major epidemics in London between 1700 and 1750, and the standard of living in the slums was very gradually rising, the city's population declined during this period. Children especially died in astonishing numbers. Seventy-five percent of the children christened between 1730 and 1749 died before their fifth birthday. Public outrage focused on their mothers. In pamphlets, papers, paintings, prints, sermons, and public debate, women were indicted for debauchery, neglect of their children, and ill-spent lives. Though alcoholic women were not responsible for this national scandal, they took all the blame. As Sandmaier writes, "The gin-drinking woman was suffering and dying from alcoholism right along with her children, yet there was an almost total absence of concern for her as a sick individual. Her alcoholism was seen only through the prism of her motherhood."

In America by the 1800s, industrialization, along with the greater availability of alcohol, contributed to a rising problem of male drunkenness. When the churches called on crusaders for the temperance movement, women responded energetically. Among them were wives and mothers made destitute by their husbands' alcoholism. This was a time of many contradictions. The crusade for temperance was driven by white, middle-class, Protestant women under the umbrella of the church. It took on the rhetoric of conventional morality: drinking was wicked and degrading; alcohol swallowed up families and individual souls; alcohol ruined men and threatened women's virtue. These women of the temperance movement spoke as exemplars of the idealized femininity Victorian culture had promoted. Pure and innocent, guardian angels of the hearth and home, they used prayer, hymns, and the force of moral virtue to oppose the evils of alcohol. Ironically, these women had to leave their homes and organize politically to do their crusading, and this gave them the skills they would soon need to fight for the right to vote. The two causes were not explicitly allied, however, and many prim, proper crusaders opposed women's suffrage. In 1884, the National Women's Christian Temperance Union endorsed woman suffrage as "a necessary weapon for home protection." In other words, it was hoped that voting women would help outlaw alcohol. In fact, the right to vote, won in 1920, followed hard on the heels of the Volstead Act of 1919, which instituted national prohibition.

The association of female purity with abstention from alcohol is centuries old, but the hundred-year battle for prohibition in America rigidified the notion that alcohol is the natural enemy of women. Naturally, the stigma attached to women who drank—particularly to excess—intensified during this era.

In the years since the Volstead Act, trends in American women's drinking have varied with the political climate. Prohibition was barely achieved before women started drinking again. The war and women's employment, a new openness about sex, the right to vote, and the preoccupation with alcohol brought by prohibition all created a climate more open to women's drinking. Alcohol consumption declined during the Depression, only to rise again—in America and in many parts of the world—after World War II.

THE POWER OF PERSISTING ATTITUDES

IN THE 1970s, American media reported an "epidemic" in women's drinking. These reports were not supported by data, but it's true that by 1983, a higher percentage of women in every age group were drinking. These numbers declined in the 1980s—but not as markedly as the decline in the percentage of male drinkers. On the basis of a survey conducted in 1992, the National Institute on Drug Abuse estimated that 40 percent of American women had used alcohol within the past month, compared with 56 percent of men—not a huge gap, and among younger women, it's narrower still. Surveys in Britain and Australia suggest that women there are drinking more heavily. Even where drinking has been considered unacceptable for women—in Africa, Central and South America, and Asia—there is evidence that women are more likely to drink; this is seen as a result of "Westernization."

Today we are at a complicated and confusing place in our attitude toward women who develop drinking problems. There are signs that the stigma of being a female alcoholic is breaking down. Younger women are less likely to hide their addiction. Since the early 1990s, women under thirty have been presenting themselves for treatment in numbers almost equal to men. The recovering women I spoke with seldom mentioned overt prejudice against them because of their sex. Yet it is easy to underestimate the power of persisting beliefs that women alcoholics are unnatural, unfeminine, and more revolting and pathetic than their male counterparts—and the harm to women who internalize this view.

The recovering women I interviewed told me about this in many different ways, but none more explicitly than Sonja, seventeen years sober at the age of fifty-eight and leading workshops for recovering alcoholics in Houston: "A drunk man with a lampshade on his head is cute," said Sonja, "but a drunk woman is a slut and a whore and a piece of trash. I don't know if it will ever really change. In mixed groups, the men will say things like, 'I just hate a drunk woman, there's nothing more disgusting,' and the women will hang their heads and say, 'Oh, yeah, that's true.' They feel it. That's why they drink in the closet."

When I interviewed Sonja, she was mourning her daughter Naomi, who had died of an alcoholic hemorrhage. After two months of sobriety, Naomi had drunk one more time, though her doctor had warned her it would kill her. On the death certificate, where it asked if the death was alcohol-related, the doctor checked "no."

"I guess he thought it was shameful," said Sonja. She pointed out that when so many elements in society reinforce old notions, it tends to keep them alive.

The negative stereotyping of alcoholic women may be more prevalent in some age groups and some parts of the country, less prevalent in others. It has an uneasy relationship with the custom of moderation in drinking for women—who still consume, on average, half of what men do. This custom has been helpful to the degree that it has protected women from alcohol problems. But the prejudice behind this custom has also stigmatized women who drink too much—and "too much" is often defined by gender roles.

In many places—on college campuses; at happy hours, whether at home or in bars where women drink freely with men—one might almost imagine that the double standard regarding women and alcohol has disappeared. In fact, the shift is only on the surface. When alcohol interferes with women's family responsibilities, or when women's problems with alcohol become conspicuous, according to Richard and Sharon Wilsnack, "the attitude of society is likely to shift from indifference to outrage and an attempt to punish rather than treat the woman's drinking problems." Women are still held to a higher standard than men.

Part Two

On the Job
and in Families

3

Marriage and Partnerships

DRINKING PARTNERS

IT HAS BEEN KNOWN FOR SOME TIME THAT DRINKING rates are highest among the divorced and never-married. Recent news reports about how marital status affects our drinking patterns have turned certain assumptions on their head and have probably made a lot of women smile. When a marriage dissolves, men with drinking problems begin to have more of them, and women begin to have fewer. (We always knew who benefited more from marriage.) A closer look at the statistics suggest what common sense might predict. Happy marriages offer a degree of protection from drinking problems, and stressful relationships can exacerbate them. Alcohol can also turn a happy marriage into an unhappy one. Alcohol, again, operates as cause and effect.

Researchers have long believed that a woman's partner had a strong influence on her drinking—essentially, that husbands led their wives into alcoholism. Newer, longitudinal research—following women's drinking over time—suggests that this isn't true. Instead, it appears that "like marries like." Heavy drinkers get together in part because their habits correspond. Since men are more likely to drink in general, female alcoholics are much more likely than male alcoholics to have a spouse who drinks (49 percent compared with 6 percent). Women who live with a partner but have never married are at the highest risk of drinking problems. They have the highest rates of intoxication, of drinking and heavy drinking, and of symptoms of alcohol dependence. Researchers suspect that these women go into their relationships with a heavy drinking habit.

Although these statistics are interesting and suggestive, they should be interpreted cautiously, since they do not distinguish between cause and effect, and age differences may confuse the picture—younger women are more likely to have drinking problems and to be "never married." Furthermore, among black women neither age nor marital status is related to problem drinking.

STRUGGLES FOR LOVE AND POWER

ALCOHOLISM IN either partner exacerbates the inevitable issues of gender and power that exist in any romantic relationship. Frank, the husband of a woman in recovery, told me that his wife, Ellen, started drinking abusively when he accepted a high-profile job in a small city. The position required that he and Ellen host a number of dinners each week and attend numerous functions. Under pressure from Frank, Ellen agreed to put her career on hold, but she soon became unhappy. "It was a disastrous move for us," said Frank in retrospect. Before a year was out, Ellen's unhappiness evolved into full-blown depression, and she started drinking from the time she got up in the morning. Tension rose between them, as each partner blamed the other for their problems. They talked about divorce. After treatment, Ellen stopped drinking altogether, but the couple never fully reconciled until Frank left his job and they moved to another city—neutral territory, where they could reestablish equal footing.

Frank encouraged Ellen to get treatment, and ultimately, he was willing to make compromises to support her recovery. Sometimes, though, a man plays a role in maintaining his wife's addiction. When two drinking partners get together, the dynamics are especially volatile and complicated. Stephie, from Atlanta, told me a story that I heard echoed by other women. She and her husband, Ryan, drank together from the time they met, though Ryan never became alcoholic. When sober, Stephie was vivacious and outgoing, and very capable, while Ryan was shy, reserved, and uncertain. After their two children were born, Stephie wanted to return to school, but Ryan didn't see the point. He wanted her to stay at her low-level job. He also wanted to make all the decisions in the family, and he became furious when Stephie refused to go along. By this time, Stephie was drinking as much as two bottles of wine a night, and Ryan had discovered that he could control his wife with alcohol. He kept her supplied with alcohol and offered it to her at vulnerable moments, or when he wanted sex, especially when she was trying to quit.

"He used my weakness against me," said Stephie. "He used my problems to maintain the status quo. He knew as long as I was drinking, he had all the power. I was dependent on him financially, and I couldn't walk out or he'd get custody of the kids. That was the big club. He had me under his thumb, and that's God's honest truth. There's no way to sugarcoat it and make excuses. People say, 'He really loved you; he was afraid of losing you,' but that's a sick kind of love if you're willing to let someone suffer and suffer."

Stephie has been sober for fifteen years. To her own astonishment, she has surmounted the enormous anger she felt toward her husband for promoting her drinking when she was all but dying. She and Ryan are about to celebrate their twenty-fifth wedding anniversary. "I think the turning point came when I told him I hated him for what he'd done to me, and asked him, 'Why would you not help me?' He put it into words and told me to my face that he'd been so afraid of losing me, he'd rather have me drinking than gone. It tore him up to admit it. When he finally saw it, he was in a lot of pain about it. It bothers him to this day."

Clinicians have noted that whenever a couple has alcohol problems—whether the man, the woman, or both partners are drinking—

there tend to be struggles over who has power in the relationship. Same-sex couples are not exempt. Michelle, a lesbian from rural Louisiana, described how she drank to bury her resentment about having the "typical female role" in her relationship, while her partner made the major decisions and took charge of the finances and property. "Whatever Hannah wanted, that was okay, and if I didn't like it, I just drank some more," said Michelle. Typically, Michelle wasn't conscious of her anger while this was happening: "I was so disconnected from my feelings I didn't know what was going on. I don't think I ever realized that I had choices."

Often, problems simmer below the surface of a relationship. If you ask either partner, he or she will tell you everything is going fine. This can be especially devastating when the woman's drinking problem goes unmentioned or unnoticed, and the damage multiplies at home and in her body until her alcoholism is so advanced that it can't be ignored any longer.

DAPHNE'S STORY

DAPHNE AND PAUL fell in love during their junior year in college. Most of their friends considered marriage a long way off. "Instead of saying they were in love, they'd say they were 'in like,'" Daphne told me. One of the reasons she loved Paul was his unabashed enthusiasm—especially for her. He called her his Greek goddess. Her mother was Greek, and Daphne has flowing black hair and olive skin. "My friends used to say that he rolled his eyes like a lovesick dog. He didn't bother to disguise it." Daphne and Paul were known for their sense of fun and whimsy, and both had a weakness for romance. Their proposal plans were in the works for weeks. On the appointed day, Paul took Daphne to a picnic on a hill, where a table was draped with a white cloth, and a basket held champagne, bread, pâté, grapes, and cookies. After a toast, he led her to the top of a nearby tower, where, looking out at the green-gold hills, he asked for her hand in marriage. When they descended from the tower, a crowd of friends were there to cheer, and the toasts began in earnest.

After college, Daphne got her master's degree in computer science and landed a good job consulting for a large business, while Paul went on to law school. Eight years later, when Paul took a demanding job with a law firm, Daphne became pregnant and gave up her career. They both felt strongly that one of them—Daphne—needed to stay at home. They despised the modern world of day care, not to mention the youth culture of violent cartoons and tacky spin-off toys. There would be no TV in their lives; there would be stuffed animals, books by A. A. Milne and E. B. White, homemade Greek pastries, apple picking, beekeeping, cartwheeling, music—a child's paradise. They moved to a country house, and Paul commuted to the city.

Daphne adored her baby boy, Lewis, and was committed to her way of life, but she began to get lonely. She felt guilty for missing the work she'd given up and for wondering how high up the ladder she'd be by now if she hadn't left. She found herself growing irritated with Lewis; she had a hard time coping with his constant demands. But she told herself that motherhood involved self-sacrifice; everyone knew that. She was happy for Paul, whose career was flourishing, and proud of her role as his supporter. Her tender touch helped him withstand the inevitable blows to his ego at work. She threw herself into creative homemaking, growing organic vegetables and canning them for winter, exposing her son to music and art, finding innovative ways of cutting household costs. Each evening, when Paul returned home at seven-thirty, he found a candlelit dinner and the table set for two. They waited to eat until Lewis was asleep, and until they had some wine together, as they'd done since they were married. Daphne found herself waiting all day for that time with Paul, when they shared their days, and the wine took away her weariness and made her feel loving and warm.

When Lewis was three, Daphne went off birth control. She imagined that when the household was fuller and noisier, she would feel more complete. The years went by, though, and she didn't get pregnant. Her sense of isolation grew. She hardly enjoyed Lewis anymore. It was an effort just to take him to the park, just to pick him up after school. She began to have disturbing physical symptoms, including fatigue, a declining interest in sex, and periods of clumsiness when she was likely to bump into doorframes. Paul became alarmed and urged her to see a neurologist.

Daphne did not connect these episodes to the tall glass of vodka she drank on her own each night before her husband came home. She didn't tell Paul about the vodka; and when she went to consult the neurologist, he didn't ask about her drinking. When I commented about how many doctors have a blind spot when it comes to women's drinking, she replied, "If he'd asked, I would have told him about the wine I drank at dinner. Two or three glasses every night."

The neurologist did ask Daphne about her moods, and she confessed to feeling blue a lot of the time, for no particular reason. After further discussion, he referred her to a psychiatrist, who prescribed antidepressants. The psychiatrist described potential side effects—dry mouth, heart irregularities. Though he suggested she not drink caffeine or alcohol, Daphne knew people who were on antidepressants and still drank, so she decided that this advice was optional. At the end of their session, the psychiatrist reassured Daphne about the marvels of modern medicine. Depression, he said, could be cured.

Her symptoms didn't go away. Paul started coming home early from work so he could help with dinner, clean up, and put Lewis to bed. "I was like a wounded bird," Daphne told me, "and he took care of me." He still called her his one and only love. Although his friends said their attraction to their wives cooled off after a couple of years, his knees, he said, still went weak in her presence. Daphne saw him as powerful and protecting, devoted and tender, a true gentleman. In contrast, she felt more and more fearful and inadequate. She tried hard to cope with her depression, joining a gym and exercising harder, joining a church, and reading inspirational books.

When it fleetingly occurred to her that she could have a drinking problem, she let the thought pass without investigation. After all, she never drank before four or five o'clock. She never got drunk. She didn't do all those things that alcoholics did, like keeping tiny bottles of liquor in her purse or getting up in the night to take a swig. She did take a prescribed tranquilizer at three in the morning, however. Occasionally she stopped drinking for a week—not even wine at dinner—just to test herself, and she found that she could do it. She regarded this as another sign that she didn't have a problem. Alcohol was a helpful friend, an ally in her battle against depression. If she couldn't destroy the enemy, at least she could cope with it. Alcohol could help.

The act was getting harder to keep up, however. Paul became convinced that she had an undiagnosed disease—and she also thought this could be the case. She began to feel desperate for some sort of solution, especially because she had lost all interest in sex. She hadn't had an orgasm in years, and this was beginning to take its toll on Paul. She suspected that he might be having an affair, but when she confronted him, he denied it vehemently. At his urging, she began to see a string of doctors. She felt hopeful each time she submitted to a new series of tests. Each time the results came back indicating there was nothing wrong, her anxiety redoubled.

One night when she and Paul were at a friend's home for dinner, she overheard Paul describing her problems. "She has trouble with her balance," he was saying. "If you didn't know better, you'd think that she was drunk." She felt a threatening sense that something was about to be taken away from her. She let the feeling pass.

Four months later, Paul came into the kitchen with his face pale. He'd been taking out the trash, and the plastic bag had split open. Empty vodka bottles had spilled onto the driveway.

Daphne cried in indignation, never imagining, she said, that Paul could be so unfair. Yes, she was drinking a little more, but she'd never hidden it and she did not have a problem. Alcohol helped her cope. It took the edge off her desperation, and he was cruel to suggest that she give it up. She could not admit, even to herself, that her fatigue and unhappiness might be due to alcohol. Drinking no longer made Daphne feel high, no longer gave her a feeling of warmth or coziness. Now all it did was allow her body to feel *normal*, and insulate her from despair. She didn't drink for fun. She drank to stay alive.

Her marriage now deteriorated into screaming matches—plates

flying, windows crashing. The more Daphne drank, the angrier Paul got and the more he tried to control her. Daphne was terrified, and increasingly worried about what all this was doing to Lewis. Finally, with a profound sense of failure and shame, she checked into an inpatient rehabilitation center. Once she had been Paul's Greek goddess, his love, his inspiration. Now, knocked from her pedestal, she was a common drunk. Her mother, who had never taken more than a sip of wine, was in a state of disbelief; her father stopped talking to her.

At the treatment center, doctors agreed that Daphne suffered from depression as well as addiction. After detoxification, they decided that she should stick with her current antidepressant, which probably hadn't worked because she was drinking. She was educated about the disease of alcoholism and encouraged to talk about her feelings of loneliness and shame, and about how she had used alcohol to fill a hole inside her. Paul came for family week and confronted her with his anger about how she had lied to him for so long. She told him she had been afraid to ask for help, afraid that he would abandon her if she didn't live up to his image of the perfect wife.

When she returned home—frightened, but eager to be reunited with her son—Daphne's biggest fear was about having sex without alcohol to loosen her up. Looking back, she couldn't remember any sober sex. Even in college, she and Paul had always drunk first. When Paul didn't press her for several weeks, Daphne finally approached him, praying it would be better than she thought. "But it was bad news," said Daphne. "I just couldn't feel romantic. I was nervous and shaky, and there was still anger between us." In addition, Daphne was ashamed of what she and Paul had done in bed when she was drunk. A few times, she had even let Paul tie her up. It had seemed funny and playful at the time, but now the memory made her feel degraded and dirty.

Her anxiety rose during several weeks of avoiding sex. She started wondering if sobriety would ruin her marriage altogether. At treatment, she'd been educated about preventing relapses, and she had learned ways of coping with certain "triggers" to drink. At four o'clock, the time when she used to reach for the vodka, she went to the gym instead. In the morning, when Paul and Lewis had left for their days and she felt empty and vacant, she went to an AA meeting. But she felt there was nowhere she could talk about the problems in her sexual life.

After three months, Daphne picked up the bottle again. Although she hid it carefully, and made new rules about how much she would drink and when, the harder she tried to control it, the more she was compelled to drink. Secretly, she blamed Paul. He was pressuring her for sex. Though he'd thrown out the vodka, he insisted on keeping the bourbon in the pantry, because he liked a glass at night, and, he said, *he* didn't have a drinking problem.

She became obsessed with his behavior, convinced that he was seeing other women. (As it turned out, she says, he was.) One night when he came home late, she stood at the top of the stairs and screamed at him. Lewis came out of his bedroom. In front of her husband and son, she threw herself down the stairs.

Physically, she escaped with a couple of bashed teeth, but this was the turning point for Paul. The following week, he moved out of the house with Lewis and told her he wanted a divorce. Daphne panicked, sure she would lose custody of Lewis. She started drinking the moment she got up in the morning and could hardly drink enough to stave off symptoms of withdrawal.

Not long afterward, she discovered that she was pregnant. She told Paul, hoping to persuade him to move back in. Instead he begged her to get an abortion, terrified of having to raise a child with fetal alcohol syndrome, as well as Lewis. Daphne refused. She'd been wanting this child for years, and she was going to have it. She tried harder to stop drinking, but she couldn't. Paul became frantic. He threatened to move away with Lewis, and never allow her to see him.

In the end, said Daphne, her body had the sense to miscarry.

When she woke up in sheets full of blood, she wanted to drown in her misery and shame. She had disgraced herself. She had destroyed her family and killed her baby, the one good seed that was growing inside her. Now all she wanted was to disappear from the face of the earth.

Dependency and Power

MANY OF DAPHNE'S experiences are common among female alcoholics, highlighting themes that will recur throughout this book:

- Her depression and her alcohol problems were entangled in complicated ways.
- Her drinking went unnoticed and misdiagnosed.
- She took dangerous combinations of medication and alcohol.
- Her sexual dysfunction both contributed to her drinking and was made worse by it; and her treatment—which in Daphne's case was very good—still failed to address her sexual problems.
- By the time she sought treatment, her alcoholism was well advanced and had infected every area of her life.

Daphne's story makes me think of Fillmore's statement that when women have alcohol problems, "Everything tends to go wrong at once."

Daphne's focus on her partner as the primary source of her self-worth is also typical of women with alcohol problems. Many clinicians believe that the key difference between addicted men and addicted women is the prevalence of "codependency" among women, who are frequently enmeshed in unhealthy relationships, sometimes, but not always, with an addicted partner. Describing codependent women who are also alcoholic, Dr. Josette Mondanaro wrote, "These women are exquisitely tuned in to the needs of others. Their satellite dishes are aimed outward, vigilantly scanning the horizon and picking up the needs of others. What is missing is a second satellite dish that should be turned inward, scanning their internal territory, focusing on their needs, feelings, and desires."

These women's extreme dependence, their attempts to rescue or control, and their undeveloped sense of self can undermine their efforts to get sober. "It's why we need gender-specific treatment," says Elizabeth Zelvin, a psychotherapist in New York City who specializes in addictions and women's issues. "When women have poor boundaries, when they look outside themselves for their identity, you have to integrate these issues into their treatment or they may never be able to stay sober."

In the past, codependents and alcoholics were often assumed to be two distinct groups, and the typical codependent was seen as the non-addicted wife of an alcoholic man. The term soon came to refer to all of an alcoholic's family members, including adult children. The inadvertently "enabling" behavior of the codependent was at first seen as a response to living with an out-of-control drinker. As one member of Al-Anon—the organization for families of alcoholics—told me, "If you have measles, you can't help getting spots, and if you live with an alcoholic, you can't help getting codependent. All of a sudden, you have your nose in the other person's business, and you don't even notice that your own life is falling apart."

Since the 1980s, codependency has been considered a "disease" in its own right, having its own symptoms and often preceding any involvement with an alcoholic partner. Yet the very familiarity of Daphne's story—the way her life gradually constricts as she takes on conventional female roles, the way she loses herself in the process—calls into question the usefulness of a disease category that describes so much of the female population. Indeed, the concept of codependency has come under attack in recent years. Some point out the double bind of women who are first socialized to put other people's needs ahead of their own and then told that this habit is pathological. Negative associations have been compounded by the experience of some women in Al-Anon, who say their martyrlike impulses were reinforced by the emphasis on being cheerful ("I will make up my mind to be cheerful every waking moment of this day," reads *One Day at a Time*, an Al-Anon book of daily meditations), on not being angry, and on looking to the self for happiness to the point where the reality of intolerable circumstances—an abusive partner, for instance—was ignored. Other women report nearly opposite experiences: they were encouraged by group members to "throw away the baby with the bathwater" by walking

away from important relationships and commitments that the group
considered codependent.

While some feminists fear that codependency itself is an oppres-
sive construct for women, others, including Elizabeth Zelvin, make a
plea for the usefulness of the concept and its potential to empower both
women and men. "It provides such a helpful set of tools," Zelvin told
me, "and it's cheaper than therapy." She points out that people in
recovery from codependency are nearly always confused about personal
boundaries—what's martyrdom, what's selfishness, when you should
walk away and when you should stay put—and naturally, some Al-
Anon members will distort its principles when they are "disease-side
up instead of recovery-side up." Most of the time, she says, groups like
Al-Anon provide tremendous support in working these issues out sen-
sibly. For desperate people coming to these meetings, the idea of codependency as a disease is usually felt not as a stigma but as a relief. The
concept helps to differentiate between what you can't control—a past
marked by the effects of an alcohol-dependent system—and what you
can control in your own internal life.

"The first principle in Al-Anon is to keep the focus on yourself,"
says Zelvin. "When my clients in therapy express a fear of being 'selfish,' I tell them you have to build yourself up; but once you're filled up,
out of the overflow, you will have a lot to give. The other principle is
detachment with love. 'With love' is important. It means you can be
compassionate and still have boundaries. It means you're allowed to
care for others without going down the tubes with them, or being in
constant emotional turmoil because you can't save them. When applied
correctly, these principles save the lives of very desperate people."

As Zelvin's perspective suggests, even now the concept of codependency is evolving, largely in response to feminist voices within
the recovery movement. In particular, relational theory is being applied
to the treatment of women. Such theorists as Jean Baker Miller, Nancy
Chodorow, and Carol Gilligan have challenged the concepts of autonomy and independence as the ultimate in human development, suggesting that women's psychological development evolves within

growth-enhancing relationships, with healthy interdependence as the goal. "In this light," says Zelvin, "we can reframe the concept of co-dependency. Instead of seeing it as a failure to separate, we can see it as a series of misguided attempts to connect to other people. Women are *good* at making connections. Because of the nature of their development as well as their socialization, they're good at relationships. But this talent exists side by side with its distortion: the idea that a woman is incomplete without the people she connects with. When a woman believes that, she gloms on to another person for her whole identity, often someone who can't meet her needs because he can't meet his own. Codependency is what happens to the capacity for relationship when it is used destructively."

Some other specialists in the field have reframed codependency in ways that emphasize cultural socialization and power dynamics. Charlotte Davis Kasl, a psychologist who is the author of *Many Roads, One Journey: Moving Beyond the Twelve Steps*, suggests the term "internalized oppression," and defines codependency as "a disease of inequality—a predictable set of behavior patterns that people in a subordinate role typically adopt to survive in the dominant culture. Codependency is a euphemism for internalized oppression and includes traits of passivity, compliance, lack of initiative, abandonment of self, and fear of showing power openly."

Similarly, in their book *The Responsibility Trap*, the family therapists Claudia Bepko and Jo-Ann Krestan speak of overresponsibility instead of codependency. Bepko and Krestan address emotional and functional overresponsibility and underresponsibility within alcoholic relationships. They note that these concepts will be familiar to those who attend Al-Anon, which emphasizes that alcoholics need to take responsibility for themselves, and that partners are most helpful when they focus on their own behavior instead of caring for the alcoholic. In family systems theory, the assumption is that a fully responsible adult will tend to his or her own physical and emotional needs and ask directly for help from others. In contrast, someone who is emotionally overresponsible sees the other person's needs as more important than his or her own and will focus on meeting them, often without having been asked. The emotionally underresponsible person expects sensitivity and recognition from others without making his or her needs known, and blames others for his or her problems. With regard to tasks, the overresponsible person will take over other people's work or direct it from the sidelines; this typically prompts underresponsible behavior from others.

Overresponsible people pride themselves on being the only ones who know how to get things done and take care of others. They feel important and powerful—but they also feel intensely angry because they can never be dependent or expect to have their own needs met. Like their underresponsible partners, they rely on external validation to feel valuable. Since they can never achieve perfect control, they are plagued by anxiety and a sense of worthlessness.

Traditionally, women are socialized to be caretakers, overresponsible for anything relating to home and family—emotionally and in terms of tasks—while men are socialized to be overresponsible in the "instrumental dimension"—meaning that they feel pressure to do something in the world and to make money. Both women and men are socialized to be underresponsible for themselves in different ways: women by ignoring their own self-interest and depending economically on men, and men by relying on women for physical and emotional comfort.

Bepko and Krestan note that in families with alcohol problems, sex roles have typically become very rigid. "It's tempting to assume that recent social changes have freed men and women from conventional expectations," says Bepko, "but when you work with families in recovery, you find that stereotyped attitudes are very much alive and well. Generally speaking, the families who have made a successful transition to new attitudes and behaviors are not the ones who end up needing treatment." When they do, says Bepko, you'll generally find that the changes in their attitudes about sex roles are on the surface. Traditional assumptions about how we will feel and behave as a female or a male are so deeply ingrained in all of us that there is often lingering guilt or uneasiness when we "fail" to meet those expectations.

Bepko goes so far as to define addictions as "disorders of power."

She explains that when couples relate within the framework of a hierarchy instead of a partnership, and struggle with issues of power and dependency but see no way to work out their conflicts, alcohol may be "invited into the system to correct it," either by suppressing feelings of inadequacy and anger or by quietly shifting the power dynamics as couples adapt to the new context created by drinking.

Though alcohol problems always aggravate issues of dependency and power, and play themselves out within the context of family roles, Bepko stresses that alcoholism is, at its core, a disordered relationship between the drinker and the drink. It begins with an effort to control some aspect of oneself by means of an external agent. Ultimately, this external agent renders the person powerless. For many women, this process is echoed in relationships: a woman drinks to rebel against her role, only to find that her alcoholism has landed her under her partner's thumb. In a widening circle, she may drink to dull the acute frustration all women feel if they are cut off from power in a culture where men are privileged.

To one degree or another, power struggles take place in all relationships. If this competition is seen as unacceptable, alcohol may enter the scene, driving the problems underground. Alcohol disconnects people from their feelings, allowing them to deny the drinking problem and the struggles that are arising because of it. Alcohol deprives a woman and her partner of an opportunity to work toward a mutual relationship and newer, more healthy expressions of dependency and power.

KEEPING THE SELF IN LINE

DAPHNE AND PAUL, though young and educated and part of a changing world, were living in a fantasy of a traditional marriage. Each was strongly invested in an image of the self that corresponded to stereotypical assumptions about women and men's identities. Daphne wanted to be a perfect homemaker and mother and an alluring sexual partner. Paul was her access to the larger world, and his love for her was what made her an important person. Paul wanted to be a gentleman, respected in his work, a devoted husband and father, a keeper of moral standards, a good provider, and married to an adoring woman. Alcohol was their friend and ally, allowing them to support their illusions about themselves and each other.

Daphne used alcohol to drown out her feeling that she was not a "natural mother." Typically, her fears for Lewis prompted her to get treatment for herself. She used alcohol to suppress her resentment of Paul: "All of his goals were in harmony," she told me. "The better lawyer he was, the more he felt worthy as a husband and father. Everything *I* wanted was in conflict." She was not, at the time, consciously aware of her longing for power in the world, since in her mind, that power properly belonged to Paul. She suppressed her jealousy and anger and noticed only that she was weary and depressed—feelings that both she and Paul considered more acceptable in a woman.

Conflict about gender roles has been a consistent theme in the literature on women and alcohol problems. As you might expect, the way this conflict has been framed has changed over the years. Well into the 1970s, the scientific literature referred to women alcoholics' "deviant sex role adjustment" and "defective femininity," the assumption being that the problem was the woman, not our expectation that she fit into a constraining role. Equally, men were said to drink because they wanted to enhance their feeling of masculinity and power, not because they might find the masculine role a burden they would like to shed. More recently, there has been a growing appreciation of flexible gender roles, the assumption being that women and men function best when they are at ease with both the "female" and the "male" aspects of their personalities, and can integrate them into their behavior and their experience of self. Claudia Bepko notes that in her clinical work, wherever alcoholism plays a role within a family, there are problems achieving this androgynous integration. Instead, feelings that run counter to traditional sex role expectations are neither acknowledged nor acted on. Behavior is polarized, and "males are pitted against females in a relationship that is overtly defined as a cooperative partnership, but covertly becomes the emotional equivalent of war."

In this context, alcohol can be used to suppress feelings that are deemed unacceptable. When she was sober, Daphne got irritated, angry, and resentful; but alcohol told her she was warm, relaxed, happy, loving, and sexy. This was in keeping with Daphne's ideal, and in keeping with Paul's ideal for Daphne. The more he praised and idealized her, the more pressure she felt to keep up the show, and the more fraudulent she felt inside.

Alcohol can also provide a face-saving way to express unacceptable feelings. When Daphne took to her bed and Paul came home early from work, her "illness" gave her an excuse to give up the traditional female role of being the family caretaker, bolstering Paul's ego, and feeling responsible for everyone. This in turn allowed Paul to take on the nurturing role, and to express a feminine side of himself without challenging his self-image. Later, when there was out-and-out war between them, Daphne could explode in a drunken rage without having to acknowledge that she was also angry when she was sober. The status quo was maintained, but only because alcohol prevented any overt challenge to the power structure.

Within a supposedly stable power structure, with Daphne and Paul presumably agreeing on the traditional arrangement in which the male is dominant, there were subterranean battles over which of the two was "on top," playing out in very complex ways. For instance, Daphne depended on Paul's idealization of her to make her feel important, but she also resented it as a covert form of control, a way of telling her how she *ought* to feel and behave. His not noticing her drinking confirmed her belief that when he looked at her, he saw only what he wanted to see and didn't care who she really was. In a sense, Daphne's "illness" was a way of getting power over Paul: it kept him at home, where all his attention was focused on her and Lewis. At the same time, his overresponsibility made her feel like an incompetent child and allowed her to slip further into alcoholism. She felt angry, confused, and trapped. If she pulled herself together, she would no longer be the center of Paul's universe, and by now she feared she could not survive without him.

In a complicated tug of war, Paul and Daphne competed with each other as caretakers. At different times, each tried to heal the other's wounds with love and attention, so that, whole and healthy, the other would be capable of giving perfect love in return. Both were angry when this didn't work, and each blamed the other for a neediness that came from within. Daphne's resentment gave her another excuse for drinking, and drinking was also a gesture of defiance, a way of escaping Paul's control. Their problems escalated.

Daphne was, in a way, saying, "You don't own me, and you can't make me stop drinking." Typically, Paul reacted to her rebellion by telling her that she was bad and needed help. By taking a position of moral superiority, he reestablished his power. Daphne drank more, reasserting her independence. Paul tried harder to control her.

Daphne accused Paul of sabotaging her sobriety by pressuring her for sex and keeping alcohol in the house. But if there was truth in her accusation, it doesn't follow that Paul was a villain. In cases like these, says Bepko, the partner is hanging on for dear life and will grasp at "any available experience of control in an otherwise chaotic and very frightening emotional climate." Paul's whole sense of himself may have been at stake. The wronged hero was a role he could seize in order to restore his self-esteem. He could take pride in his selfless behavior while caring for Daphne and Lewis; he could feel good, responsible, and competent at a time when family life was veering out of control. Since taking charge was a matter of necessity, he could deny any wish for power.

Ultimately, says Bepko, in such cases, it's all going in one direction. The woman's drinking makes her increasingly dependent, more in her partner's power. The power structure won't change unless the drinking stops, the alcoholic dies, or the partner leaves.

Five years later, Daphne and Paul are still picking up the pieces. Daphne has been sober for two years. She shares custody of Lewis with Paul, who is now married to another woman. She plans to reenter her profession; and on most days she feels a sense of hope and possibility.

The hardest task has been to value her sobriety for her own sake, and to believe that her life is worth fighting for. She works to build a firmer sense of self, but it hasn't been an easy road. "Paul had this big, warm, exciting orbit, and I wanted to stay inside it, even if it kept me spinning," she told me. "No matter how awful it got, I felt safe when I was in his sphere." Her divorce from Paul brought her to despair. Seeing him as a heroic father (he had full custody for three years) and herself as a failed mother, she had little motivation to stay sober. Her emotional fusion with Paul also made it easy to resent him and kept her locked in the old power struggle, which didn't stop with the divorce. Gradually, she saw that the cycle was killing her, and that she needed to step outside it. "Whenever I relapsed, it was usually because I was focused on Paul instead of myself," she said.

At first, focusing on her own feelings in therapy and at AA filled Daphne with fear. She said, "It felt like falling through a void." Her experience, according to Elizabeth Zelvin, is common among recovering women. "They're confronting all the feelings of sadness and loss and fear and loneliness and not being safe, of not knowing how to be a healthy adult who operates in the world. A lot of women describe it as a void, a black hole. There's no self at the beginning of recovery; it has to be built from the ground up. Without the alcohol, they think there's nothing there to help them cope, so becoming aware of any feeling is just terrifying."

AA helps Daphne by giving her practice focusing on herself. She's working through the twelve steps with the warm support of her sponsor. At meetings, the "no cross-talk" rule means that nothing she says is challenged, and this provides a feeling of safety. The stories of other alcoholics give her some perspective on her life. In therapy, she has come to see how her passivity and reliance on others helped her get through childhood with a father who expected adoration from his daughter, and how these traits were encouraged by the old-fashioned ideal of wife and mother. It helped to understand that she was not alone. To one degree or another, most women struggle with these issues.

"Things are definitely getting better, and I'm taking responsibil-

4

Mothers:
A Message from the Owl

*When my son Michael was sixteen, he was working after school,
and one day I went to pick him up. I'd been drinking. I had to
make a left turn onto the road where he worked, and I fell
asleep waiting for the light to turn. The owners of the corner
store called the police because traffic was piling up behind me.
Michael spotted the car and ran over—I was in the ditch, I
don't know how I got there—and he said to the cop, "Don't
worry, I'll take her home." And he did. That corner store had
fresh corn that fall, and I was going to go buy some for dinner.
Michael said, "Mom, I don't think you want to go there," and
he told me what had happened.*

    Every time I think of this I shudder.

MARIANNE, AGE SIXTY-FIVE,

SOBER FOR EIGHTEEN YEARS

ANY WOMAN WHOSE CHILDREN ARE BEYOND A CERTAIN
age knows what it's like to fail them. We want to buffer our children
with unconditional love, to watch them grow in competence and joy, to
shore up their roots in the soil of our acceptance. But even the proudest
mothers see their own shortcomings reflected back at them. We hear
our own angry words coming back at us from a child's mouth; or we
watch a daughter lose a friend because of her bossiness, and realize that
we've kept her under our thumb; or see a son belittle his girlfriend, and
it dawns on us that we have not insisted on being respected by our hus-

band and children. A mother may behave "perfectly" but find that her children hide their feelings, having read her buried pain. We try to protect our children from suffering, but they discover suffering in part through their experience of our own limitations.

All mothers know, as well, how hard it is to come to a mature acceptance of these limitations, and a realistic sense of where our responsibilities to our children begin and end. On some level, we expect to be judged by our children's health and happiness. Children come into the world with both a father and a mother (whether or not both are present), as well as extended families, religious communities, schools, a peer group, and a broader society; but our mother-blaming culture reinforces a tendency to imagine ourselves as completely in control. In all the examples of "mother failure" above, the mother-child dyad is just one factor—how might the picture change if we asked questions about the larger family? Too often, we don't ask questions before laying blame at a mother's feet. It's as if mothers are omnipotent, when in fact they're only one link in a chain.

When a woman has failed her children in small or large ways because of alcohol problems, her guilt and confusion increase exponentially. Her self-condemnation is echoed and reinforced by the reaction of people around her. Despite changing roles, women—especially if they have children—are expected to be more loving, self-sacrificing, and virtuous than men. A mother who has passed out on the kitchen floor with a hungry baby in the next room will probably see herself as a monster. Only another drink can blunt her feeling of remorse.

"Woman needs to give. She cannot help herself." So goes one theory. "Woman's primal driving force is love and the service of those she loves." Since no woman is an endless fount of nurture, this myth of the perfect mother becomes a whip to punish women. In particular, an alcoholic woman, who probably can't manage to put her children first, will be judged unnatural, unfeminine, a failure in her most basic role. Thus we see simplistic news stories about addicts who have "lost their maternal instinct."

Though mothers who drink can look as if they "care more about alcohol than their children"—a frequent accusation—clinicians who work with these women say their guilt is enormous, sometimes so large that they defend against it with all their energy. This can make them look as if they don't care at all. "When a woman's shame gets intense, when she feels threatened or inadequate as a mother, you'll see her retreat," explained Sandy Klevens, a chemical dependency counselor. "The families don't get it. They just think she's a bad mom. She may be doing a bad job because of her addiction, but she cares. She cares enormously."

This was certainly true of the women I interviewed who drank when they had children at home. "I was hung over when I went into labor," one mother told me, "and my daughter took three days to be born. They told me it was because I'd been drinking vodka . . . When she was born, I was so ashamed, I couldn't look at her." I wondered if the hospital staff recognized her shame, or if they thought she wasn't interested in her baby.

Another mother told me about giving her ex-husband custody of her daughter, because she drank too much to care for her properly. The decision was so painful that she convinced herself she'd been tricked by her family—she could not face her own responsibility. Fifteen years later, tentatively sober, she cried as she told me the story: "My own mother abandoned me," she said. "If there was ever one thing I didn't want to do in my life, it was abandon my own daughter."

Marianne described how her twelve-year-old son retreated to his basement room whenever she was drinking. "He was a lonely kid for those years," she told me. "When I got home from treatment, if I laughed, he'd come near me to see if he could smell alcohol on my breath. I felt so sorry for that boy."

Ideally, a woman learns to distinguish between appropriate guilt—guilt over behavior for which she tries to make amends—and the shame that cripples her and keeps her in the cycle of addiction. I asked the family therapist Claudia Bepko how a woman makes that leap, how she comes to terms with any harm she's done to her children.

"She needs concrete strategies for making amends," Bepko replied. "If the children are old enough when she's in recovery, she can sit down with them and tell them the truth. So much of her relationship with them when she abused alcohol will have been based on lies. It's so freeing to be truthful, and to tell them, 'I'm sorry.' Truthfulness is healing in relationships between parents and children."

As for letting go of shame, "You do that in community with other women," said Bepko. "You can't heal shame in isolation. There has to be community. You see that other women are forgivable; therefore you must be too." Bepko said that when her clients don't feel comfortable in twelve-step programs, as many don't, she tries to bring them into some kind of group therapy.

The healing power of a group leaves some women awestruck and profoundly grateful. Amy, a sixty-three-year-old artist from New York City whose story appears in Chapter 8, kept repeating to me, "I don't understand why I was cured. There's a sense of mystery about it." Her cure was encompassing. Not only is she sober—with no impulse to drink—but she has shed a lifetime of anxiety attacks about her health. "Before treatment at Betty Ford, I would say I have been really anxious all my life. And it went away!"

"That's astonishing," I said.

"You're telling me!" she replied. "I wouldn't dream of drinking over the things that make me anxious now, and they make me half as anxious."

She was awed by how open she became to other people—the staff, the other women—and the sense of belonging to deeper and deeper layers of community, culminating in family week, when all three of her daughters flew out to participate. Each daughter went off with a group of nine others, working on her own issues—"It was about them, not about me, which none of us had expected"—while Amy traveled to the three different groups. Each daughter confronted Amy with the pain and difficulty her drinking had caused. "By this time," said Amy, "all of us had allies of our own." Her daughters' connection to the families of the patients was "profoundly moving" for each of them, said Amy, and this deepened her own sense of community. In her time at Betty

Ford, she broke through her isolation and recognized how much she shared with other people.

"Each one of my daughters said that she had had no idea why I didn't just stop, but she had come to understand that I *couldn't*, that I wasn't just a powerful person who was being difficult. A lot of the guilt washed away at that point.

"I don't know why it worked," she repeated. "I have no idea."

ANGER AND BLAME

AS I WAS writing this book, many people who heard about it had stories to offer me. By far the most passionate conversations I had were with men and women whose mothers or mothers-in-law still struggled with alcoholism. They told me tales of unbelievable neglect, callousness, and cruelty—truly these women sounded like "the most difficult woman in the world"—and revealed their own deep and persistent feelings of hurt and bitterness.

One man's story stood out in particular. I'll call him Jack. His wife, Jack told me, cried all the time because of her eighty-year-old alcoholic mother, Marie, whose affairs she had to manage, and who never had a kind word to say. The scenes she caused were endless and became the stuff of legend. There was the time she boarded a commuter train from San Francisco to El Cerrito drunk during the evening rush hour. Before her brief commute home was over, she had managed to throw up on two businessmen and terrorize a young mother, whose baby she kept wanting to hold. Then there was the Christmas dinner at her daughter's house in Pasadena when Marie knocked all the food and champagne glasses off the table and the next day blamed her behavior on "the worst gas attack I've ever had." There was the time when she took in a family of illegal Mexicans, worked them to the bone, and then, in paranoia, accused them of stealing and persuaded Immigration to send them back to Mexico. She drank a bottle of wine a day when she was on the wagon, and half a gallon of gin every two days when she wasn't.

When Jack's wife was young, Marie had the money to hire cooks

and nannies. She never paid the family any attention, except to criti-
cize, to tell her daughters they were fat and couldn't do anything right.
Marie's husband—a well-regarded real estate developer in the Bay
area—devoted his life to taking care of her. When he died, she said,
"I'm glad that bastard's dead." She never visited after the birth of her
grandchildren. She could never remember their names, often confusing
them with her sister's grandchildren. Astonishingly, she had so far sur-
vived every alcohol-related illness you could think of—cirrhosis of the
liver, fibrillations of the heart, phlebitis, blood clots in her legs and
lungs, deteriorating vision and hearing, and two emergency trips to the
hospital when a long-standing stomach ulcer began to hemorrhage.

Jack's anger on behalf of his wife was deep and genuine. His own
family life—he and his wife have two young daughters—was profoundly affected by the ongoing emergencies, and by his wife's pain
and self-doubt. He asked me not to broach the subject with his wife,
since the shame she felt in childhood has never dissipated and she
would be upset with him for bringing it up.

Clearly, it is no favor to anyone to minimize the burden on families of alcoholics, or their legitimate anger, or the damage alcoholism
does to a person's character. Jean Kirkpatrick, the founder of Women
for Sobriety, the women's self-help recovery group formed as an alternative to AA, wrote, "Years of drinking narrow the personality without
the drinker's awareness. We become subjective, egocentric, demanding, self-pitying, resentful. We are wrapped in a cocoon, aware only of
self with no relation to others or the outside world. We weren't like
this to begin with, but the insidiousness of alcohol's effects made us
this way."

Families affected by alcoholism know that, in the words of Alcoholics Anonymous, "It is not caused by weakness of will, immorality or
a desire to hurt others," but especially if there is a relapse, or when their
own hurt redoubles, the need to blame reasserts itself. This may be
most true when the alcoholic is a mother.

"When a mother is the substance abuser, children take much
more license in terms of attacking and shaming and holding her to

account, much more so than they're likely to do with a father," said Claudia Bepko. "You'll find that true even when the father is the alcoholic: children tend to blame the mother for the husband's drinking." Bepko said some children want to see the father as the good guy no matter what he does, and there's usually more fear of his aggression and violence. "And kids feel more betrayed by a drinking mother than they do by a drinking father. That's cultural. So much of the responsibility for family life rests on the mother, and you get angrier at the person you're more dependent on."

I asked Jack if there was anything positive, anything at all, that he could say about his mother-in-law. He paused for a long time before saying, "Her intelligence is not completely blighted. You can see glimpses of what she might have been had alcohol not gotten in the way. She has a prodigious memory that comes and goes. She knows everything about California history, and she once thought of writing a book about the Victorian architecture of San Francisco."

My further questions yielded this. Marie was an only child whose mother died of cancer when she was four. Her father died in a car accident when she was in her teens. An alcoholic, he'd wrecked his car many times before the crash that finally ended his spree. As a young woman, Marie was a pistol. She moved from Salinas into San Francisco on the small bit of money her father had left her, and there she became a prominent architect. In fact, she was one of the first women to make a mark in this male-dominated field in the Bay area. Her first marriage failed during World War II. After that, she gave up her career to marry again and have children. Her alcoholic drinking began, most likely, during her first marriage.

Her husband, said Jack, would have been a major developer if his wife hadn't been a drunk. As it was, he devoted himself to trying to keep her from doing embarrassing things in public. For twenty years he picked up all the pieces. At age eighty-one, he couldn't take living with her any longer and moved to a house around the corner, but two or three times a day he came and continued to pick up the pieces, even when he himself was dying of cancer.

Family members of problem drinkers who attend Al-Anon learn that what looks like virtuous behavior—picking up the pieces after an alcoholic—can actually help maintain an addiction. In a circular inter-action, the drinker becomes less and less responsible, and the non-drinker overfunctions. "It gets to look like a saint and a sinner," says Bepko, "but in effect, the overresponsible person is complicit in the problem. And you have to wonder why somebody would continue being an overfunctioner and sustaining a great deal of anger instead of taking a position."

I am not Marie's daughter, and so, I suppose, it is easy for me to be moved by sympathy for her as well as for the family she helped wreck. From Jack's account, it seems Marie had many risk factors for alcoholism: a family history of alcoholism and a chaotic childhood, including the early loss of her mother. After making her way in the world as an architect, she gave it all up to get married. Though there are no comparable studies of women in that era, today's data show that such "role deprivation" correlates with alcohol problems in women. And what about the husband who picked up after Marie during their entire marriage and, it appears, martyred himself for his family? Did he have anything invested in his role as a saint? Jack's account sug-gests family dynamics of overresponsibility and underresponsibility. It sounds as if his mother-in-law has given the others a very good run for their money and has energetically enacted her role of villain; but as Bepko suggests, it makes sense to stop blaming and see her as one player in a larger system.

MOTHERS AND DAUGHTERS

LIKE HER MOTHER and her grandmother before her, Pepina, thirty-four and sober for nearly six years, has an altar in her house consisting of a table covered with a white cloth, holding a cross, white candles, a vase of white flowers, and a big cup of water with ice, for the spirits when they get thirsty. (She lives in Florida and her air conditioner is broken, so the spirits, like corporeal beings, get thirsty rather often.)

She practices the religion of Santeria and, like her mother, prays to Saint Barbara and the Merciful Hearts of Jesus. "I'm not a Bible thumper," she told me, "but I believe the Book has answers." She opens it at random, when she's struggling inside, to see what wisdom she might fall upon. She keeps an eye on the cup of water. If it gets murky, something bad may happen: time to wash the cup and start out fresh. Pepina's mother is clairvoyant, and Pepina too has dreams that foretell the future.

Pepina's mother, Gloria, has had a lonely life. Abandoned by her mother when she was a baby, she was raised on a farm in Puerto Rico by her great-grandmother, married "young and naive," and moved to America, where her husband abandoned the family after three daughters were born. Her new husband, Pepina's stepfather, confined her to the house and forbade her to work, while he openly slept with other women. "She still doesn't know how to write a check," Pepina told me. "He closed her up, kept her uninformed. She started drinking out of loneliness. I think it's unusual for a Puerto Rican woman, but she was so naive, and she just didn't know any better."

Pepina treasures her connection to her mother through their shared religion, but their closeness has not always been healthy. "I think I actually lived her life," Pepina told me. "I went through everything she suffered with my stepfather. We were best friends, and she told me everything."

They also fought a lot. "We *still* do," said Pepina. "My mother was extremely strict and overprotective, and I was rebellious. At the same time, she drank so much that when I got home I would find her asleep, and I would have to make the meal for my two sisters. I was a little adult, a mommy from the age of thirteen."

In her book *The Motherline,* Naomi Lowinsky points out that every daughter needs to identify with her mother and to differentiate from her. When these poles become too extreme—when a girl feels a need to be identical to her mother or to reject her completely—she has trouble differentiating between "me" and "her" and therefore has trouble developing an identity. Pepina's mother was unable to respect her separate needs, and Pepina was caught in a double-bind: she felt pressure to become her mother and, as a reaction, a violent wish to reject her. Since her mother had strict standards about sexual morality, Pepina acted out by having casual sex.

This conflict was painful, but it eased up when the pair began to drink with each other during Pepina's teenage years. "We became best friends again," Pepina told me. "We'd laugh and tell each other stories and hug each other, and stop fighting for a little while." Worried about her mother's isolation, Pepina—as soon as she came of age—got her mother out of the house by taking her to bars.

Tied to her mother yet longing for a life of her own, at twenty-two Pepina found a man to drink with who would take her mother's place. This was the beginning of a painful odyssey of alcohol, sex, and drugs, with ramifications that are still playing out. Ten years later, sober for four years, Pepina finds herself back in Florida with her two-year-old son, living near her mother, learning at this late point in her life how to let go and still to stay close. Since her mother continues to drink, this largely involves drawing boundaries around their relationship. Pepina will see her mother only when she's sober.

Several recovering women told me about drinking with their mothers. As they became young women, alcohol came into these mother-daughter relationships in insidious ways. Since drinking removed inhibitions, it allowed the pairs to connect emotionally in ways they did not when they were sober—or at least to imagine they were connecting, since bonds formed in the haze of alcohol often appear on reexamination to have been more about an alcohol-induced general aura of good feeling with little actual communication or connection. As with warring marriage partners, alcohol can take the edge off conflicts between mothers and daughters and give them a sense of oneness with each other; but it can also get in the way of the letting go that is necessary to the growth and well-being of each. The women I spoke with who drank with their mothers were still struggling to separate emotionally and to gain a clear sense of autonomy.

JILL'S STORY

EVEN WOMEN WHO don't drink with their mothers may drink as a way of identifying with them. Jill had her first drink when Zoë, her closest friend and deepest connection, a woman whom she considered her second mother, committed suicide because of alcoholism. Away at school, Jill was overcome by grief. "It was September," she told me, "and I was an hour away from home. I didn't drive. It was my first semester. Zoë was a wine drinker, and I wanted to know why she drank, what it felt like, why she kept doing it." Her roommate told her to buy a bottle of wine, and she'd share it with her. Jill bought a bottle of Riunite. After a few glasses, she was tired and able to sleep for a little while. "I thought, 'Okay, it gives you the feeling of being relaxed. That's why people drink.'"

Identification with a person we have loved and lost is a normal part of grief. As Judith Viorst observes in *Necessary Losses*, it can be a way of "taking in the dead, by making them part of what we think, feel, love, want, do." Sometimes, identification can take a self-destructive form—as it often does for the children of alcoholics. Jill's next few years were tumultuous. She began to drink heavily. She transferred from one college to another and eventually dropped out altogether on the second anniversary of the death of her "second mother." Drinking was a way of holding on to her grief, as if she were trying to keep Zoë alive in this way. When she was twenty-seven, her real mother died; then her father died when she was thirty-three. She relied on alcohol to help her through each loss.

Again, there's something so compelling about the mother-child bond that we are tempted to look at it in isolation. For me, Jill's story illustrates the point. She talked a lot about the loss of her second mother, and when I wondered why she needed a second mother so badly—what about the first?—she began by saying her mother was alcoholic and was confined to a wheelchair because of discoid lupus. As a child she took care of her mother, physically and emotionally. Very close, they cuddled and teased and played. Every night, Jill would spread Pond's cold cream on her mother's face and bring a steaming washcloth, watching as the contours of her mother's face took shape beneath it, before she gently wiped the cream away.

"But when I was eight," said Jill, "my mother rejected me."

She said this abruptly. I asked her what she meant, and she told me that one morning her mother announced that Jill should not touch her anymore, or tell her that she loved her. It seemed that her father "didn't like" their relationship.

"I abided by her wish," said Jill. "But I didn't know how to handle it, so I put up a wall." Never again did the two of them discuss the matter, and never again did they put their arms around each other. "Except once," said Jill. When Zoë committed suicide, Jill's mother and father came to her college to give her the news. Jill's mother sat on the bed next to her, and intuiting the worst, Jill started sobbing before a word was said. Her mother hugged her for the first time in a decade. "She touched me that day," said Jill, "but that was as far as it went."

I was so stunned by this rejection, and the consequences it clearly had for Jill, that it took me some time to get the bigger picture. Gradually, Jill explained how frightened her mother was of her husband, who had terrifying bouts of violence. Jill still believes her father could have killed either of them; she put herself in danger when she defended her mother in their quarrels. Looking further back, Jill's father had been hit by a car crossing the street when his own alcoholic mother sent him out to a grocery store. He was three years old at the time. His head injury might have been a factor in his sporadic violence. He died of a seizure, shortly after Jill was married. His death prompted in her an overpowering wish to go back to school and do something that would have made him proud, but she was terrified of failing. "More than anything else," Jill told me, "this fear of failure tipped me into alcoholic drinking."

Jill's story provides another example of how diverse and complex are the factors promoting drinking. Her familial vulnerability seems to be a matter of biology and behavior influencing each other—with drinking creating chaos and fear and physical injury, which elicited more drinking, which elicited more chaos, until the process acquired a momentum of its own. Biological, social, psychological, and cognitive factors interacted in a kind of dance.

But Jill's sobriety also demonstrates that a high-risk background, including traumatic life events, does not lead to an implacable fate. After generations of trouble, she has examined her own position in the cycle and, with help from AA and a therapist, has learned how to step outside of it.

DRINKING DURING PREGNANCY

FETAL ALCOHOL SYNDROME (FAS) affects one to three of every 1,000 babies and is the leading known environmental cause of mental retardation in the Western world. It is caused by regular, heavy drinking and perhaps even by occasional bingeing. Infants and children with FAS suffer from growth deficiencies and physical anomalies, especially facial abnormalities. In a long-term follow-up study published in 1992, the French physician who first described FAS in 1968 has found that mental retardation and serious psychological and behavioral problems follow these children into adulthood.

The effects of moderate or light drinking in pregnancy are not at all clear. Some investigators have found low birthweight in babies whose mothers drank an average of only one drink a day; others have not seen such an effect even when mothers averaged four drinks a day. Some researchers report slightly earlier deliveries when mothers drink moderately; others find no such association. Many researchers report that mothers who drink even a little are more likely to miscarry, though many others find no relationship between drinking and miscarriage. Some investigations point to such neurobehavioral problems as hyperactivity and decreased sucking in the babies of moderate drinkers, and some have found reduced Apgar scores (which measure a baby's well-being after birth), but here too results are contradictory.

Presumably because the stakes are so high, the U.S. surgeon

general has responded to these inconsistent findings by urging women to abstain from drinking during pregnancy. In the United States, all alcohol beverage containers must, by law, have a label warning of potential birth defects if women drink during pregnancy. The U.S. Department of Health and Human Services cautions that "There is no known safe level of alcohol consumption for a pregnant woman." European countries have tended simply to recommend light, infrequent drinking by pregnant women, but even in Europe the tide may be turning. In January 2000, the British medical community published a statement urging pregnant women to abstain from alcohol.

Many women will want to avoid even a small risk to their unborn child, if all it means is abstaining from alcohol. Yet it's worth nothing that an uncritical focus on the effects of light drinking allows politicians and policy makers to blame light-drinking mothers for unexplained damage to their babies. Especially when these women live in deprived areas with poor health care, other harmful factors could well be responsible. We know that African-American women who drink the same amount as white women are at seven times greater risk for having a baby with FAS, and Native American populations (taken together) have an incidence of FAS more than thirty times that for whites. Though genetic influences could be a factor in vulnerability, researchers report that most frequently it appears in populations with low socioeconomic status, regardless of race. Our long history of scapegoating impoverished, addicted women should warn us to take a broad view.

PROSECUTING PREGNANT WOMEN

MIDDLE-CLASS WOMEN who are addicted to alcohol or drugs deal with mother-blaming primarily on a psychological level. Poor minority women, by contrast, are increasingly faced with more concrete consequences of society's inability to deal with addiction in women in effective ways. Since 1985, prosecutors have used drug tests to charge more than 200 pregnant and postpartum women in thirty states—

nearly all of them African-American—with child abuse, delivering alcohol or drugs to a minor through the umbilical cord, and drug possession. These charges have been mostly overturned, but in October 1997, South Carolina became the first state to uphold the prosecution of women for child abuse for their conduct during pregnancy. Some prosecutors use the threat of jail or loss of child custody to try to force women into treatment.

There appears to be an odd inconsistency at this moment in our history. In 1995, the National Institute on Drug Abuse budget included $88.2 million for women's health, and it is funding research and innovative treatments for addicted women. At the same time, federal cutbacks have resulted in the closing of treatment centers, and insurers have limited the type of treatment they will pay for.

In general, our society is moving away from treatment of addicted mothers toward criminalization. "The political swing of the country is becoming more moralistic," says Elsa Sorenson, supervisor of a women's unit at a substance abuse treatment center for more than twenty years. "Treatment is no longer available to anyone who needs it. There are federal cutbacks, and treatment centers are closing down, while jails are being built all over the place. We're incarcerating people instead of treating them."

The threat of prosecution and of losing child custody have frightened many women away from seeking treatment. One of these is Louise, a forty-two-year-old African-American, sober for seven months, who in our interview stressed her attention to her children. "Even if I was drunk," she said, "I focused on my kids. Before I got ready to drink, I would feed them. Before I got ready to go out, I would make sure they were going to be taken care of. Even if I did get sloppy drunk, I always focused on them." Louise—whose story appears in Chapter 12—was raped three times before the age of fourteen, and she has fought depression all of her life. She described going to a doctor a year ago when she reached the end of her rope: "I told the doctor I was giving up. I didn't want to be here anymore. I didn't want to be in this world. She knew I was dead serious. My blood pressure was sky-high.

She had to lay me on the table. I was just crazy. She said, 'Do you truly want to stop drinking?' I told her, 'No, I don't.' I said, 'Alcohol helps me; it helps me with the pain; it helps me, period. It's like my blanket. I've hid behind it so long, I don't think I could give it up. But I'm willing to try because of my kids and for myself.'

"She wanted me to get treatment; she said I needed that. But I told her I can't, no. My kids, I said, they need me. I can't do it. That would kill me quicker than anything. Because here—one thing I know, if you have any kind of problem, the state will get involved, and they'll be trying to take away your kids."

Louise was in no danger of having her children taken away. She and her children had moved in with her sister, who was taking good care of them. The doctor eventually persuaded Louise to accept outpatient treatment. When I interviewed her, she was still very shaky. Her psychiatrist was urging her to check into a hospital to deal with her frequent night terrors, but Louise remained wary, saying, "I'm still thinking about my baby."

Having young children often deters women from seeking or continuing treatment. Those who rely on family and friends to provide child care and transportation often exhaust their support system. As a group, substance-abusing women have fewer financial resources than men, and this is another obstacle to child care and treatment. In a painful irony, treatment providers are now losing pregnant women who are afraid of being charged with criminal behavior, and mothers worried that their children will be taken away. As a result, these mothers and their children are falling through the cracks.

PARENTING SKILLS

MANY ALCOHOLIC WOMEN devote whatever resources they have to caring for their children. Certainly not all of them abuse or neglect their children, nor are they all as ineffectual as Jill's mother. Yet treatment providers note that some women with severe substance abuse problems may not have developed the skills they need to raise their children effectively. Depressed mothers, who are tired and unmotivated, may have trouble accomplishing daily tasks. Women who have been physically or sexually abused as children frequently develop relationships with abusive men and are then unable to protect their children. They are also at higher risk of neglecting their children or becoming abusive themselves. One study showed that whether or not they have been abused, mothers who currently abuse alcohol are more likely to physically abuse their children.

A woman's sobriety may be threatened by problems with disciplining her children—especially as they get older and more difficult to manage. One recovering woman who struck me as a very effective mother told me that her hardest problem on returning home from treatment was dealing with her rebellious teenage daughter, who, while her mother was actively drinking, had gotten used to getting her own way. She'd say to her mother, "Who are you to tell me what to do? You're just an alcoholic." If mothers have not themselves experienced a healthy childhood, if they have not internalized adequate ways of loving and disciplining children, it takes training and education to interrupt intergenerational cycles of addiction, violence, and mental health problems.

Parenting programs are by no means the norm at inpatient or outpatient treatment centers. "They create another unit of cost," explained Dr. Camille Barry, acting director of the Center for the Substance Abuse Treatment in the Department of Health and Human Services. "But in the last five years, we've become especially concerned about these wraparound services—parenting classes, child care, transportation, issues of safety and nutrition—because more often than men, women with substance abuse problems have basic unmet needs."

Even when treatment centers can provide parenting support and education, the situation is complex. A woman in recovery may have multiple needs, many of them urgent; she may be overwhelmed by having to address parenting skills at the same time that she is dealing with depression or a history of sexual abuse or a current abusive situation. With so many competing concerns, it can be hard to prioritize and address them.

Yet these concerns need to be addressed, and, said Dr. Barry, clinical experience suggests that a full range of services helps women enter into and stay in treatment. Par Village is a long-term residential treatment program in Saint Petersburg, Florida, that allows children from infancy to age ten to live with their mothers while the mothers are in treatment. Shirley Coletti, president and founder of Operation Par (Parental Awareness and Responsibility), finds that children are a woman's best motivation to get sober. "It's awfully hard if you do have kids," Coletti told me, "because it's a lot of work to get treatment, perhaps go to school, and take care of your children, all the while having thousands of eyes on you, watching your parenting and coping skills. Nonetheless, the women who have kids do as well as or better than those who don't. A woman who comes into the program having lost custody will do okay in her first weeks, but she'll do much better when she gets her kids back."

Coletti noted that when women return home after having been in treatment without their children, there's always a point at which they get overwhelmed by all the pressure, and many relapse at that time. "Our idea is to get them over that hump while they're still in treatment and still have our support." This program, based on what's called the family unification model, seems to work; at an eighteen-month follow-up, 85 percent of the women who finish the program are still clean. Coletti notes that comprehensive programs in general are having outstanding success rates.

Other innovative ways of meeting women's needs are springing up across the country. In San Francisco, the Women's Alcoholism Center offers residential treatment for low-income alcoholic women and their children, with separate treatment for the kids, to help them with issues of trust and encourage them to be children instead of caretakers. The center is funded by private and public sources such as foundation funds for child care and city funds for low-income housing. The women either work, go to school, or do volunteer work. They receive four hours of treatment each day during the first three months, including AA meetings and classes on parenting, money management, and coping with stress. The minimum stay is six months; the maximum is a year.

The Hazelden Women and Children's Recovery Community opened in 1997 in a suburb north of Minneapolis; its mission is to support women with children in early recovery whose next step is independent living. Some of the women come straight from treatment (sometimes but not always at the Center City campus of Hazelden); some have just completed a stay in a halfway or three-quarters house; some have gone home and discovered that they need more help to stay sober. At the recovery community, these women support themselves, paying for rent and child care as well as a $100 monthly participation fee. This is difficult for most of the women. Though they vary in their earning potential—some have professions to which they can eventually return—these women often have past bills and poor credit. There are weekly two-hour group meetings and weekly one-on-one meetings with the staff, who do advocacy work for the women and help them with issues ranging from parenting and relationships to financial and legal problems to starting a car on a frozen morning—"whatever needs to be talked about to maintain recovery," said Sandy Klevens, coordinator of the Women and Children's Program. "We're more a warm, supportive environment, a therapeutic community. The staff lives in one of the apartments, and the women and children pop in to see us." The Recovery Community has apartments for up to twenty women and their children. The usual stay is a year, but many women choose to stay longer.

THE BEST MOTIVATION TO GET SOBER

IN THIS DISCUSSION of mothers with alcohol problems, it's important to remember that most mothers who drink do so responsibly. The only risk factor for alcohol problems that has been linked to motherhood is the "empty nest" syndrome—some women cope with the loss of their mothering role by turning to alcohol. As we have seen, when mothers do have alcohol problems, children are often their best motivation to get sober.

Rachel is a Native American of the Ojibwa tribe, so soft-spoken that as we sat together in a little lounge at the Minnesota Indian Women's Resource Center, I had to strain to hear her. Her story is a good reminder that even women who see no value in their own lives, who don't believe they are worth the challenge of getting sober, can often look beyond their pain and see the faces of their children.

At the age of twenty-one, Rachel gave birth to a daughter, Angela, who was blessedly normal in spite of the fact that Rachel had been drinking throughout her pregnancy. Two years later, she became pregnant again. This time, more aware of the danger, she immediately quit drinking and smoking, but she spent the full nine months feeling miserable. "Looking back," Rachel told me, "I believe I was in withdrawal for a lot of that time." As soon as her son was born, she started smoking marijuana with her husband, though she did not resume drinking until she finished breastfeeding.

One sweltering August afternoon when little Curtis was four weeks old, Rachel and her husband were smoking marijuana in their duplex. When Rachel checked the baby's cot, he was lifeless, and she realized that he had stopped breathing. She snatched him up and ran outside in a panic, her husband right behind her. Fuzzy-headed, out on the sidewalk, they passed the baby back and forth between them, neither of them having the slightest idea what to do. An upstairs neighbor thrust her head out of a window and yelled, "What's wrong?" Rachel yelled back, "He quit breathing! Call an ambulance!"

The neighbor said, "Run him to the hospital!"

Rachel shook her head, remembering. "We were only half a block from the hospital," she said, "but we were stoned, so we didn't know what to do."

Fortunately, the baby was breathing by the time Rachel reached the emergency room—the running seemed to help him. But the trouble wasn't over. "My son was in intensive care all night, and they were talking about doing a spinal tap. Through this whole emergency, my husband was home sleeping because he was so stoned. I had no one there with me." It took a year of hospital visits and tests for the doctors to discover that the baby was severely allergic to smoke. That first night, frightened and alone, keeping vigil over her child, Rachel had a lot of time to think. She began to realize that her highest value was to be a good parent, and she wasn't.

Her journey to full sobriety was a slow one, and it began with a decision—made that night in intensive care—never to touch marijuana again. She'd been drinking heavily since the age of fourteen. She hardly remembers her ninth- and tenth-grade years, because she drank so much. Giving that up wasn't easy or quick.

One afternoon when her son was three, he came downstairs from his nap and announced to Rachel and her mother that a man with great big eyes had been knocking on his window. "We thought it must have been the owl that we'd seen down at the corner, and to Ojibwa people, as for many tribes, owls are messengers of death. My mom absolutely flipped out, because my son had been so sickly, and if an owl comes to your window, that's a death sign. I'm an educated person, but when you hear those stories from the time you're a little kid, it doesn't matter how educated you are.

"Ojibwa people also believe that our children come from the Creator. Babies are still so close to him that if you're not doing right by them, the Creator could take them back at any time. We cherish and treasure our babies.

"When the owl came to my son's window I was really distressed, and I had to find a way of working with my fear. I decided this owl could be there to remind me that we never know when someone will die, we never know how much time we will have with anybody. You need to love the ones you're with, because they are gifts from the Creator, and an owl can be a reminder of that." Not long afterward, Rachel sought treatment for her alcoholism.

Seventeen years later, Rachel's office desk is lined with pictures of owls, and when we went to lunch, there was a little stuffed owl hanging from her rearview mirror. "I had to put it in the trunk when one of my Ojibwa friends freaked out," laughed Rachel. "She's grown and educated, but she couldn't drive in a car that had a messenger of death in it. But me, I'm focused on the positive reminder to cherish the people around me, and my time on earth."

Rachel's path to true sobriety was not immediate. Like many alcoholic women, she was preoccupied with her husband's more obvious addiction, and that preoccupation reinforced her own denial. Looking back, she sees these two frightening experiences with her son as transforming. They gave her a clear view of her life and told her what really mattered. Although she felt appropriately guilty for the way her drinking put her children at risk, the motivation to change certainly did *not* come from feeling ashamed or being shamed by other people. It came in transformative moments when she gained an insight into something larger than herself, and a reason to get her life in line with what she valued. Her love for her children allowed her to tap into her own resources of strength and imagination, and the wisdom of her tribal culture.

5

Teenage Girls and
College Women

*I slip in and out of feeling lost. I don't
know where my place is in the world,
or what I should be feeling.*
— KRISTINA, AGE EIGHTEEN

WHEN KRISTINA LOOKS BACK ON HER EIGHTH-GRADE
year, one scene stands out in her mind. It was winter in rural Vermont.
She, her boyfriend Tim, and a gang—all boys—were walking down the
street drinking Tennessee Tea (a flavored Jack Daniel's) from a fruit
drink can. Lately these boys had taken her into their group. She was a
shy kid, and she loved the attention. The sun was making slush puddles
on the sidewalk, and she was feeling good. The guys were chanting
"Drink! Drink! Drink! Drink!" She took a swallow with every com-
mand: Kristina the partier, the fun girl to hang out with, in the most
fun year of her life. The next thing she knew she was on her back in a
dirty snowbank, laughing boys towering over her. Tim had taken off her
pants and was having sex with her.

"I guess it was rape," Kristina told me, "but it didn't hit me for
three years." We were sitting in a corner of a bakery—her choice of a
place to meet. She was eighteen and had an elfin look, her feathery hair
pushed back with a headband studded with jewels—bright blue, setting off her blue-green eyes. Two little diamonds chips studded each

ear, and her nails were layered in green and black with drizzles of pink on top. She clutched her arms over her stomach. At moments when she relaxed, her flannel shirt opened, and her T-shirt bared an inch of belly. By her junior year, Kristina had stopped drinking and had joined a recovery group at school, where the counselor urged her to forget about Tim. "But I couldn't do it. I was angry, but I wanted Tim to like me. I begged him to get back together, but he wouldn't talk to me."

She glanced away. "I have a little problem with alcohol right now," she said. "It all started that eighth-grade year."

My heart sank. Before our meeting I knew that Kristina had almost died from an alcohol overdose when she was just fifteen. Kristina later told me that she was saved by a girl—"a sweet little puppy girl, the opposite of me"—who got her parents to drive her to the hospital. Shortly afterward, she ran into trouble when she wouldn't give a boy money to buy drugs at school, and he slammed her head into a window. Not badly hurt but nearly hysterical, Kristina ran to the school counselor. In the hour that followed, she revealed the names of "all the bad druggies" she knew. The "druggies" threatened to hurt her if she wasn't gone by the next day. Kristina left on the bus that afternoon and never went back.

Her parents sent her to a new school, where she gained a reputation for "freaking out" if anyone so much as mentioned getting drunk or smoking marijuana; this is why I'd been told that she was sober. With the help of a school counselor and a peer-based recovery group, she had indeed stayed sober for three years. When she graduated from high school, however, she lost her counselor and her support group— and at college, socializing centered on binge drinking and casual sex. "College was quite an influence on me as far as alcohol goes," Kristina said wryly. Now in her second semester, Kristina was clearly not yet out of the woods.

We stopped talking for a while as a mother with a toddler settled in at a table near us. Kristina watched as the mother spread out a sheet of wax paper and dumped a cup of Cheerios on it for her little boy to play with while she sipped her coffee. "I still feel terrible about how I lost my childhood," Kristina said. "I didn't have one. It was sex, drugs, and alcohol way too early. I was never a carefree kid." Yet, she said, having been through trouble so young, she had gained maturity, and this was compensation. "I feel more healthy and wholesome. . . . I've learned to respect myself and my body. . . . I'm glad I've changed."

Kristina was trying hard to *make* herself mature, healthy, and wholesome. It was as if, by declaring it, she might make it so. She floated ideas—as many adolescents do—then stepped back to see if they seemed true. Watching her hands twist in her lap, I wanted to believe that she was already purified by fire. In the end, Kristina herself must not have been convinced. Her face fell, and in a small voice, she told me she was having trouble with mood swings. She was proud of herself when she stayed sober and attacked herself when she slipped. She really didn't want to drink or smoke. Sex was "not safe for me at this point," she said. Nonetheless, she often had unplanned sex. "When it gets so hot, I just don't care," she said. She was struggling to be good, but she felt as if the devil were reaching his hand out across a line and trying to pull her over.

Her parents still believed what she had told them when she was in ninth grade: that she'd tried alcohol on four occasions, culminating in the visit to the emergency room. If she had told them the truth, they wouldn't have believed her. They thought she was a little angel.

"I slip in and out of feeling lost," she said. "I don't know where my place is in the world, or what I should be feeling. . . . I'm feeling bad about myself this year."

"How do you deal with that?" I asked her.

Her eyes teared up. "Basically, actually, I just cry."

WHEN GIRLS ARE INTRODUCED
TO ALCOHOL

KRISTINA'S STORY was raw and unfinished; her efforts to shape herself were brave and tentative. Her development was precocious on the one hand and stalled on the other, and her voice was simultaneously rebellious and muffled. Though she spoke in understatements, her pain was palpable. Her feeling toward me vacillated. In one interview she

invited me into her deepest confidence; in the next she drew back, as if
my closeness worried her.

She is, of course, one of many adolescents having trouble navigat-
ing the tortuous path from childhood to adulthood. In the best cases,
adolescents lose and then regain their equilibrium. It's a time of turmoil and conflict, out of which, ideally, a mature identity emerges. The
developmental tasks of this period—moving from dependence to relative independence, learning to manage emotion and to live with
ambivalence and ambiguity, balancing self-expression and respect for
others, dealing with authority, solidifying a sexual identity, developing
a capacity for intimacy, establishing personal values, and maintaining a
sense of competence—are daunting for any child.

For girls, there are particular challenges. A study by the American
Association of University Women found that though 60 percent of elementary school girls were happy with themselves, by high school that
number had dropped to only 30 percent. As we know from this and
other studies, adolescence is a time when girls' self-esteem typically
takes a nosedive. Mary Pipher's book *Reviving Ophelia: Saving the Selves of
Adolescent Girls* helped focus national attention on the way so many girls
"crash and burn" as they enter adolescence, and on the cultural factors
that contribute to their loss of "preadolescent authenticity"—that time
when they knew what they wanted and what they felt. Girls come of
age in a culture that sees the female body as a marketing device and is
obsessed with an ideal of model-thinness. From the media, the hallways
at school, and the marketplace, they learn to objectify themselves and
become detached from their own feelings. Girls know that they have
more choices than women ever did before, and many are told that nothing stands in their way. Yet women's consciousness of themselves as
equal to men is in its very early stages. Our lives are still influenced by
cultural beliefs that are thousands of years old. It's charming and in
many ways a good sign when girls believe that sexism is a thing of the
past, but that belief can backfire during adolescence. Having left their
tomboy days behind, they feel pressure to conform to a feminine ideal,
and they begin to sense the ways that women are still valued less than
men. They're not likely to see this as a cultural phenomenon. Instead

they internalize the problem, believing that there is something wrong with them.

Pipher writes about the gap between "girls' true selves and cultural prescriptions for what is properly female," and notes that, sadly, "just when they most need help, they are unable to take their parents' hands." For years the common wisdom was that teenagers need to withdraw from their parents. Established developmental theory minimized the importance of the parent-child bond, stressing instead the teenager's need to develop self-reliance. In 1969, John Bowlby, an influential developmental theorist, challenged this model in his book *Attachment and Loss*. He argued that attachment itself is a basic instinct, even more pressing than the need for nourishment and/or the need for sexual expression. More recently, drawing on the work of Jean Baker Miller, Nancy Chodorow, and Carol Gilligan, relational theorists have suggested that although everyone has a need for intimate relationships and autonomy, girls, who perceive themselves to be similar to their mothers, develop a sense of self in the context of that relationship and are more attuned to connection. Boys must develop an identity different from their mother's and are therefore more focused on the need for self-reliance.

Relational theory suggests that girls and women are most likely to develop a secure identity by means of growth-enhancing relationships. For girls to develop within the context of their attachments, not only do they need support and solace, but they also need their parents to recognize a new voice within the family and to adjust their decision-making process to accommodate an emerging adult. Such recognition allows continuing development by supporting the formation of new relationships based on mutual care, respect, and influence. Ideally, in the face of a culture that militates against the confident assertion of a feminine voice, girls learn to state their own needs as well as respond to those of others. They come to experience themselves as agents of their own thoughts and actions, and gradually, as they become women, take full responsibility for themselves within a network of relationships in which they give and receive support.

Reality, of course, falls short. Today many girls hear, "You're smart and talented; you can be anything you want" on the one hand; and on the other, "Be thin, be attractive, don't show off, be cheerful, make other people feel good, dress nicely, be good and unselfish, think of other people first." Amid conflicting pressures and the usual tensions of adolescence, it's difficult for a girl to identify her own needs and wishes. It can be hard to sort out her sexual feelings from the pressure she feels to be sexual, hard to like a self that can't meet the feminine ideal, hard to let go of working on herself long enough to enjoy herself in work and in play.

Today, when the mean age of the first drink for girls is less than thirteen years old, and regular drinking begins, on average, at age fifteen, a girl is likely to be introduced to alcohol just at this highly sensitive point in her development.

TODAY'S TRENDS:
HOW OFTEN, HOW MUCH, HOW EARLY

Teenagers

In 1999 the National Institute on Drug Abuse conducted a study called Monitoring the Future, which polled 45,000 high school students. According to these students' reports, 25 percent of eighth-graders, 49 percent of high school sophomores, and 62 percent of seniors have been drunk at least once, and many more have tried alcohol.

Since adults use alcohol, and since part of an adolescent's job is to test boundaries and proclaim independence, some of this drinking is "normal." It isn't always a red flag signifying that a child has been derailed from healthy development. Kids drink and try tobacco and marijuana out of curiosity about what adults are doing. They do it to fit in and be like other kids. Some experimentation with alcohol is virtually universal in adolescence; it isn't all pathological or self-destructive. In fact, research has linked drinking in adolescence with enhanced social functioning, less loneliness, and more positive emotional states in early adulthood.

Generally speaking, the drinking habits of adolescents, like those of adults, are subject to demographic and cultural influences. The percentage of teenagers who drink is higher in the Northeast and North Central regions of the United States, and lower in the South and West. National studies of adolescents find alcohol use highest among American Indians, followed in decreasing order by whites, Hispanics, and African Americans, with Asian Americans drinking least of all. Among Hispanic students, Mexican Americans drink much more heavily than Puerto Rican or Latin American students. The largest gender disparity in drinking habits is among Asian Americans: in this population, girls and women drink considerably less and less often than boys and men. All these differences are probably due to cultural influences. It appears, for instance, that among ethnic minority communities, family values have a very strong influence, whereas in the majority population peer clusters rival family influence. Ethnic families who have been in the United States for two and three generations begin to have drinking habits that look more like those of the country at large.

Researchers believe that religiosity in teenagers, regardless of their faith, makes them less likely to drink. When drinking habits of different religious groups are compared, it appears that Jewish teenagers are likely to drink, but less likely to drink excessively or to develop alcohol-related problems. Being Catholic increases the odds that an adolescent will drink and drink heavily (an influence that affects girls more than boys). Though Protestants as a whole have lower drinking rates, Episcopalians, Lutherans, and Presbyterians become drinkers more frequently than children from more conservative denominations. There seems to be no association between drinking and the parents' socioeconomic status.

Studies of the drinking habits of particular populations provide useful information for efforts to prevent substance abuse, but the results—which are often tentative—can lead to harmful generalizations. For instance, the misperception that Jews are rarely alcoholic can reinforce the denial of Jewish alcoholics, their families, and their doctors, and it may also contribute to a Jewish alcoholic's isolation, whether she is actively drinking or in recovery.

Use of alcohol and drugs is also susceptible to fashion: the "neohippie" trend in the 1990s may be partly responsible for the dramatic increase in the use of illicit drugs during those years (leveling off since 1997), and the slight reduction in use of alcohol. Teachers and kids will tell you that habits follow the lines of social groups and cliques. A teacher of creative writing at a high school in Fort Collins, Colorado, explained, "The ones who do alcohol here in Fort Collins are the 'good kids,' the ones in student council and on football teams; and the 'cowboys and cowgirls' who live on farms and ranches outside of town. The kids who dress in strange clothing, get piercings and tattoos, go to poetry readings and foreign films—the creative kids—are more likely to do drugs." She added that generally speaking—unlike kids at the school in Los Angeles where she used to teach—the kids in Fort Collins are not consumed by alcohol and drugs. "They're outdoorsy kids; they go mountain climbing, hike canyons, go to reservoirs."

In many areas, the social life of teenagers does center on alcohol. Two girls from a suburb of Washington, D.C.—both honors students, neither of them showing other signs of trouble—told me that their weekend parties begin on Friday at lunch, at school, when they sip wine coolers out of soda cans. Typically, they each drink five beers on a Saturday night. Girls in Vermont told me about kegs of beer at massive high school gatherings held at least once each weekend in isolated fields or homes where the parents are away. According to two girls from my neighboring town of Middlebury, Vermont, the number of students who choose not to drink at all is very small, and "they're not necessarily who you'd expect." The honors students, the athletes, and the popular kids all tend to drink. It's hard for students to choose *not* to drink and feel good about it. One girl said ruefully that she'd thought about quitting her lacrosse team but decided not to, "because at lacrosse practice, and on the bus going to games, is the only time I can be with all my friends when we're not drunk."

The national averages for binge drinking among teens are uncomfortably high. In the Monitoring the Future study, about 15 percent of eighth-graders reported having five or more drinks in a row in the two weeks before the survey; for sophomores, the figure for bingeing was 26 percent, and for seniors, 31 percent. As one girl told me frankly, "At our age, the only reason to drink is to get drunk." Binge drinking in college is strongly predicted by drinking in high school.

College Women

Binge drinking is the number one health problem on college campuses. Something in the campus culture must be awry when, each year, college students spend more on alcohol than they spend on books, soda, coffee, juice, and milk combined. The number of students who abstain from drinking altogether has increased somewhat since 1980, but students who drink alcohol appear to be drinking more and more frequently.

The public has become aware of this problem through dramatic, highly publicized alcohol-related deaths resulting from overdoses and accidents. Several studies document alarming habits among students. In 1997, at the Harvard School of Public Health, Henry Wechsler conducted a survey of a random sample of students at 116 four-year colleges in the United States. Forty-four percent of students had binged in the two weeks before the survey—39 percent of women, and 49 percent of men. Half of these had binged three or more times during this period. (A binge was, again, defined as four drinks in one sitting for women, and five for men.) Since 34 percent of people of this age who are not college students are also binge drinkers, the discrepancy is significant, though not overwhelming. The statistics become startling when one looks at drinking in fraternities and sororities: two of three fraternity and sorority members are binge drinkers; among those who live in Greek houses, four of five are binge drinkers.

Because binge drinking among college students is so common, some people object to treating it as pathological. Instead, they see it as normal life-stage behavior that, typically, students will grow out of. It is true that most people who are binge drinkers in college will eventually modify their habits, particularly as they take on adult responsibilities such as a job, marriage, and children. There are problems, however, even in the short run.

Weschler's study found that college binge drinkers are five to ten times more likely than drinkers who do not binge to drive after drinking. Binge drinkers are eight or more times more likely to fall behind in their schoolwork, miss classes, forget where they were or what they did, have accidents, and damage property; and frequent binge drinkers are twenty-two times as likely to experience five or more of such alcohol-related problems. Eighty percent of students who live on college campuses but do not binge report such secondhand effects as date rape, having property vandalized, being the victim of an assault, or having their sleep and study interrupted.

Students who enter college with any sort of vulnerability to alcohol problems are at special risk. Most of their classmates will escape the most severe consequences of problem drinking. Most will survive the occasions when they drink and drive; most will get through school and go on with their lives. They may, in their thirties and forties, look back on their college drinking with humor and amazement, and perhaps say a prayer of gratitude for having lived through it without hurting themselves or others. For them, abusive drinking may indeed be a developmental stage from which they emerge without noticeable harm. Twenty-five percent of students, however, come to college with a family history of alcoholism. They enter a culture in which abusive drinking is taken for granted. A survey at one northeastern university found that most students do not view consuming up to nine drinks in a row as problematic and only the classmate who reaches for the tenth drink is seen as abnormal or deviant. Those who are in any way predisposed to alcohol dependency, whether through genetic vulnerability, a history of trauma, or a lack of confidence which makes it difficult to resist social pressure to drink, and those who find in alcohol relief from internal and external pressures, may remember their college drinking as something that started out as fun but led to tremendous suffering.

As many as 360,000 of the nation's 12 million undergraduates will ultimately die from alcohol-related causes, more than the total number who will be awarded advanced degrees.

What can people do?

Studies of college students suggest that those who drink imagine *everyone* is drinking, and in part, their exaggerated perception of how much other students drink drives their own behavior. When they form a more realistic picture and understand that many students do abstain, they feel more comfortable making other choices. Some colleges offer substance-free housing, where students who wish to avoid the drug and alcohol scene sign contracts agreeing to abstain. Also, drinking rates do vary at different colleges. Prospective students and their parents can attend admissions meetings and ask if there are surveys about drinking; they can inquire as well about the influence of Greek organizations on student life. It's wise to look at a calendar of campus events to get an idea of the social events, especially student-sponsored events, that are likely to be alcohol-free.

Some schools that are intent on reducing alcohol-related problems have instituted a controversial measure—they notify parents the first time a student is caught drinking or has caused any trouble because she was drunk. It's best, however, if the college responds to infractions not just with disciplinary measures but with education. Behavioral intervention, where available, can be particularly effective. In one research trial, heavy-drinking students who took an alcohol skills training program (teaching them how to refuse alcohol, for instance, and how to measure what they drink) reported significantly less drinking one year later. In a more recent study, a single motivational session offering heavy-drinking freshmen feedback on drinking practices resulted in fewer alcohol-related problems over the first two years of college. An "Alcohol Alert" bulletin warns, "Prevention, early detection, and timely intervention are vital if we are to reduce the number of alcohol-related problems on college campuses today."

RISKS OF DRINKING FOR GIRLS
AND YOUNG WOMEN

AS STUDIES DOCUMENT how widespread teenage drinking is, researchers have begun to question whether there might be medical risks specific to this age group. For instance, alcohol suppresses growth hormones: might bingeing or regular drinking prevent an adolescent from achieving full adult height? Nutrition is another area of concern. The typical teenagers' diet is often insufficient to begin with, and nutritional needs increase during adolescence. Alcohol further reduces the metabolism of carbohydrates, proteins, and fats, and it impairs the absorption of vitamins and minerals. In turn, these nutritional deficiencies may make teenagers more vulnerable to additional adverse effects from alcohol. There is some evidence that drug use may increase a young person's risk of illness later in life by causing a decrease in physical hardiness during adolescence. Alcohol has also been shown to depress antibody production and reduce the number of infection-fighting white blood cells, potentially damaging the immune system. Certain health-related consequences—for example, liver injury and neurologic dysfunctions—are due more to individual vulnerabilities than to long-term chronic drinking. Adolescents who abuse alcohol show elevations in liver enzymes and poorer language function. Studies of teenagers in treatment report alcohol-induced ulcers, appetite changes, weight loss, eczema, headaches, and episodes of loss of consciousness. And in February 2000, scientists reported the first concrete evidence that heavy drinking can impair brain function in young people. Dr. Sandra Brown, who led the research, noted, "Significant brain development continues through adolescence," which means that "alcohol may have quite different toxic effects on adolescent brains than on those of adults."

For girls and young women, alcohol takes an even heavier toll. Because more of the alcohol they drink is absorbed by the body, they can reach acute intoxication well before a boy. The absorption process is affected by the menstrual cycle, so that the effects of a particular amount of alcohol are hard to calculate. Alcohol can prevent ovulation and increase levels of testosterone; the consequences to girls are not clear, but high doses of alcohol have been found to delay puberty in female and male rats. Like older women, girls who drink compromise their immune system and put themselves at greater risk of alcohol-related liver damage and breast cancer. Girls and young women who drink heavily are particularly likely to smoke and use illegal drugs, often at the same time.

Half of all teenage girls are dieting on any given day, and dieting further enhances the effects of alcohol. Eating disorders are so widespread in America that they are considered almost normal. The medical complications of eating disorders include menstrual and reproductive problems, low bone-mineral density resulting in fractures and osteoporosis, gastrointestinal problems, cardiovascular abnormalities, dental decay and disease, obesity, and fluid and electrolyte imbalance. When you add the effects of alcohol, the health hazards increase exponentially.

The medical effects of alcohol are worrying, but accidents, homicide, and suicide are still the number one threats to girls and young women who drink. Half of all motor vehicle fatalities among fifteen- to twenty-four-year-olds, and half of all murders, involve alcohol. Those who drink are also more likely to smoke cigarettes and use other drugs.

Most frightening, teenage girls who drink more than five times a month are almost six times more likely to attempt suicide than those who never drink (26 percent versus 4.5 percent). They tend to have difficulty with impulse control: they're more likely to drop out of school or be expelled, to get into car accidents, and to run away from home. They are more likely than heavy-drinking boys to be depressed. In a study of 133 adolescents with alcohol dependence and 86 controls, the alcohol-dependent girls had nearly twice as many symptoms of depression as boys. Girls who drink are more vulnerable to sexual and physical assault than girls who don't drink. According to the national school-based Youth Risk Behavior Survey of 1993, girls who drink are five times more likely to be sexually active, and their partners are a third less likely to use condoms. These girls' early sexual activity puts them at risk of HIV infection, and at high risk of catching human papilloma virus (HPV), which causes cell changes that can lead to cervical cancer.

Depression, suicidal thoughts, impulsive behavior, and even symptoms of bipolar and borderline personality disorder can all be induced by drinking. Yet research has found more and more convincing evidence that alcohol is rarely the sole cause of trouble for teenage girls. Drinking tends to be one piece of a larger picture. As with women, girls' coexisting disorders, particularly depression, tend to precede their drinking, and they report significantly more "negative events" in their social networks than boys do—meaning friends or family members in a crisis that affected them badly. The overwhelming correlation between traumatic events and alcohol problems holds true for both boys and girls. In a study of adolescents, of whom 132 were alcohol-dependent, 51 abused alcohol, and 73 served as controls, researchers found that traumatic events involving interpersonal violence were common among the group with alcohol problems but rare among the control group. The adolescents who were dependent on alcohol or abused alcohol were six to twelve times more likely to have a history of physical abuse and eighteen to twenty-one times more likely to have a history of sexual abuse, with physical abuse more common among males and sexual abuse more common among females.

Many clinicians and researchers believe that girls with a drinking problem are less likely than boys to get the help they need. This is in part because of a difference in their coping styles. Studies have confirmed what people know from experience: boys are more likely to turn their aggression outward, whereas girls are more likely to turn against themselves. When boys break the rules in visible ways, they get attention and sometimes help.

Patrice Selmari, manager of the Chemical Dependency Unit at Hazelden Center for Youth and Family, believes that girls who are substance abusers are still slipping through the cracks. "The girls are much more apt to be diagnosed with depression or other mood issues, and have their chemical dependency overlooked. The guys act out angrily—they'll even act out their depression. They put their fists through the walls and get noticed." Shirley Coletti, the founder of Operation Par in Saint Petersburg, Florida, concurs. "Young ladies are allowed to get further in their addiction and dependence before anyone identifies their problem. We find scores of excuses for girls and women—everything from 'she's having her period' to menopause! It's denial on the part of society not to believe that young women, just like young men, can get seriously involved in alcohol and drugs as early as junior high school."

Since drinking is so widespread among adolescents, it is hard to determine when a girl is headed for trouble. Counselors who deal with chemical dependency need to do a thorough assessment, asking where the girl is in her development, how alcohol and drug use may have stunted her growth, where she stands in school and in her relationships with family and friends. Bingeing is so common among college students that it can be particularly hard to make distinctions. Patrice Selmari says that an adolescent needs treatment when her initial experimentation has evolved into a regular pattern of use—perhaps every weekend—and she is drinking specifically to alter her mood. "We think of this as stage two," says Selmari. "At this point, there's usually some evidence of tolerance building up, and the peer group may have changed so that about 25 percent are new friends who are also drinking or using drugs. At stage two, if you make a contract with your child not to drink for thirty days, she probably wouldn't be able to do it." Parents need to be especially concerned if their daughter seems chronically tired, has cut down on extracurricular activities, has become defensive, is skipping school, or is paying less attention to her schoolwork and her personal appearance.

Traditionally, girls have been protected from many of the risks of alcohol because they start drinking later and drink less heavily; but this gender gap is breaking down. Since 1995, Monitoring the Future studies have found that adolescent girls and boys are equally likely to drink. Boys are still more likely to drink heavily, but girls are catching up.

Girls and boys in the eighth and tenth grades were equally likely to have consumed five or more drinks consecutively on at least one occasion in the two weeks prior to the survey. There is some evidence of a convergence of drinking patterns among male and female college students, particularly if quantities are corrected for body weight and water.

While older women tend to hide their heavy drinking, girls and young women today are most likely to binge with a group of young people. Daughters are fifteen times more likely to begin using alcohol and drugs by age fifteen than their mothers were.

Getting drunk at an early age is an alarming development for both girls and boys, because among whites (though not among blacks) it is a very strong predictor of problem drinking and multiple addictions. Thirty years ago, women typically began drinking later in life than men, and this may partly explain the higher number of male alcoholics. Now that girls and boys take their first drink at the same early age, some researchers predict an upsurge in the number of women who become dependent on alcohol. Other researchers are less alarmed, noting that women's biology and sex roles may still slow down their drinking when they get married and begin to have children.

Yet there is no denying that adolescence is a high-risk time for developing behaviors that lead to addiction, and an early start with alcohol extends this high-risk period. An analysis of results of a survey on alcohol published in January 1998 found that more than 40 percent of respondents who began drinking before age fifteen became dependent on alcohol at some point in their lives, compared with 24.5 percent of those who began drinking at seventeen, and 10 percent of those who began at twenty-one or twenty-two.

And the age at which use, abuse, and addiction begin is getting even lower, taking doctors, clinicians, and researchers by surprise. "It floors everybody when nine- and twelve-year-olds get involved with alcohol and drugs!" said Dr. Camille Barry, acting director of the Center for Substance Abuse Treatment, Department of Health and Human Services. Clinicians describe girls arriving for treatment with their backpacks loaded with needles and drug paraphernalia in one pouch, and a worn stuffed animal in the other.

Since emotional development is largely suspended when girls start using alcohol and drugs—if regular use begins at age twelve, then emotional development is arrested at age twelve—older girls and young women who come to treatment seem like children. (We'll consider this aspect of alcohol abuse below.) Patrice Selmari told me she recently made an intake assessment of a twenty-year-old woman and mistook her age: "I thought she was fourteen! She told me, 'I'm just a little girl who likes to play.' And she was—she had a bouncy, young walk, she wore sparkly makeup like young teens do; her hair and clothes were like a kid's; and she told me that she loves to blow bubbles. She'd been using alcohol since she was eleven, and inside, she's still eleven years old. In interactions with her peers, if any kind of conflict or sadness comes up, she gets up and walks away. She just wants to play."

STALLED DEVELOPMENT

WHEN TEENAGERS RELY on alcohol or drugs to ease anxiety, they lose the opportunity to develop healthy strategies for managing mood swings and making friends, and to develop skills that lead to sturdy self-confidence. This stalling of emotional development and growth at the point when hard drinking begins is one of the main negative effects of dependence on alcohol. When girls turn to alcohol for help because their resources are depleted, it depletes their resources further and delivers them back to their problems—which now may be bigger than before.

Kristina's story suggests this circular process. When I interviewed her, and asked her to start anywhere she liked, she began by saying that when she was one year old, her father left the family and "took off with a bunch of different women." Her mother, a fundamentalist Christian who was a former model, didn't know about these women. She idealized her husband. "My dad was a saint; she believed that," said

Kristina. Her mother allowed him to pop into and out of the family's life, believing they would one day reunite.

Kristina didn't think her father was a saint. He took her and her sister along on his dates with other women and made her lie to her mother. It took nine years for her mother to figure out that he was cheating. She divorced him and turned to other men. To this day, said Kristina, her father is stringing her mother along and trying to control her.

"I really love my mom because of all the shit she's been through," Kristina told me. "My father thought that she should wait on him hand and foot. He didn't like it that she worked long hours at her shop . . . I understood her, and my father didn't understand.

"I hated my father. I hated him for hurting my mom so much. She's really vulnerable, very submissive to men, and I have to watch out for her."

Though tremendously protective of her mother, Kristina revealed that by her early teenage years, she was quietly furious with her mother for allowing herself to be subjugated and for being so preoccupied that she could not see her daughter's emotional needs.

Such anger in adolescence is not unusual. During the teenage years, new cognitive skills that the celebrated Swiss psychologist Jean Piaget called "formal operations" allow adolescents to think symbolically—which means, among other things, that they can think about their own and other people's thinking. The psychologist David Elkind has described how this new skill allows the adolescent to reconceptualize her past and her future. With the appearance of formal operations, writes Elkind, "Young people can conceptualize and attribute motives to their parents' behavior that they only intuited before. Many painful memories of childhood are resurrected and reinterpreted in adolescence. Hence young people begin, in adolescence, to pay their parents back for all the real or imagined slights parents committed during childhood that were suppressed or repressed—but not forgotten." Much of adolescents' anger and acting out, says Elkind, has its roots in childhood experience.

Kristina came to adolescence with a powerful sense of having been wronged. She resented being used as a pawn by her father. She deplored the way that, as a "half-time dad," he still dominated her family. She perceived her mother as distracted, working long hours, and never inquiring about her daughter. Said Kristina: "She never asked, 'How are you, sweetie?' or 'What did you do today?'"

Under the stress of this difficult family situation, Kristina was not ready to meet the challenges of adolescence. Isolated, lonely, and angry, she was unable to assimilate strong contradictory feelings; unable to soothe herself when she was feeling bad; unable to form a realistic picture of her parents; unable to trust her own potential to grow in health, competence, and wisdom; and unable to have intimate relationships.

If she couldn't do this for herself, there was another way at hand. Wine coolers, beer, vodka, Tennessee Tea—any of these gave Kristina a ready-made identity and instant access to a social group. She didn't have to develop communication skills; she only had to join in the group's drinking. "I felt really good, like I was part of something," she said, noting that if anyone at school gave her a hard time, a guy from her group would talk to that person, "and maybe scare him." Even now she added, "Nice to have that kind of acceptance."

The sense of belonging that alcohol can initially bring is a common theme among alcoholics—as is the loneliness that invariably follows. As another young woman said to me, "I used to have long, soulful conversations with my friends. I thought we communicated best when we were drunk. Now I realize we only communicated our drunken selves, and the next day we didn't remember anyway." Kristina too eventually felt isolated, especially after being threatened at school, and it became clear that her friendships were based on nothing more than alcohol and sex. Instead of giving her a lighter, funnier, happier identity, the blurry good feeling of being drunk hid Kristina's true self: it had no air to breathe and no space in which to develop.

Not surprisingly, she placed her self-worth in the hands of a boy—a boy who was willing to steal sex when she was all but unconscious. Desperate for his approval, she pursued him when he walked away from her, writing him letters and calling. In effect, she replayed the drama of her parents' relationship, with herself in her mother's role. This fact was not lost on Kristina, who commented, "I had seen my father humiliate women all those years." Kristina's use of alcohol made her vulnerable to sexual and physical assault; essentially, it perpetuated the emotional context of her early family life.

Similarly, Kristina's drinking initially eased the painful clash between her love and her hatred for her mother, keeping her from the difficult but liberating insight that ambivalence is part of being human. During our interviews, she struggled with this problem in several different contexts. Noting that her mother still doesn't know how precariously balanced she was for all those years—doesn't know about the early sex, the constant drinking, the marijuana and the speed—Kristina said she would probably never tell her. She first said scornfully, "She doesn't seem to care much anyway," but then, a few minutes later, added sadly, "I could never tell my mom, because it would break her heart." Such painful swings of perception often dominated Kristina's emotional life. "I change with the weather," she told me. "One day I'm antidrugs and alcohol and think people who use them are a bunch of fucking losers; other times I talk to them and think they're really cool." Her attitude toward her previous boyfriends and teachers also vacillated. Naturally, it was hard for her to make and stick to decisions.

At our last interview—nine months after our first—Kristina wore a little chain necklace that said "God loves you," and she carried an oversized paperback student Bible. Now nineteen, she had made a decision to take time off from college. She was going to Spain with a youth group, and she needed time to clarify her objectives. "My priorities are changing," she said. "Church is becoming more important to me, and my studies. I have things I want to do." She intended to go back to school and become a Spanish teacher.

She had made certain gains since we first talked. She was more conscious of her mixed feelings toward her mother. Her mother had offered her wine on Christmas Eve—told her the bottle was in the fridge—and Kristina had been angry. "I love her to death, but she's confusing," she said. She'd lived with her sister over the summer and had confided in her about her experiences in eighth and ninth grade, which she had thought she'd never do. "Still," she said, "she doesn't really know me. In our family it's almost a game: you have to figure out who the person is." She told me she was proud of her newfound independence, and of the fact that she was dealing with her problems on her own.

Kristina told me that she and a new friend, a boy, had made a pact that when they wanted to drink or smoke marijuana or have sex, they would leave the scene and pray. She was making a valiant effort to get a grip on her behavior. This is typical of people struggling with alcohol problems, and it is often part of a compulsive cycle that goes from making rules about drinking to breaking those rules to feeling guilt and remorse and back to making new rules. I hoped Kristina's new religiosity would be a real source of strength, and not just another scramble to control herself.

HURRIED CHILDREN

IN YOUNG PEOPLE, stalled emotional development can be combined, heartbreakingly, with precocity and pseudo sophistication. In *The Hurried Child*, David Elkind argues that our culture fails to protect children from the pressures of adulthood. Our children are growing up too fast, he says. They are pushed too early into achievement and sex, and they are exposed to violence in the media before they are confident about learning to master their own aggressive impulses. A veneer of knowledge and sophistication can make them seem wise beyond their years—their vocabulary sounds streetwise and savvy—but they are still children inside. Because they mimic adult ways of relating, their isolation and sadness cannot be seen. When the protection of childhood is over too soon, children can become overwhelmed. Here too, drugs and alcohol are both a cause and an effect. Drugs and alcohol promise sophistication, maturity, and escape from pressures, but the pressure to use them creates its own anxiety. ·

Elkind's analysis makes me think of Nell, whom I have known since she was an eager-to-please ten-year-old. From a distance, I've watched her transformation from an awkward preadolescent into a glamorous and outwardly confident young woman, preparing to go to an elite college, and dating an older man.

When Nell and I met in a restaurant in Manhattan on a cold spring day, she was eighteen, and two months' out of inpatient treatment for addiction to alcohol and cocaine. I got to the restaurant first and went inside because of the cold wind. I kept glancing out the big restaurant window, and when no one arrived, I went outside to check. In a corner of the building, I found Nell huddled in an oversized jacket, pale with cold, smoking a cigarette. She looked about fourteen. The wind whipped her blond hair over her face. She had come in a taxi from the apartment where she lived alone.

Inside, with steaming plates of food in front of us, she took off her jacket and recovered her assurance. If only she could ever drink again, she told me—she knew she couldn't—she would want a Stoli martini. That was her favorite, or sometimes Stoli and cranberry with lime. She'd learned to like grappa on trips to Europe. She preferred a vodka martini in winter, dry with three olives and a splash of vermouth. A Tom Collins was good in the summer, or a screwdriver if it was lunchtime. She liked the bar at Grand Central Station, and "very fancy hotel bars." Her parents allowed her to mingle with their guests at cocktail parties, a drink in hand, and she felt "very adult and included."

To Nell, whose mother is a well-known writer, the grown-up world sparkled with celebrities and yachts and gallery openings. She always wanted to be older than she was. She ran with an older crowd of New York kids who knew who Nell's mother was, and, said Nell, "They liked me more for it." Alcohol was part of the scene, a way of claiming the rights of adulthood and achieving status. Nell drank regularly from the age of thirteen. "It was wonderful," said Nell. "I had been overemotional and sloppy, and I had crushes on boys who didn't like me, but when I drank, none of that happened. I was invincible. Nobody could touch me."

By the time Nell was sixteen, her drinking was taking her to places where many adults would have a hard time coping. She traveled frequently to Atlantic City. She dated a married twenty-seven-year-old fashion designer, who took her to shows and introduced her to his friends. At a Rauschenberg triple opening, Nell met an artist who offered her cocaine. He was glamorous, and Nell was interested. By that time, her tolerance for alcohol had increased to the point where she couldn't get high no matter how much she drank. Also, she said, "I was becoming a sloppy drunk"; she wasn't functioning well, wasn't showing up when she was supposed to, wasn't caring for her appearance. She thought cocaine would help her function better. It did—for a couple of weeks. "I also thought it would help me get a handle on my drinking," said Nell, "but once I picked up the cocaine, I never put it down."

Nell's effort to get a grip on her drinking by turning to drugs was irrational but not unusual. By getting high on some other drug, you cut back on your drinking for a while, and alcohol then works better when you go back to it. Today, the vast majority of adolescents who abuse alcohol take other drugs concurrently, most commonly tobacco, marijuana, cocaine (including crack cocaine), and psychedelics. They often use one drug to mitigate or counteract the effects of another. Nell, like many teenagers, became an expert at manipulating the effects of various drugs, including alcohol, cocaine, and clonazapam, a third-generation Valium that she took to help her sleep.

These drugs in combination are potentially lethal, but obviously Nell was not thinking about her health. She slept with "weird people" and couldn't remember who they were. Physically, she felt terrible: she was exhausted all the time; she shook when she didn't drink enough; her nose was tremendously painful from sniffing cocaine, and it bled frequently. Twice she overdosed, her heart pumping wildly, her head pounding, her body drenched with sweat. Still, the drugs kept her from experiencing her own misery. "They ridded me of feeling," she said. During this time, she was also bulimic and then anorexic. "I launched a full-scale war on my body," said Nell. Her boyfriend, the fashion designer, didn't help. He took her to watch clothes fittings "to see how good a girl with a size four body looked." At five feet, eight inches, Nell dropped to 110 pounds.

Drinking and drugs got Nell into situations far beyond her ability to cope. Patrice Selmari told me, "I see it all the time. These girls grow up before they're ready. They have had adult experiences without an adult frame of reference so they haven't been able to integrate those experiences." Ironically, though Nell and her parents wanted her to go to the Center for Youth and Family, for ages fourteen to twenty-five, that center was full. Her situation was urgent, and so, once again, Nell was placed with the adults.

As Nell told me her story, I thought of the AA meetings I'd attended. Her narrative fit the arc of an AA story, which often begins with the "first drunk." (Nell's was at age three, when she drank the last drops of champagne from everyone's glass at her cousin's bar mitzvah.) The story typically proceeds through the trouble alcohol brings. Nell was a great storyteller, and she had me riveted. Throughout, she acknowledged such "character defects" as anger and self-righteousness and shook her head about her previous ignorance and denial. She recited many of the slogans of AA, for example, "Your best thinking got you here." She frequently repeated, "I'm an alcoholic." The vernacular of recovery was familiar to me from meetings, from friends, from AA literature. She spoke with the insistence of someone who isn't really sure, and at first I was saddened by what seemed like a chasm between any experience Nell might actually "own" and the language she adopted to tell her story. I'd seen that twelve-step groups tend to be dogmatic; they can encourage an unquestioning adherence to the program. Was Nell adapting to the treatment culture in a way that, once again, denied her access to her true thoughts and feelings?

Since that day, I have interviewed many women who have been in AA, and I have been impressed both by their sympathy for the girls and young women coming into the program and by the way many of them have transcended the rigidity of language and thought that characterizes early recovery. One woman, when I asked for her story, said, "Would you like the AA format?" I laughed and said, "No, the other one." She laughed too and said, "Different audience, different story."

She described being "pompous and arrogant" when she first joined the program, and being accepted anyway. Gradually, she became more flexible, more open and receptive, more secure. She spoke of her wish to be there for frightened newcomers like Nell.

Nell and I shared a taxi headed downtown—she was on her way to an aftercare meeting. She got out first, and as I watched her pick her way through traffic, looking young and tentative again, I was glad for her broad network of support: the aftercare counselor she met with one-on-one, the AA meetings expressly for teenagers. She was fresh from her inpatient treatment, and I imagined that the slogans she learned there could be a tool to keep her from slipping into old behaviors. Once her sobriety was firmly established, there would be time and opportunity for deeper healing and the affirmation of her personal voice.

ALCOHOL AND SEX

IN THE FOUR years she has worked at Hazelden's Youth and Family Center, Patrice Selmari has seen the girls seeking treatment get younger. She abhors the pressures they experience coming of age too soon in a society that judges them by their looks, glorifies thinness and supports self-destructive dieting, encourages them to please others and ignore their own needs, pressures them to be sexually active before they are ready, and bombards them with media images of casual violence against women. Internalizing these messages, girls and young women tend to carry a heavy burden of shame and guilt. They come to treatment, she says, with marked problems of self-esteem: "very different from the young man who thinks he's invincible at sixteen, who thinks he's going to conquer the world."

The pressure to be sexually active is particularly hard to deal with. Certainly girls today—not just those who drink—are sexually active earlier and with more partners. In 1995, the National Youth Risk Behavior Survey showed that 52 percent of high school girls have had sexual intercourse, nearly double the rate of 1970. Fourteen percent of high school girls had four or more sexual partners.

As young teens, Kristina and Nell had been attracted to boys and were eager to explore their sexuality. They associated sex with freedom and sophistication. Sexual intercourse came quickly, outside any kind of committed relationship, among peers for whom this was the norm. Both felt confused by a sense of violation, even though the choice had been theirs. Both were afraid of pregnancy and STDs, and Kristina was afraid of her parents' disapproval and of going to hell. Both girls were uncomfortable exposing their less than perfect bodies, and both had seen women's sexuality associated with degradation. The two girls from Middlebury, Vermont, described losing virginity as a rite of passage and said that girls often got drunk "to have sex and get it over with."

If, as girls told me, they are drinking to loosen up for sex, they are only following the example of their elders. Professors Sharon Wilsnack and Richard Wilsnack of the University of North Dakota School of Medicine and Health Sciences, who have been studying women's drinking for twenty years, found in a survey that nearly two-thirds of women who had used alcohol in the past thirty days drank to "get in a party mood" and make it easier to have sex.

Drinking to have sex implies a certain ambivalence, and among girls in particular, mixed feelings about sex are not unusual. Mary Pipher believes that junior high girls are not ready for more than kissing and hand holding: "Girls of this age are too young to understand and handle all the implications of what they are doing. Their planning and processing skills are not adequate to allow them to make decisions about intercourse. They are too vulnerable to peer pressure. They tend to have love, sex, and popularity all mixed up. And when they are sexual, they tend to get into trouble quite rapidly." Healthier high school girls still avoid intercourse, says Pipher. "Because of my work, I see the unhappiness of early sexual intimacy—the sadness and anger at rejection, the pain over bad reputations, the pregnancies, the health problems, and the cynicism of girls who have had every conceivable sexual experience except a good one. I'm prepared to acknowledge exceptions, but most early sexual activity in our culture tends to be harmful to girls."

Even as the social norms prescribing ladylike behavior are breaking down, a double standard persists with regard to both drinking and sexuality. Girls still can get a bad reputation from drinking too much or from having sex. The norms are fickle and contradictory. As Mary Pipher notes, the same girls pressured to have sex on a weekend night are called sluts at school on Monday morning. One girl told me that at a party, it's "okay to have one partner but not two."

Drinking, then, becomes a way of dodging responsibility for sex. If you have sex with someone uncool, or if it gets turned on you in the hallway at school, you can always say that you were drunk. When you are not sure of what's acceptable, or of what you actually want, drinking eases the way. Among college-age women too, drinking provides an excuse when one is needed; if you wake up next to a "loser," you can always say that you were drunk.

There is a contradiction here. On the one hand, girls and young women who drink to loosen up for sex may believe they are crossing over into a realm traditionally preserved for men. They drink, and they act on their sexual desires. In reality, they can't always tell when they are acting to please themselves and when they are responding to pressure from the boy or from their peers.

Sadly, each sexual encounter facilitated by alcohol chips away at a young woman's self-confidence. If sex was not her choice, if she did it because she was drunk, and she isn't even sure if she wanted sex at all, what happens to her sense of personal power? If she is not consciously making a decision, she has little opportunity to take responsibility. She begins to feel like a victim, subject to the pressures of her peers and circumstances, unaware of the freedom she does have to direct her own behavior and make choices.

Studies suggest that the girls most likely to drink are those whose attitudes about sex roles are more egalitarian and whose attitudes about domestic roles are less conventional. Among males, those with "macho" attitudes—who believe men shouldn't participate in household chores, for instance—are more likely to drink. Since traditional standards tolerate and even encourage heavy drinking among males, but stigmatize females for heavy drinking, it's not surprising that as the social norms prescribing ladylike behavior break down, the less conventional girls are drinking more like boys.

Unfortunately, the association between drinking and personal liberation has been picked up by the advertising industry. In an ad for Jim Beam Kentucky Straight Bourbon Whiskey, a tousle-headed young woman with a come-on look in her eyes holds a box of matches; next to her stands a bottle of Jim Beam. The slogan reads, "Get in touch with your masculine side." The ad seems to imply that drinking Jim Beam is a way of appropriating power once reserved for men, including the right to take the initiative sexually.

All this is ironic, because, as we have seen, girls and women who are drinking heavily, even when they are actively pursuing a career, are often not "liberated" in any meaningful sense of the word. Their confusion about sexuality and choice is aggravated by their increased vulnerability. Current estimates are that one-third to three-quarters of sexual assaults involve drinking by the victim, the perpetrator, or both. At one university, 67 percent of the male sexual aggressors and 50 percent of female victims had been drinking at the time of a sexual assault or another form of victimization. Under the influence of alcohol, a young woman may be less alert to high-risk situations and less capable of resisting an attack. She is also vulnerable to the widespread perception that a drinking female is fair game—as epitomized by two ads. One features a sexy woman and a bottle of tequila, with the slogan "Two fingers is all it takes." Another ad shows a drink topped with ice cream and a cherry, and the slogan, "If your date won't listen to reason, try a Velvet Hammer."

A girl who has been drinking may not see sexual aggression for what it is. When Kristina found herself on her back in the snow, her boyfriend on top of her, she blamed herself and interpreted the incident as further proof of her worthlessness.

"When working with young women who have been raped while they were drunk, I always use the analogy of an unlocked house that gets robbed," says Yonna McShane, prevention specialist at Middlebury College. "The thief is guilty of robbery and should be held accountable. The fact that I increased my vulnerability to the robbery by neglecting to lock the door does not make me responsible for the thief's criminal behavior." McShane encourages women who are assaulted while under the influence of alcohol to focus their anger where it belongs: on the man who assaulted them. "Down the road," she says, "it's also in their best interest to look at how they increased their vulnerability to danger, so they can learn from this."

In encouraging young women to hold the rapist accountable, McShane helps them define their own boundaries. Later, in examining how they increased their vulnerability by drinking too much, she helps them accept responsibility for taking care of themselves. It sounds simple: it's the task of all parents to encourage a child to recognize and to take on appropriate levels of responsibility for his or her needs. Yet as we've seen, this can seem revolutionary to girls and women, who have been socialized to take care of others first. They haven't necessarily learned to think of themselves as subjects in their own lives, rather than objects in a male narrative. They lose touch with their real feelings, and those feelings go into hiding. And shame, after all, is the wish to hide oneself.

Shame can also change its shape and find new ways to ambush girls and women in recovery, as I learned from interviewing Sandy.

SANDY'S STORY

"I LOVE a stage," said Sandy, explaining why she liked to binge between the ages of fifteen and eighteen. Her periodic planned drinking allowed her to blow off steam, to dance, show off, and have fun. One night during her freshman year at a college in Boulder, Colorado—where sorority life meant even more partying—she ran out onto a highway and was hit by a truck going thirty-five miles an hour. She lost four teeth, cut open her knee, and needed to have her stomach pumped, but miraculously, after a week in the hospital, she was otherwise okay.

Her parents, who are divorced, flew immediately to see her. Her mother returned home shortly afterward, but her father, who was not typically available emotionally, stayed with her. "He came through full force," said Sandy. "He was very shaken up, more than me." He told Sandy she should drop out of school and spend thirty days at a rehabilitation center in Seattle. Though Sandy hated the idea, she was persuaded by her father's concern. He was a high-powered millionaire attorney whom she thought of as prizing achievement and appearances above all else, yet he insisted that she quit school and get help.

At first Sandy hated rehab. She couldn't relate to the older women's stories of hiding bottles and being afraid to appear in public. The second week of the program, a counselor said: "These women you're with have been drinking for years. You have problems, red flags for alcoholism in your future. When you listen to these stories, I want you to think, 'This hasn't happened to me. Yet.'" The counselor told Sandy she should never drink again, and Sandy bawled. Not even on her wedding night? Her twenty-first birthday? New Year's Eve? "I wanted to be part of a cool group," she said. "It shocked me to think I wouldn't!" When she left rehab, it was with the attitude that she would try sobriety for a while. That "while" has lasted seven years.

Twenty-five years old now, having graduated from the University of Washington, Sandy works as a pharmaceutical sales representative. She is dynamic, attractive, and athletic, and a good role model for younger women. For seven years she has given alcohol awareness speeches at colleges, and she focuses on the benefits of sobriety. "Scare tactics don't work," she told me. "You talk about rape and death and violence, and it might be true, but the audience just thinks, 'That won't happen to me.' So I talk about how great it is not to drink. I save money and calories. I don't get hangovers. My weekends are productive. I can always go home when I want. I have no alcohol-induced behavior to regret.

"But the most positive aspect of not drinking is the practice I get being myself. Most people don't think about needing to practice this as a skill. In our society, we don't get much opportunity—alcohol lets us be comfortable, and we don't have to learn. I have had to practice for years at being myself every time I went out. In my first year after rehab, I used to sit quietly on the couch with my Diet Pepsi, and sometimes

I'd leave crying, thinking "Why do *I* have to be an alcoholic?" It's taken me seven years to gain the confidence I have at parties, and this confidence now extends to all aspects of my life. Life is better for me in a lot of ways, a lot of areas."

Sandy's friends describe her as fearless, funny, charismatic. She's a very engaging young woman, direct and appealing, with a brave way of opening herself and at the same time knowing where she stands. Yet when I asked her, as a matter of course, if she'd ever had any eating disorders, she spoke in urgent tones and revealed another side of her story.

She hated her body, she said. She was shocked that with so many wonderful things in her life she would struggle so much with food and her body. "I cried myself to sleep last night," she said. "I'm dying to go to see my counselor, but I don't have an appointment until tomorrow. Last night I took a sleeping pill to go to sleep, because I was crying so hard. Back in Boulder, when I was drinking, it was different. I felt cool because I was in a sorority, I felt like a pretty girl . . . I've never really had that sense of belonging since then. I seem to think the only way I'll really be loved is if I'm thin. My mom to this day worries about weight, and my dad always talks about beautiful thin women. He's dating a twenty-three-year-old woman, two years younger than me, and he says to me, 'Isn't she beautiful?' He's just been divorced from a stick-thin fashion designer. They were married for twenty years."

Sandy is aware of her many good sides. She's responsible, honest, smart, kind; she loves nature; she cares for others; and she has great friends. "Really, I'm a wonderful person, but I *hate* my body. I want to hide in my bed all day and dream of putting on an outfit I can feel good in. I am consumed 100 percent by one silly, silly thing while many positive things go unnoticed. I place all my importance on how I look. Meanwhile, it seems almost rational. My dad is dating skinny, beautiful women; my mom's obsessed with losing weight; my sister just lost lots of weight, and she's getting all these compliments.

"I know struggle is supposed to make you stronger, but where is the fruit? These days I feel envious of people who are dying. Their struggle is over. When Princess Diana died, I felt glad for her."

Sandy went on to tell me the most vivid memory of her childhood. She and her sister had been spending equal time with her mother and father, but Sandy hated her father's new wife, so she "complained and complained." When she was nine years old, her mother went back to court and sued for full custody. She won. It was a Wednesday night, which meant that the girls had dinner with their father. As the clock struck nine—time for him to drive them home—he sat sobbing on the couch. "I've lost my girls," he cried. He sounded unnatural—he wasn't used to crying. Sandy, sitting opposite him on an ottoman, felt pain all through her body.

Sandy swore to herself that she would take care of her father and make up for abandoning him, as she saw it then. But nothing she did was good enough. Each week she planned what she would say at Wednesday's dinner. To this day, she plans what she will wear when she sees him next. She can't let go of the fantasy that if she makes herself thin and beautiful, her father's ideal, he will shower her with affectionate attention, and she will find a man to fall in love with and marry. The reason that these things haven't happened, it seems to Sandy (although she really knows better), is roughly fifteen excess pounds of weight.

The Shape of the Ideal Daughter

THE RATE of eating disorders among girls and women is so high that it isn't surprising when girls who drink abusively have eating problems as well. Studies trying to ascertain whether alcoholic women have higher rates of anorexia nervosa and bulimia nervosa than women in the general population have yielded contradictory results, but a striking finding emerged when researchers analyzed results by age group. Seventy-two percent of female alcoholics under the age of thirty had lifetime histories of eating disorders, compared with 11 percent of all alcoholic women. Mostly their disorders involved some kind of binge-ing and purging, either bulimia or a subtype of anorexia in which girls restrict their food intake and occasionally binge and purge. These studies don't take into account the numbers of women and girls like Sandy, who may binge but not make themselves vomit, and who are consumed by anxiety about food and about their bodies.

Many of the girls and young women I spoke with had stories like this. They tried desperately to shape themselves into the ideal daughter they thought their parents wanted, by studying, dieting, and being good; they turned their anger on their bodies when their needs weren't met; they pretended to be happy when they were wilting inside. Twenty-two-year-old Kirsten, who, when I met her in Minneapolis, was worried about how she would look for her mother that night, summed it up: "Trying to be something I'm not is basically what I've been doing my whole life."

Kirsten's family was so convinced of her saintliness—"I was the angel of the family, the total model child," she said—that no one guessed she drank every single day of her college career. No one suspected even afterward, when she started passing out at work; crashed her car; and fell down a flight of steps, cracked her head, and went into a two-month coma. Another "model daughter" with whom I spoke didn't tell her parents about her drinking until she'd been in AA for two years. Still another had a father who was convinced that she was only pretending to be alcoholic. He slipped a bottle of bourbon into her car when she left for her honeymoon.

The outwardly conforming female child is praised and idealized, though ultimately disempowered. Ultimately, every girl knows that wherever there's a pedestal, there's a danger of falling off; idealization is a way of keeping a girl in line. But her counterpart, the girl who openly challenges the status quo, may have a rougher ride. In *Women, Sex, and Addiction*, Charlotte Davis Kasl notes that many alcoholic women were nonconforming children whose families punished them for varying from the ideal. Such children become scapegoats, absorbing the family's wrath. This is a harder role from which to recover, though Kasl has worked with many such women whose rebellious energy has kept them fighting all the way to recovery. The punishment of girls who vary from the ideal serves as an example to the rest.

My point here is certainly not to blame particular fathers and mothers. When patterns are so widespread, when the culture supports them to this degree, all of us participate, and all of us share in the harm. Sandy's father, a bold, outgoing man and a powerful lawyer whom people love or hate, is himself a "foodaholic," who has had his stomach liposuctioned. Nell, who thought her family cared more about her appearance than her inner life, discovered that her mother, too, was anorexic as a child. The pictures of her at that stage had been removed from the family albums. Evelyn Basoff, in *Mothers and Daughters*, recalls how she urged her daughter to wear a clingier dress to a dance, implicitly encouraging her to "market her sexuality." She had temporarily slipped back into believing that a girl finds her value by conforming to a feminine ideal. She was motivated by concern, as, no doubt, was the mother of a college girl who last week, on a ski lift, told my husband she had binged the night before and didn't feel too good. "Binged on alcohol?" he asked. "No, food," she answered. "This is my week to eat. Next week I'll drink. My mother said, you can either drink or eat. It's the secret of not getting fat."

When parents idealize their daughters, they may believe they are enhancing their daughters' confidence. Men who believe their daughters can do no wrong get a lot of positive feedback—people smile warmly at a smitten father. It can be hard to see how an image of idealized femininity drives a girl's true feelings underground, makes her flaws into shameful secrets, and encourages her to judge herself.

In my last talk with Kristina, she kept going back to the lack of honest communication in her family, complaining that if she tried to tell her mother anything that didn't fit with her ideal of a girl child, her mother would say, "That's nice, dear." Her father, too, simply didn't believe his angelic daughter could misbehave. Kristina saw her early drinking and wildness as a bid for attention. Maybe if she acted out, they'd stop what they were doing and really listen to her. She may also have been rebelling against her role.

Our interview was winding down. As the clock neared five, Kristina suddenly jumped up anxiously. "I have to go," she said. "My father will be getting off work. He doesn't know I'm here and I'm talking to you."

She had chosen this location, which was very near her father's office, even though it meant an hour's drive for her.

"I'll change names in the book," I assured her, "and any details that could identify you."

"Don't worry," she said, with a trace of scorn. "My family doesn't read."

We said good-bye. I remembered that once before, she'd said not to bother when I told her I'd change her name. I wondered if, once again, Kristina was looking for a way to get to her parents—to shake them up, and to reconnect. Perhaps she hoped that her parents, by reading her story in a book, might see through the haze of their idealizations and find out who she really was.

6

On the Job

IN THE EARLY 1990S, A GOOD DEAL OF ATTENTION WAS focused on women's difficulties juggling work, marriage, and children, and the idea got around that "role overload" was driving women to drink. Another stereotype was born: the stressed-out working woman who turns to drink for solace. In Britain, newspaper headlines from 1990 to 1994 included these: "The Women Who Drink to Another Day at Work"; "Career Mothers Driven to Drink"; "Success Drives a Girl to Drink—Lonely High Fliers Can't Share Stress."

In fact, studies have found no correlation between women's employment and alcohol dependence, nor have they found evidence that working women suffer more from problem drinking than non-working women. Women who work report no more alcohol-related difficulties—in their health or their family and social lives—than women who don't work. Instead, studies of women generally find that lack of defined social roles, or loss of social roles, is associated with higher rates of problem drinking. Researchers hypothesize that the more roles a woman has—family, marriage, paid employment—the better her self-esteem and her social support, which, in combination with her many responsibilities, discourage excessive drinking. Nor are women prone to drink because of stress at work. A study published in 1997, which collected data from 3,001 men and women, found no association, for women, between job stress and the amount or frequency of drinks consumed—results that are consistent with the findings of several other studies.

Women who are balancing many roles are not surprised to find their risk of alcohol-related problems is low. It's physically demanding to work all day, pick up children at school, make dinner, put the kids to bed, connect with your husband, and catch up on bills and phone calls, even if you have a spouse who does the dishes, gives the kids baths, and takes out the trash. Many women find that although a beer or a glass of wine at dinner seems tempting, it makes them too tired to do the evening's work. A social worker told me that the best thing she'd ever done for herself was give up the gin and tonic she used to drink while watching the news. "I was feeling that I couldn't keep up with my life," she told me. "I'm working and I have young kids, and there's always something I have to do in the evenings." One study of middle-aged working women found that they put off drinking until periods of work-related stress were over.

Yet the stereotype of the working woman who drinks begins with an observable fact. In 1993, the National Household Survey on Drug Abuse found that women who work outside the home are 67 percent more likely to drink heavily than homemakers. This is not quite the contradiction it seems. The distinction is between problem drinking and dependence—which are not elevated among women who work—and heavy drinking (sixty drinks in the last month, by today's stricter definition), which, in several studies, is more common among women who work. Women who work are also less likely to abstain from drinking altogether. Large gender differences in men's and women's drinking still persist. Employed men continue to have more alcohol-related problems than employed women—but given the great increase in the number of working women (in 1960, not even 20 percent of married women with children under six were working outside the home; in 1991, almost 60 percent were) it seems fair to say that women's relationship to alcohol is undergoing a significant change.

It may be that problems with alcohol will catch up to working

women. Generally speaking, alcohol-related problems in any population increase as consumption increases. This correlation holds true
across many cultures. We also know that at two drinks a day, a woman's
health risks increase significantly. We have no information about
problems due to women's increasing consumption of alcohol, but it
may be that statistics about alcohol have not caught up to a changing
reality.

Employed single women may be more prone to alcohol problems
than employed married women. If she has no children, a woman may
find she can use alcohol as a way of reducing stress without negative
consequences, and she presumably has more time to stop for a drink
after work with friends. A National Employment Survey found that
single women were more likely to report a connection between job
stress and "escapist drinking"—drinking to relax after work or to forget about problems at work. Also, problem drinking was higher
among single women with combined demands at work and home.

Clearly, the interactions of variables that help protect a woman
from alcohol-related problems or put her at greater risk are more complex than any existing theories about gender, work, and drinking.
Complicating factors call any generalizations into question. For
instance, a study reported in the journal *Work and Occupations* found
that though there was no direct connection between the amount of
alcohol consumed and stress on the job, lower job satisfaction does
result in a higher risk of problem drinking. Surveys of Hispanic populations in California demonstrate that ethnicity, acculturation, and
work environment are also significant factors in risk. For instance,
Mexican-American women who were better paid and worked with
mostly white employees consumed more alcohol, and were less likely to
abstain, than all other categories of Mexican-American women. And an
unwanted status—being retired or unemployed when you want to be
working, single when you'd like to be married, married when you'd
like to be divorced, or childless when you want a child—is a better predictor of problem drinking than either employment or family status
examined out of context.

As any woman knows who has never felt a measure of control over her drinking and could find in any situation a good reason to have a drink, the most wonderful job, the most wanted marriage, and the most adorable children are no guarantee against alcoholism. This being said, it should not blind us to the ways that particular contexts can support healthy drinking patterns, while others may encourage abusive drinking. We need to know more about the relationship between work and drinking, how employee assistance programs can help people who are having alcohol problems, and how managers can help create an atmosphere less likely to contribute to the development of substance abuse among employees.

WOMEN IN MALE-DOMINATED OCCUPATIONS

RESEARCH INTO WORKPLACE environments and their influence on drinking is incomplete, but one intriguing finding seems to be consistent. Women who work in male-dominated occupations are more likely to have problems with alcohol than women in occupations that are predominantly female.

Alice

A thirty-one-year-old lawyer with a claims department of a supermarket chain, Alice is frustrated by the perception people frequently have that her life has been picture-perfect, though she understands why they might think so. She comes from an educated family in Milwaukee—her grandmother went to college in the 1920s—and both of her parents had an active sense of civic duty, serving on school boards, church boards, and volunteer foundations. "Nothing bad seemed to happen to us," said Alice. "We had a *Leave It to Beaver* image." Alice was the prized daughter of her father, who told her she could do anything she wanted. She graduated near the top of her law school class and went on to land a job at a major firm in her hometown. Four years later, she is moving up in her profession and engaged to be married to another lawyer.

Her colleagues know her as a ferocious worker. At her first job, she usually stayed at work until midnight. On one occasion, having pushed very hard to complete a major project, she was told not to come back to work for two days, because she needed to take a vacation. "I looked good," Alice told me. "I went to a good school, I came from a good family, I was economically secure, I was young and high-achieving. When I came in and said I needed treatment for alcohol problems, my company was completely shocked."

Her employers were shocked in part because her performance had not been affected by her drinking, but also because her drinking looked moderate when she was compared with her heavy-drinking colleagues (most of them men). When her firm held functions at a bar during happy hour, Alice was among the lighter drinkers. Aware of how her drinking could veer out of control, she was especially careful among her colleagues. When they went on a bus trip for a conference, and everybody was drinking expensive wine, she always drank one glass, so as not to stand out among the others. And even her private binges in front of a television with a rented movie looked moderate in the context of her profession. "I absolutely felt my drinking was completely within the norm," Alice told me. "I could compare my behavior with that of other lawyers and see that a lot of people had problems, and one of them wasn't me. Among the professionals with whom I was socializing, it was standard to have a dinner party with eight people and drink twelve bottles of wine."

Moreover, said Alice, at law school she had been "almost a light drinker" compared with her peers. There was incredible pressure to drink at law school, and the other women were drinking like the men. This prestigious school is in a small town with two bars, and "we were expected to work hard and play hard," said Alice. She and her group of friends collaborated on projects and helped each other; their social and academic responsibilities went hand in hand. "In some ways, that school was preparing us to go on and network," said Alice. There were kegs on Friday for softball, and there was a party every weekend with an open bar. "It *never* occurred to me that I had a problem, because so many people drank so much more than I did. People were up all night and punching hands through windows. Others drank until three or four in the morning. I might drink six beers—a lot for 105 pounds—but it didn't look bad to anyone else."

For Alice, however, six beers were more than enough to cause problems. She got "sloppy and weepy" when she went out with men, and the next day she couldn't remember what she'd done. The bouts of depression she had suffered since college were getting worse, and her anxiety attacks were mounting. "I felt kind of dead inside," said Alice. "When I went to bed at night, I'd think: I don't care if I wake up tomorrow morning." She went to a psychiatrist who put her on antidepressants, but they didn't work, probably because she was drinking. Back in Milwaukee, she decided to get inpatient treatment for alcoholism after a humiliating evening at a wedding reception at a conservative country club, when she accepted a dare to dive naked into a lighted pool.

It was a year after her graduation from law school when she told her old classmates she was going to treatment. They became upset. "They looked at me, and knew I drank less than a lot of them. It put them on notice." Her colleagues at work were supportive but shocked. If she was dependent on alcohol, what did this say about them?

Women lawyers are increasing in number and influence, but the customs of the profession have been defined by men. Even among attorneys who graduated from law school after 1967 (when women entered the profession in large numbers), men are much more likely to be partners. Women in most positions are financially worse off than their male colleagues. As in most professions, women and men are held to different standards. An article in New Jersey Lawyer points out, for example, that a male attorney who leaves work early to be with his children is seen as a good father, while "a woman who does the same thing is often seen as a slacker."

Trying to understand why women in male-dominated occupations are at higher risk of alcohol-related problems, some researchers point to the stresses that come from built-in obstacles—the stress of competing with men on an unlevel playing field. However, the connection between work-related stress and drinking is inconclusive. A more evident factor is that opportunities to drink with coworkers are increased when the norms are established by men. Social scientists talk about "workplace culture," the shared vocabulary and understanding among workers about values, rules, conduct at work, social and working organization, and collective beliefs. This culture influences workers' behavior—including drinking—both on and off the job. Studies of railroad workers, tunnel builders, and assembly line workers, for instance, have documented social situations important in developing work-related drinking networks.

Among lawyers, especially at large and medium-sized firms, there is substantial pressure to socialize informally and formally with colleagues at events where alcohol is almost always present. Not showing up can knock you off a partnership track, for in these social contexts, lawyers make connections, showcase their strengths, and are informally evaluated by their colleagues. Firms hold dances, dinners at restaurants and country clubs, parties, and weekend retreats, where alcohol almost always lubricates the conversation. Coworkers often get together for drinks after work. For anyone predisposed to a problem with alcohol, there are ample opportunities to develop it. In addition, an attorney's life may become unbalanced, with work as the sole focus and friends belonging to the same profession. This, says the clinical psychologist and attorney G. Andrew Benjamin, is "a telescopic life." Strong outside relationships may be difficult to maintain; but without them, says Benjamin, lawyers are more vulnerable to alcoholism and depression.

Law has become known as a high-risk profession for alcohol problems, though there are no reliable data on the rate of alcoholism within the profession. One commonly cited study found that among lawyers who had practiced for two to twenty years, 18 percent developed problem drinking, and among those practicing for twenty years or more, the figure was 25 percent. Such statistics are hard to interpret because they are not broken down by gender, and men have a higher rate of alcohol problems than women. In addition, this study has been criticized for not being sufficiently rigorous. The American Bar Association itself estimates that 15 to 18 percent of lawyers abuse alcohol or drugs. William John Kane, director of the New Jersey Lawyers' Assistance Program, is skeptical about the idea that lawyers are at an especially high risk of alcoholism. "I don't think attorneys have more problems than the rest of the world," he told me, "but they do have special barriers to recovery. They have great argumentation and advocate skills, so they can keep people at arm's length." He added that if, among lawyers who drink, one in ten has an alcohol problem—the same proportion as the rest of the population—the issue needs attention.

In recent years, as this problem has entered public awareness, the profession seems intent on breaking through its denial. In 1988, the American Bar Association created the Commission on Lawyer Assistance Programs (previously called the Commission on Impaired Attorneys), and now all fifty states have lawyer assistance programs that educate the profession on substance abuse and facilitate treatment. Though reliable figures are scarce, many other occupations are thought to have high rates of substance abuse, including physicians and airline pilots, whose professional associations were the first to apply monitoring programs to protect the public and encourage rehabilitation.

In Alice's experience, frequent heavy drinking among lawyers was the norm, and in this context, her alcoholism went unnoticed. "It wasn't until I started going out with old friends I'd grown up with who'd gone into business that I started to notice my drinking was heavier than theirs," said Alice. "They didn't want to go out with my professional friends because we drank too much! That's when I started to see a discrepancy and, on some level, began to wonder if I might have a problem."

When she got sober, she found that not drinking at all in a male-dominated workplace introduced problems of its own. At first, she was hugely relieved and quite open about telling people in her firm that she had been to treatment. "I was just so happy that there was something I could do to make me stop feeling the way I felt before," she said. Lawyers in the firm continued to meet during happy hour at bars, and nobody pressured her to go. At her next job, with the state legislature, Alice's boss was protective of her once she told him she was in AA. "When we'd go out to dinner and the waitress asked about drinks, he'd say quickly, 'Alice doesn't drink!' It was a little uncomfortable, but it made me feel safer at the time." But much of the legislative work was accomplished over drinks, and Alice sometimes felt handicapped, as if she had to try twice as hard to be accepted as part of a working group.

Now in her fourth year of sobriety, Alice has taken a new job with a telecommunications company in its government relations department—where 70 percent of the employees are men—and not drinking has bothered her a good deal more. "It's not that I wish I could start drinking," she said, "but I've felt a lot more pressure. Recently we all went to a three-day conference where there was a lot of drinking. I hated having to explain, and this now weighs on my mind. I don't know how much of this is in my head, but at the conference, when people were partying at ten o'clock at night, I didn't want to be around them. I was tired, and I didn't have that kind of energy buzz you get when you're drinking. I missed out on a lot of the bonding—it happens when people are staying out later, telling jokes, finding opportunities for getting to know each other. I feel that I have to work a lot harder to compensate. In the profession I'm in, a lot of it is your personality. You need to be on, and they need to see that you relate well to others and that you can network. At parties, people impress each other with their social skills, and those skills are what you need in the government relations business. Lobbying is one of those places where social life and drinking are a primary part of the job."

Since drinking can be a symbolic expression of power, and since it is generally less socially acceptable for women, women in male-dominated jobs who do drink may be in a double bind. Should they tell jokes, communicate, and drink like a man, and risk being seen as behaving inappropriately for a woman? Or should they adhere to traditional expectations about women's behavior, and risk being seen as unassertive and inadequate? Alice's fiancé is also an attorney. Recently they went to a Christmas party for his firm. "A lot of people were drunk. A lot of men got sloppy," said Alice. "But the men who got obnoxious—you could see that people thought it was funny, and they didn't lose respect. But the one person who stood out was a woman, and I've heard repeated comments about her ever since. She was not any more sloppy than the guys—just loud and slurring her words, kind of hanging on people—but everybody noticed her."

A working woman who drinks too much is more noticeable than a housewife who drinks at home. Historically, women with alcohol problems tended to quit their jobs before being identified by employee assistance programs. Today, they are more likely to stay and seek treatment, and perhaps this is evidence that the stigma associated with drinking for women is lessening, at least a little bit.

It isn't easy to find the right balance. An effective state legislator from Missouri told me that she always orders one scotch with the men, then quietly switches to water, which gives her an advantage in negotiations. Although Alice struggles with the image she projects by not drinking, she feels she has it easier than her husband, who is also in recovery. "I stand out less when I don't drink," she says. "I'm not drinking like the other lawyers, but I'm abstaining like a woman. When he doesn't drink, he doesn't fit either the typical behavior of a lawyer or the masculine stereotype." Alice notices, too, that there seems to be less pressure on the older women lawyers to drink. "A lot of women attorneys at that party who had young children weren't drinking. I felt that because I'm younger, there's more expectation for me to drink. I'm still in that party stage of life."

While an occupational culture can influence drinking and put a woman more at risk of developing problems, there's no simple correlation, and again, it's risky to make generalizations. Dana, whose dependence on alcohol landed her in treatment in her late twenties, pointed out that it's hard to separate cause from effect. She drank heavily in college, and even more heavily when she started work at a bank. "The way the bank worked, I was a team leader, with the salespeople under my direction. We entertained clients to try to get their business. You'd go to a steak house for lunch and drinks, go to receptions before an art opening or a play. I was single and worked downtown, and I got paired up with men. I was the hostess. The men drank like sailors, and I got right in there with them." But Dana doesn't blame her drinking on the atmosphere at work. "Bankers aren't notorious for swinging from chandeliers," she said. "I was seeking my own level, and I managed to find the frat house in a conservative industry."

Some female-dominated occupations may also put women at higher risk of heavy drinking and problem drinking. Nurses and flight attendants, for instance, are subject to many risk factors. Studies of women in England and Wales have shown high rates of mortality from alcohol-related causes among hairdressers, bar staffers, and women in artistic and literary occupations.

DRINKING ON AND OFF THE JOB

WHEN WORKING WOMEN do have problems with alcohol, what happens to them and to their jobs? How are they treated by their employers and fellow workers? What are their chances of getting help?

In a study of 301 white middle- and upper-income alcoholic women from outpatient and inpatient treatment centers in Michigan, Edith Gomberg asked about drinking in the workplace. Fourteen percent of those in high-level occupations, 21 percent in middle-level occupations, and 36 percent in lower-level occuations reported drinking at work. All the alcoholic women reported that much of their drinking was done at home, though those in their twenties reported more drinking in public places. Some anecdotal evidence suggests that employers are more likely to protect female workers who have alcohol problems, concealing these problems as long as possible. (One woman, for instance, told me about the boss who simply had her lie down on a couch until she sobered up.) The latest studies, however, find no evidence of gender differences in treatment referrals, except that in the previously cited study of employee assistance programs, women's referrals were more likely to come through the recommendation of a coworker or a boss than through a formal evaluation process.

Though federal cutbacks and managed care have meant that many women are not getting the kind of treatment most appropriate for them, a positive effect has been a new emphasis on early detection of alcohol problems. This trend is a result of the realization that prevention and early intervention are much less expensive than treatment of an established problem. The changes are by no means universal, but in some workplaces the norms are shifting. Dale, a computer programmer, said that only nine years ago she worked with a group of people who put in twelve-hour days, and who would bring wine into the computer room after hours. Now, she says, "Nobody drinks on the job, and nobody laughs at excessive drinking. There's a new level of concern and an awareness that help is available."

High-achieving women like Alice are not generally at risk of alcohol problems—in one study, women with a professional or graduate degree were least likely to have had five or more drinks at one sitting on two occasions in the past month. But high-ranking female executives may be more likely to be drinkers than women of comparable age and education in lower-level jobs. A study conducted in 1992 found that among employed women, those in higher-status (managerial and professional) occupations had a higher prevalence of drinking—though not of alcohol dependence. This may be another aspect of drinking in male-dominated work environments. High-status women with drinking problems were four times more likely than high-status men to quit their job.

Alcohol, Sex, and the Workplace

THE MOST explosive situations at work develop when a woman's drinking coincides with a habit of using sex to get power, control, and physical affection.

Kelly, now thirty-seven, grew up in a wealthy suburb where her material needs were met in plenty, not her emotional needs. "My parents were Germans raising American children," she told me, "and they had no idea how to manage us. My mother was ultracontrolling and moody—I don't think she liked being a mother. She hit us all a lot, but I was the most rebellious and the most pissed off and the most willing to say it, so I got singled out for a lot of her abuse. I used to sit there and let her beat me, until my brother told me, 'If she touches you, you need to hit her back.' One day she did, and I exploded. I pounced on her, I beat her, I clobbered her—she ran to her room or I swear I would have killed her. A normal mother would have had me institutionalized."

Kelly never received encouragement and praise from her mother and father, or the parental strength and protectiveness that all children need. Without this care and acceptance, she could not learn to love herself. Instead, she grew up hungry for attention from other people, some form of proof that she was real and that she mattered. At the age of twelve, she discovered that alcohol temporarily filled up her emptiness. At about the same time, she discovered that her stunning good looks gave her power over men. On the surface she was vital and attractive, full of fun and mischief. When men fell for her, it gave her a heady feeling. Sex was a way of getting the attention she so desperately craved, and it substituted for genuine attachments.

Although she drank heavily and took drugs, Kelly did well at college. Afterward, she went to work at an insurance company in New York "in their little blue-blazer section." It was trouble from the beginning. Her reputation for drinking and easy sex grew. One colleague in particular, "a pretty snazzy salesman," used her to entice his clients. "I wasn't on this salesman's team," Kelly told me, "but whenever he had to entertain clients I was always invited. I was young and pretty and I laughed and drank a lot. There was always a chance that some dopey, stupid client would think I'd do anything to close a deal. My colleague played that card pretty heavily." After such an evening, Kelly couldn't always remember what had happened. "I'd go to people in the company, totally ashamed and full of remorse, trying to find out."

As her addiction got worse, Kelly tested the limits of her power over men, and her fantasy that she could get away with anything. "It's not that I was trying to sleep my way to the top," said Kelly. "I was just so crazy I didn't know what I was doing." The last straw for her company came at a business dinner: drink in hand, she whispered to her boss, "I'm interested in fucking your friend." The friend was another of her bosses. The next day she was fired.

This was the early 1980s. It is interesting to note how different this story would sound if Kelly were a man. For so many years, if a male employee propositioned a female employee at a cocktail party—a familiar form of sexual harassment, usually with the male in the position of authority—it would have been shrugged off. If the drinking looked like a problem, the offender might have been urged to get treatment instead of being summarily dismissed. The sexual overtures would be explained away as "just being drunk." In Kelly's case, her drinking was an additional insult, heaping shame upon shame.

Kelly has now been sober for fourteen years, but she still feels humiliated when she remembers this incident. Though she has sorted through many of the problems in her life, on some level, she said, she thinks of herself as a "slut," and she can't get over that. Describing her struggles both while she was drinking and in sobriety, she spoke in terms of her bad behavior, her shortcomings, and the things she needed to "work on" in herself.

Kelly is devoted to AA: "What's not to like? It's fun! People make you laugh at all the miserable shit you've been through, they ask how you are, and they care." She also remarked, though, "The people who have a harder time in AA are women. A lot of women don't ever really recover." In particular, she said, she and all her recovering women friends struggle with relationships, and with shame about their sexuality.

Kelly's framing of her behavior as a personal problem, stemming from character defects which are part of the disease of alcoholism, reflects her immersion in the twelve-step philosophy. This model encourages her to make a disciplined effort to change, and that is its lifesaving power. She continues to be cheered and supported by AA meetings. I never questioned the importance of AA in her life, but hearing about her bouts of self-loathing through many years of sobriety, and her redoubled efforts to "fix" herself after every disappointment, I began to wonder whether she, like many women, might be helped by another perspective. I wondered whether Kelly's sense of shame may seem insurmountable because it reflects her internalization of attitudes she grew up with, ideas about what it means to be female in a society that both covets and despises women's bodies. Was it really all her fault that she had chosen the role of *femme fatale*, or does she have reason to be angry about prevailing attitudes that lead so many women to conclude that their bodies are their best means to power? Might it not be appropriate—and freeing—for Kelly to be angry at that colleague who used her sexual availability to clinch his business deals? And what about the company that tolerated this but did not tolerate her propositioning a man who had power over her? Kelly spoke of her failed relationships as if she were always in the wrong and the man always in the right. Was her focus on individual, spiritual, and emotional progress encouraging her to accept all the blame in situations where blame should be shared?

Walter Brownsword, who is on the staff of the University of Vermont Counseling Center, notes that many addicted women believe they were born with a basic fault, as if they were a "demon seed." For them, the disease concept, which is meant to be freeing, sometimes backfires. "They hear it as, 'You've got this dormant thing in you that's going to torture you for the rest of your life,'" said Brownsword. He finds it helpful to get his clients thinking critically about what they believe it means to be a woman or a man in our society, the conditions that led to their negative view of themselves, and the context in which they learned to avoid themselves and pay no attention to their needs. Just as, in early sobriety, the disease concept allows many alcoholics to stop blaming themselves because they see the physiological basis of addiction, a deep understanding of the social and cultural context of women's self-loathing may be critical to women who wish to be free of it.

Sharon, a secretary and single mother from Las Vegas, identified with the women Brownsword describes. Sharon got sober in AA, but for many years, she said, "I was still in hell. There was a guy at one of the meetings I attended who used to introduce himself by saying, 'I'm Mike, and I'm a degenerate drunk.' That pretty well summed up how I felt during my eleven years in AA." When Sharon heard about a sixteen-step empowerment group that took a different approach, she decided to give it a try. There, she was encouraged to look at the shame she had experienced growing up with a stepfather who was a drill instructor in the military, who liked to comment on women's stupidity, and who called Sharon a "stupid Polack." "My mother was terrified of him, and we walked on eggshells around this man. My idea of a woman? Fear and service."

Sharon came to understand that she had been set up to feel bad about herself, and that her drinking was a defense against depression. "That understanding gave me back my power," she said. "Very simply, I realized that I could make my own decisions. The power within me was truly there. I had energy and rights. It made me feel free. Instead of feeling defective, I knew how I got where I had been, and that it wasn't really my fault."

Dale, a forty-eight-year-old computer programmer in Washington state, came into her own within the framework of AA. Her lowest point came when she was fired after one week as a secretary, because, as she was told, she "didn't have enough self-confidence to do the job." Today she is a high-ranking employee, earning a generous salary.

Dale also risked her livelihood by mixing drinking, sex, and work, though her story is different from Kelly's. Her alcoholism didn't develop until she was in her late thirties, and at that time, the only man she'd slept with was her husband. When he left her for another woman, she started drinking heavily and taking Valium. Two years later, she began affairs with two men at work. One, a consultant for her company, was married, had children, and was twenty years her senior. Since he lived in Georgia, the two met for secret weekend trysts at places across the country. "He'd pay for my airfare, and I'd fly to meet him," said Dale. Meanwhile, her boss—a Mormon with four children and a fine reputation—became infatuated with her. The two began meeting secretly. "We talked and fondled—it was an 'everything but' relationship," Dale told me. "He thought I was just wonderful. He couldn't communicate with his wife, but he liked my mind and my energy and my interest in life. I was passionate, and he liked that, too. We would neck like teenagers in a parking lot. Once the police came by and checked us out—just like in high school."

Dale would get drunk with her lover from Georgia, but her boss didn't drink, and she never drank around him. Mostly, she drank alone at home. "If I'd been in a decent state," said Dale, "I never would have let this happen. It's not something I ever could have imagined doing before, and not something I can imagine doing now."

Her situation came to a crisis when her lover in Georgia developed prostate cancer. She'd seen him on New Year's Eve, and he was dead in July. During that time he called her every day, from the hospital and from home. His wife called Dale and said, "I know he loves you. He's talking about going to live with you. Please talk him into waiting until he's well." Dale recalled, "He wanted to come out here and live in the woods with me and my kids!" Three weeks before his death, his wife called back and asked Dale not to talk to him anymore—it was too hard on her and on him. "I heard about his death from a friend," Dale said sadly. "I felt as though I deserved all that pain."

This was a turning point. Dale decided to grieve without any distractions. She cut off her relationship with her boss. After a frightening blackout—she woke up with her ten-year-old son beside her and didn't know when he had come into the room, or who had written the notes she found beside her—she never had another drink.

Dale believes that her loneliness, her drinking, and her affairs were all interconnected, part of the larger problem of her wounded self-esteem. "It's a pretty low blow when someone leaves you for someone else," she said. "I thought this woman my husband loved had something I did not. In my sick mind, I thought, my husband may have left me, but I must be okay because I am able to attract these two married men. It's a powerful feeling to think that a married man will choose you to spend time with over his own wife, and risk his job."

At the time, Dale was not aware of this motivation. She was in love with the consultant from Georgia, she had fun with her boss, and she treasured their physical closeness. "I didn't have a conscious feeling of power, but it played a part. A smart man who is successful in his field pays attention to you—it's a tremendous ego boost when you feel worthless. It's a great feeling to have someone risk his marriage for half an hour with you after work.

"It's been six or seven years since I felt that worthless. . . . The way I acted was out of character for me. Now I have such compassion for other women when it happens to them! I haven't known anybody who's had a series of affairs like that and healthy self-esteem. It's all tied up and related."

Indeed, at that time Dale was hardly capable of thinking of her best interests. She could think only of the potential consequences for her boss. If their relationship had been discovered, he would have been badly hurt, "professionally, as well as personally and in his marriage." She never gave a thought to the risk she was taking. Only now, looking back, does she see the danger. "I was risking my livelihood, that's for sure. I was a single parent making just enough to support myself. The only other person in my office was a longtime friend of my boss, and she was loyal to his wife. Either she or I would have had to leave, and it probably would have been me. I don't know what would have happened to me."

Dale has used her eight years of AA membership to achieve not only sobriety but also satisfaction in her career and in a new marriage. Most important, she has rebuilt her confidence; she no longer depends on external validation, because she believes in her soul that she is worthy.

Interestingly, Dale attends two different AA meetings, each for a different purpose. One, she said, is mostly men, many of whom are newly sober. At this meeting there is a certain grit, a life-and-death fervor, which she appreciates. At the other meeting, all the participants are women who have been sober for a while, and the word "alcoholic" often doesn't come up. The women focus on helping each other with problems that arise at work and at home. During our interviews, Dale twice remarked that, compared with many of the people at her AA meetings, she was "coming from a different place." I wondered if her ability to thrive within AA was related to her clarity about her own perspective.

It is worth remembering that the recovery movement itself is vast and contains many conflicting impulses and social currents. For all its emphasis on personal transformation, it has not escaped a feminist-influenced consciousness about women's issues, and this awareness may be getting stronger. Something is shifting when, as noted earlier, a lawyers' magazine points out that the profession's attitude toward women attorneys makes it tough for them to seek help for addiction. Indeed, in the last two years community recovery support programs have sprung up across the country. Unlike AA (which, as they point out, must remain "apolitical"), these organizations endorse and oppose specific causes related to preventing addiction, to treatment, and to recovery; advocate for policy changes; and work to reduce the stigma of addiction.

It remains to be seen what course these organizations will take, but the trend looks promising for women. For example, the Woman's Consortium, which is based in New Haven, Connecticut, is an advocacy group that works on behalf of women with mental health problems, especially those with addictions. Conventional treatment, which emphasizes breaking through an alcoholic's denial, is often not relevant to poor women who are not able to meet their basic needs and who are most often victims of trauma. The consortium puts pressure on the government and on treatment providers to address these women's trauma, assist with housing and transportation for them and their children, and offer job counseling. It's an approach that looks realistically at the role of social context and personal experience in these women's addictions and sees their medical, emotional, social, and spiritual needs as part of the same picture. Instead of resigning itself to crisis management, expecting these women to live from relapse to relapse, the consortium hopes to empower them so that they may become confident enough to tend to their own needs and contribute to the workplace and their communities.

Part Three

Take Two
at Bedtime:
Drinking as
Self-Medication

7

Love Hunger

IN THE TESTIMONIES OF WOMEN ALCOHOLICS, ALCOHOL is often referred to as an actual partner in a relationship: "Alcohol was my true love; I never went to bed without Jack Daniel's." Caroline Knapp, in her memoir *Drinking: A Love Story,* writes:

> *Our introduction was not dramatic; it wasn't love at first sight, I don't even remember my first taste of alcohol. The relationship developed gradually, over many years, time punctuated by separations and reunions. Anyone who's ever shifted from general affection and enthusiasm for a lover to outright obsession knows what I mean: the relationship is just there, occupying a small corner of your heart, and then you wake up one morning and some indefinable tide has turned forever and you can't go back. You need it; it's a central part of who you are.*

Like the touch of a lover, alcohol brings ease, warmth, excitement, and oceanic feelings. It melts away self-consciousness. It offers courage. It brings out wit and charm. Many drinkers—not only alcoholics—savor the rituals of drinking: ice in a bucket, wineglasses and tumblers, and special recipes, like vermouth passed over a glass of gin for a perfect martini. Expectations about how alcohol will affect you are a significant factor in the development of drinking habits. Several women with whom I talked remembered the excitement of their parents' cocktail hour: the hors d'oeuvres and gin-soaked olives, the way their mother's laugh changed and her spirits lightened, their father's joviality, the way the kids were suddenly allowed a longer leash but still wanted to play nearby, in the aura of beneficence and humor.

Over time, for an alcoholic, a drink becomes not just a positive experience but a necessary one. She begins to organize her life around alcohol. Anything that gets in the way—relationships or obligations— may be dropped, because she believes she can't survive without it. Meanwhile, as tolerance develops, the initial comfort alcohol brought may have dropped away. Now she needs to drink to stave off withdrawal pains. The hypnotic lover becomes a demon lover, consuming time and energy, giving nothing in return. "I think of alcoholism as possession," I was told by a man whose wife is actively drinking although the courts have ordered that she cannot be with their children alone until she achieves three months of sobriety. "It's like a slug at your brain stem that's indifferent to human life. It wants only to preserve itself. It will ride its host and won't interfere except insofar as it is threatened. Then it saps your emotions and your mind. It takes over your will. It urges you to give up everything you used to love, so you can keep it alive with drink."

Often, women are introduced to alcohol and drugs through a romantic relationship; when the relationship fails, the alcohol and drugs fill the gap. Because of this, and because unhealthy relationships with men frequently undermine women's recovery, a new model is developing as a way to conceptualize women's addiction. Taking off from relational theory (which, as described in Chapter 5, stresses relationships as the framework and context for women's growth), this model sees the essence of addiction in troubled relationships, where love for a drug increasingly cuts the drinker off from connections to human beings. Diane Byington, Ph.D., who has a private practice in psychotherapy in the Denver area and has written on relational theory and addictions, says, "When women are in relationships with men where they're offering everything and not getting much back, the relationship to a drug starts to seem a lot more appealing—it feels a whole lot safer." Men also retreat from human relationships to relationships with objects or experiences, and they often understand what Byington is suggesting when she asks if they have a relationship with their car. She finds that talking about what makes a relationship mutual and fulfilling allows clients to realize how isolated they have become. "Recovery is about ending the relationship with alcohol and drugs and rebuilding essential connections: to yourself, to a higher power, and to other people."

Some recent research lends credence to the relational approach. In an article analyzing data collected over ten years from a representative sample of 696 American women, Sharon and Richard Wilsnack evaluated how well women's personal and social characteristics predict their drinking behavior. They found three specific patterns of predictors of problem drinking. The first, confirming much other research, relates to adverse childhood experiences; the second to a lack, loss, or impairment of interpersonal ties; and the third to these women's expectation that alcohol would make them more self-confident and less sexually inhibited. "The common denominator of all three patterns is women's relationships," Sharon Wilsnack told me. "Even early experiences such as sexual abuse, which is a powerful predictor of drinking problems decades later, may be important largely because of their long-lasting effects on women's relationships. It could be that the current bad relationships fuel the drinking." Wilsnack cautions, "All of this is interpretation, but the relationship theme makes sense." Many of the Wilsnacks' findings support this perspective. Drinking alone, for instance—"the solitary, norelational variable," Sharon Wilsnack jokes—was a predictor of a range of drinking problems. Perhaps most persuasively, women who reported having a single confidante over a long stretch of time—even women predisposed to alcoholism by a range of high-risk factors—were unlikely to develop alcohol problems.

It's not possible to sort out cause and effect here. Most likely, cause and effect work in a reciprocal fashion. Alcohol abuse gets in the way of relationships, but if you are grounded in a sustaining relationship, you aren't as vulnerable to alcohol's pull.

Sometimes, the relationship between romance and alcohol is not what it appears. When women drink to tolerate a difficult relationship, economics can be the hidden factor. Sarah, for instance, who had just completed four weeks of inpatient treatment when I first spoke to her, told me she felt good for the first time in fifteen years. The staff had advised her to go directly to a halfway house for at least three months, because they believed that if she returned right away to her boyfriend, Sam, she would surely drink. Sarah believed that those three months would undo her relationship altogether, and so she went back to Sam, the love of her life, and resumed drinking eight weeks later.

She was not, as it first seemed, simply blinded by love, though she spoke of her great need for Sam, and she clearly felt affection for him. She was also concerned about her ability to care for herself. She had a history of panic attacks that had gotten her fired from several jobs. She would open her mouth to speak, but no sound would come out, and she would flee. Sarah was afraid of slipping, as she said, all the way into the gutter. Sam was abusive and goaded her into drinking, but he supported her.

Women's relationships are also complicated by the way alcohol affects sexuality—both psychologically and physiologically in contradictory ways. Many cultures throughout history have associated alcohol and other intoxicants with enhanced sexuality. The truth is that physiologically, alcohol—especially in large doses—diminishes sexual arousal by reducing the blood flow to the genitals and decreasing the intensity of orgasm. Alcohol can also affect the hormonal cycle and deaden the senses. Yet women generally report that drinking enhances sexual pleasure. Why should this be so? It may be that some women's anxiety about sex overwhelms their capacity to enjoy it while sober. For them, the disinhibiting effects of alcohol may more than compensate for its negative effect on blood flow. It may also be that some of the general excitatory effects of alcohol get interpreted as sexual excitement, or even, as one study suggests, that alcohol increases women's testosterone level, which may heighten sexual arousal. Finally, the age-old belief that alcohol heightens sexual excitement may be more powerful than women's own experience. In a study at the University of California at Los Angeles, Linda Beckman and her colleagues asked sixty-nine female volunteers, aged eighteen to thirty-four, to keep a daily diary through two to three menstrual cycles, recording all they ate and drank and all their activities. Afterward, when the women filled out a retrospective questionnaire, they reported that alcohol stimulated them to initiate sex. Their daily diaries, however, showed no such association. These women had just finished observing themselves under a microscope and yet were unable to interpret accurately what they had observed when it did not match preconceptions about alcohol-induced sexual assertiveness. This should not surprise us. When our culture tells us that something is true, we tend to see it even when it is not there.

In spite of women's reports that alcohol enhances their sexual enjoyment, however, sexual dysfunction—lack of interest or enjoyment in sex, few or no orgasms, or pain during intercourse—remains a robust predictor of continuing alcohol problems. This reflects more than alcohol's negative effects on sexual function, since for many of these women sexual dysfunction *preceded* heavy drinking. Researchers suspect a spiral in which women drink because they believe it will help them loosen up, but the alcohol dulls their senses and makes them less sexually responsive, which increases their anxiety and their wish to drink to loosen up.

Drinking, then, may look like a way of managing one's sexuality, of tolerating a relationship that is distasteful, or altering oneself to make a relationship work. It can also coexist with the hungry pursuit of romance, which has its own relentless cycle, similar to alcoholism: pleasureful anticipation, an initial high, and then a crash—emptiness, shame, and desolation, and an urge to seek relief by pursuing another romance.

Sophie's Story

Sophie is a forty-six-year-old dancer, now sober for six years. She thinks of her twenties and thirties as "gray, foggy stretches of time alternating with big bursts of drama." She had a tendency to engage in "wildly tempestuous affairs with totally inappropriate men"; the members of her dance company would comment, "Who needs *Dynasty* and *Dallas* when we have Sophie around?" Tall and jaunty, blond, with a toothy grin and natural warmth, she has a way of attracting "difficult men"— but it's easy to see how anyone would be attracted to her.

The daughter of a teacher and a social worker, Sophie had "a conventional, small-town, WASP upbringing." Though her parents drank very little, Sophie's father was volatile. He could be adoring, but he could also break into sudden rages that terrified his daughter. Sophie became tense, eager to please, and somewhat prone to depression. An excellent student, she went to college at the age of sixteen. She was very hard on herself and never satisfied with her work. "No wonder I became a dancer," said Sophie. "It's a perfect profession for a perfectionist. In your body and in your movements, you always fall short of the ideal."

The first man Sophie got involved with—she married him in her early twenties—was twenty years her senior and, like her father, volatile. He was also an alcoholic. "A tumbleful of vodka with a little tomato juice was his idea of a Bloody Mary. And for the seven years we were together, I drank whatever he put in front of me. It made me less self-conscious and inhibited; I felt funnier, prettier, warmer. Alcohol *works*—at least in the beginning." She recalls long, soulful conversations with her husband: "I thought we communicated best when we were drunk—though I didn't remember anything the next day."

Like so many women, Sophie was introduced to alcohol by a lover. Her drinking started in the service of a relationship, then gradually took over and replaced the relationship. Sophie's husband deteriorated quickly from using alcohol and drugs. She watched him desperately trying to find a balance between barbiturates and alcohol—taking one for energy, the other to calm himself down. "It seems incredible to me now, but I really didn't know what the problem was. I knew that *something* was wrong. I told him, 'I feel like I'm on a sinking ship, and I have to get off, or I'm going to go down with the boat.'"

Finally, Sophie left him. Soon afterward—as if she'd been a prophet—she heard that he had drowned while swimming in the ocean. He had probably been drunk at the time.

At age thirty, Sophie was alone for the first time in her life. "It was intolerable to me. I've heard the phrase 'attachment hunger,' and it rings a bell for me—I had it in spades. That's when I bought my first bottle of alcohol, all on my own. It was a bottle of gin." The gin distanced Sophie from her painful feelings, the longing for romance and affection, and the fear that, on her own, she was only half a person. It also gave her a focus outside herself, a focus that became a preoccupation and then an obsession. Even as, unconsciously, her fears began to grow, she began an internal dialogue that many of the women I interviewed spoke about, familiar to drinkers in denial: the hundred ways of proving to herself that she did not have a drinking problem. "I put the gin on the shelf, and I said to myself: this will last a week. That seemed an acceptable amount to drink. I made it last exactly a week, and immediately bought another."

During this period, Sophie was touring with her dance company and doing some teaching. Her work acted as a control. She didn't drink until the evening, and if she woke up sick in the night, the thought of having to dance or teach in the morning kept her from curing herself with another nip. She learned quickly that whatever she had in the house she would drink, so she bought half-pint bottles, poured a third down the drain, and drank the rest. At this level of consumption she avoided bad hangovers, and to her, it proved she was not an alcoholic.

On her dance tours, she'd keep a bottle of gin in her handbag. When she put the bag through the X-ray machine at an airport, she'd be embarrassed by the outline of the bottle. The other dancers thought this was funny—and as it ended up, three of the seven women in her company became full-blown alcoholics. "We were traveling so often," recalled Sophie, "and when we'd get in late at night, it seemed as if there was nothing to do except have a drink. We weren't doing drugs, thank God—we couldn't afford it."

During certain blissful periods—a few months or a year—a new man could fill up Sophie's emptiness. In the arms of her newest love, her boundaries melted away. Merging with a man, she was whole and complete. She felt safe and grounded. But as soon as any ambivalence entered into the relationship, she began to panic. She clung to romantic expectations of a perfect love. She could not tolerate the complication of her own or her partner's feelings—no anger was allowed, and no jealousy. Any leveling off of passion was extremely threatening to her. She saw no compensation in the return of ego boundaries, no freedom in the ability to turn her gaze elsewhere. For anyone, it's frightening to see past the idealized image of a partner to the actual person. The compensations of mature adult love—support and companionship, acknowledgment and even celebration of difference—should make up for the loss of full-time rapture. For Sophie, the sense of her personal boundaries falling back into place plunged her into fear. She was right back where she had started—running away from the recognition that, in the end, no other human being could take responsibility for her, and no human being could make her safe.

When each relationship ended, she'd "go scurrying off to a new therapist." Her mood swings and erratic behavior might have alerted a counselor who was knowledgeable about alcohol problems, but none of these therapists asked about Sophie's drinking, and she never told. Meanwhile, the alcohol that "worked" in the beginning now made her maudlin and depressed, weepy and hopeless. Her anxiety—which she thought she was curing with alcohol—deepened.

Sophie, like so many alcoholic women, focused on her lovers' problems with alcohol to keep herself from seeing her own. Lying in bed next to her new man one night, the two of them clutching their heads after too much gin, she had a little glimpse of truth: "I knew why *he* was clutching *his* head, and I said to myself, wait a minute—I'm in the same boat he is."

Not long after that, she had a dinner party in her one-room apartment, and at about ten P.M. she excused herself to lie down on her bed—two feet from the table—for a minute. She passed out. When she revived at three A.M. and found that the guests had gone, she was mortified.

A few days later, another dancer called Sophie and told her she wanted to go to an AA meeting, because she was afraid she was an alcoholic, and asked Sophie if she would come with her. "I graciously consented," said Sophie. "We went to the meeting. I kept going, but my friend never went back.

"I still didn't believe I was an alcoholic. I kept going as an antidote to my loneliness. I was riveted by the honesty of the sharing. A woman there sort of appointed herself my sponsor, and to please her, I managed to stop drinking for ninety days. Then I celebrated with a drink, saying to myself, I guess I'm not an alcoholic if I can stop for ninety days. But I got another ninety days together, and then another."

Sophie never had another relapse. While she was freeing herself from the impulse to drink—understanding at last that no cure for loneliness could be found in a bottle of gin—she still believed in the power of a man to fill her life and make her feel complete. Instead of protecting herself during this difficult transitional time, she followed a new lover to London. "A job for me came up at the same time, and I thought it was meant to be." When the relationship broke up, she found herself alone in a foreign city, disoriented and frightened. "I nearly died of loneliness," said Sophie quietly. "I didn't know it was possible to feel that desperate."

Sophie now believes that it was herself she was missing in those days. Having experienced herself as a satellite of her volatile father, she unconsciously revived those dynamics by finding new men to revolve around. They became the sun and she the moon, absorbing and reflecting their light, power, and energy. When the relationships came apart, and the sun was gone, she entered the dark. She didn't know where to go for energy and power, except to another man.

Sophie is a graceful, vivacious woman, but she had no knowledge of how to get access to her own resources and be nourished by them. Instead, in a process psychologists call projection, she attributed many of her own positive qualities to the men she adored. For as long as she could, she merged with those men in order to repossess her own powers.

Relationships are doubly difficult when partners are stalled in their emotional development. Sophie still experienced herself as passive, instead of the agent of much of her misery and the source of her own strength. Her focus on men prevented her from becoming familiar and comfortable with her own needs and confident that she could manage them. Her wish to merge with a man arose from a part of herself that felt like an abandoned child.

In discussing teenage girls, we noted that women and men with alcohol problems are often stalled in this way, especially if they began drinking before they consolidated their identity. In this respect, alcoholics are not necessarily different from the many people without a drinking problem who grow up with a deficient or negative sense of themselves, shaped in part by their childhood environment and reinforced and re-created in unhealthy relationships with schools, teachers, and adult partners. A person who is not in the grip of some compulsive behavior can, if she chooses, carry on with a wounded sense of self; but the alcoholic, if she wishes to stay sober, will probably need to confront her pain and sadness. Getting sober is only the first step. Next comes the difficult work of healing, of identifying old patterns and letting them go, and starting over like a child, reclaiming one's own voice and accepting one's own feelings.

Sophie spoke of her first years of sobriety as the most difficult period of her life. In London, she "lived at AA meetings," leaning on other recovering alcoholics. This dependence was qualitatively different from what she had experienced with her lovers and with alcohol. Now, support involved not a fantasy of merging, but rather learning to trust other people and allowing them to see her weaknesses and strengths. Feeling accepted at AA, she gradually became more accepting of herself. She became aware of how self-critical she was, and as she began to let go of her negative judgments, a more compassionate attitude rose in their place.

Years later, the circumstances of her life haven't changed much, said Sophie—she's still single, still dancing, still teaching—"but I'm much happier. I have sane relationships with men, and I don't mind living alone. I don't wake up shuddering with anxiety. I used to think I had to have alcohol to enjoy sex, but without it, sex is better."

At the moment, Sophie is struggling with the process of putting her mother in a nursing home, and she's upset and sleepless. "Probably anybody would be. But I've learned I can get through hard times without drinking. I swim instead, a few times a week; I go to meetings; I get myself a massage. I'm still prone to obsessive thinking and compulsive behavior; I could still drink if I ever forgot how terrible it is. I go to meetings two or three times a week to remind myself. They calm me down. Sometimes when I go I'm bored and tired, and I sit there with my eyes closed. But for an hour, I acknowledge that I have this problem, and everything in my life depends on my staying on top of it.

"Drinking keeps you from growing up and dealing with life on life's terms. It's a constant avoidance technique. One of my lovers and I used to say that the others were grown-ups and he and I were adorable children who shouldn't be expected to tend to the business of this world. It was a seductive way of thinking, and my lover—a writer— could capture the magic of that childlike perspective in his work. But now I don't *want* to be a child any longer. I'm not running from responsibility. I do my part, and I like that."

For Sophie and many other women I interviewed, their alcohol problems, painful as they were, became an opportunity to transcend the rigid structure of identity and to experience peace, connectedness, and gratitude. Their new lives are not about miracles but about opening up to a whole range of experience, including such negative feelings as ambivalence, anger, and sadness—the feelings they used to try to medicate. The first months (and sometimes years) of sobriety can be agonizing. Alcohol used to provide a barrier against discomfort, but now that is gone. It takes enormous courage, enormous faith, to wait it out, holding on to the promise that the agony will subside in time, and you will learn how to manage your feelings. The pain and the cravings may never disappear altogether. But although you may initially feel beset by hornets, eventually it is possible to brush them off.

SEXUAL SHAME AND ISOLATION

WHEN DRINKING has been part of a larger picture of failed relationships, early sobriety can plunge women into a period of intense shame. They are likely to condemn themselves. Instead of locating the problems in destructive relationships, they tend to blame their own deficiencies. Certainly it is appropriate to look inward and assess one's own capacity to change, but this perspective shows only part of the picture. Sophie's relationships—in which the man's needs were her preoccupation, she needed a man to complete herself, and romance was "forever after"—followed a familiar cultural script. Women tend to feel enormous shame as they attempt to come to terms with their failed relationships, taking all of the blame and hurt upon themselves and letting their partners—and their culture—off the hook.

Tamara's Story

Tamara is a lively, articulate, attractive thirty-seven-year-old with a husky voice and a gift for vivid speech. When she got sober, she was stricken with shame about her "promiscuity," a loaded word in alcoholism research. In early studies, male alcoholics were said to have "numerous sexual partners," while female alcoholics were "promiscuous." The behavior was the same, but the negative value judgment was aimed at the women only. Tamara described her self-loathing by telling me of a woman she had just read about. In a psychotic state, this woman killed her sleeping daughter to protect her from people who were coming to steal her and take her into slavery. "They put her on medication and gave her therapy every day," said Tamara, "and gradually she came out of her psychosis. Then she began to realize the horror of what she had done. She'd killed her own daughter, and she had to live with that! I hadn't killed anyone when I was drunk, but getting sober and coming out of the fog, I realized—oh, my God, all the really horrible things I had done, the impression I had made on other people, and the pain I'd caused." She felt helpless in the face of her self-loathing. "I didn't have coping strategies, but I still had all the problems that led me into my addiction. I felt a tremendous amount of sexual shame."

In fact, Tamara had little interest in sex when she was drinking, but she used men for access to alcohol and drugs. "They adored me; they thought I was beautiful. I would meet them at bars and attach myself to one, who would be sort of like an island for me. Home base. I felt a little bit safer than when I was on my own. They'd buy me drinks. I rarely had any money." Focused entirely on her addiction, Tamara would have preferred to avoid sex altogether. "But if things didn't go quite right, that's where I ended up. I'd lead someone on too far, and I'd feel obliged to have sex with him. Or the person who took me home would have ideas, and I'd be too drunk to fight it. Today they'd call it date rape. At that time, if they wanted to screw me, there was nothing to stop them."

While she was drinking, Tamara ran away from any man who had a crush on her. When she was sober, the roles were reversed. She became the pursuer, and any man she hooked up with ran away after one or two dates. "No wonder," she told me. "I never said anything truthful to any of them. I told lies to boost my self-esteem—that I was filthy rich, for instance. They'd see that I was nuts, and leave." Tamara felt used, degraded, ashamed, and very, very lonely. She spent hours each day fantasizing about romance, marriage, "and just someone who wouldn't run away from me!" Young and beautiful, she had no trouble attracting a new man for one or two nights, and she fell into each man's arms with the fervent hope that he would rescue her. When the man left, her self-recrimination intensified, and her fantasies picked up and led her into bed with someone else.

Her actions may seem hard to comprehend. It makes no sense to try to cure sexual shame by sleeping with another man, just as it makes no sense for a remorseful drinker to reach for another drink. Yet such behavior is part of a common self-destructive cycle that picks up speed when a person feels cut off from any sense of hope. When there is no real connection to self, lover, family, or community, shame and isolation intensify, and so does the need for psychic numbing, which compulsive rituals create. Said Tamara: "I replaced booze with sex."

Tamara's loneliness stretches back to her difficult childhood with an emotionally absent father and a depressed mother who mostly ignored her but often flew at her with her fists. She now sees her drinking, her use of drugs, and her "revolving-door" relationships as desperate attempts to break out of an isolation so painful that she considered suicide. "I always felt haunted, just haunted," she said. As she grows in her understanding of what makes a mutual relationship, she also looks more kindly on her past behavior, seeing her addiction and her indiscriminate sexuality as a drive to connect, before she understood how to do so in a healthy way. Alcohol was a substitute "best friend," she told me, and, "Sex was an attempt like all other attempts to get out of myself and try to make some connection with the world."

Now, although she has been sober for thirteen years, she still struggles with relationship problems. Not long ago, her fiancé broke up with her, saying that she was too disorganized and that he didn't always feel loved. Painful as this was, it prompted a period of real growth, and Tamara is optimistic. "I've had an enormous amount to learn about relationships," she told me. "I've had to learn how to be receptive to love, how to listen, and how to be honest. Each relationship has brought me further along."

Tamara relies on AA meetings to stay sober, but she attributes her gradual progress with relationship problems to hard work in therapy. As we have noted, though AA is referred to as a "program for living," women may need another context in which to come to terms with specific life problems, especially when they involve sexuality. (Unfortunately, sexual problems are often not dealt with in treatment centers either.) Some women find the support they need at same-sex meetings within AA. Others that I interviewed turned to Women for Sobriety, because its members are all women, and because this organization tends to be more open to discussions of factors contributing to addiction. Any woman with continuing relationship problems or repeated relapses may benefit from the support of a trained professional as well as a recovery group.

LOVE AND POWER

UNDERLYING SOPHIE'S and Tamara's stories about love hunger is another, paradoxically related, theme: women's need for power. This theme has received attention in relation to the male drinker's psyche, as in David McClelland's book *The Drinking Man* (1972), in which he theorized that men drink to boost an illusion of power over others. The more McClelland's subjects drank, the more they fantasized about sexual conquest, physical prowess, aggressiveness, and personal influence. McClelland's subjects were all men, but—typically—his results were assumed to be valid for women also. Analysts who conceded that women are less likely to fantasize about conquests were simply reinforced in the assumption that women are less vulnerable to alcoholism than men.

The terms of the debate about alcoholism, gender, and power have changed over the years. Sharon Wilsnack, who was a graduate student of David McClelland's, was disturbed by references in the scientific literature to alcoholic women's "deviant sex role adjustment." She began her own research in 1972 with studies of female social drinkers and problem drinkers, and she reframed the issues surrounding power and dependency into an analysis of conflicts generated by the narrow range of acceptable behavior in women. When I asked her about the most recent work on drinking and power, she laughed and said, "It's an idea that won't give up," but conceded "there's *something* in it." As we saw in Chapter 2, anthropological studies have reported that men's drinking is designed in part to demonstrate their masculinity, that is, their stamina, self-control, independence, and willingness to take risks—a finding that bears some relation to McClelland's early work. Also, as described in Chapter 3, feminist family systems theorists have noted that problems of dependency and power are prevalent in the intimate relationships of alcoholic couples.

It's more consonant with a traditional notion of femininity to speak of women's need for intimacy than of their need for power, but the obsessive drive for union may in fact involve both. Sophie, for instance, had little faith in her own resources, so she projected them onto men; she felt energetic, cheerful, and productive only when she was in the early stages of falling in love and she and her lover experienced an illusion of merging with each other. This is a drive for "relationship" only in a distorted sense. More precisely, it is a drive to repossess the power one has given away. When an early romance wore off and ego boundaries fell back into place, Sophie felt depleted and the relationships fell apart. She would then look around for another magnetic, mercurial man, an object for her projection, a man whose power she could share and thereby restore herself.

This phenomenon is familiar to students of developmental theories. For example, in one normal stage of development, the infant has an illusion of merging with the mother and sharing in the mother's perfection. The dawning recognition that the mother is a separate being destabilizes the child. Children may revel in their emerging powers, but they will also long to restore the symbiotic union with the mother whenever the world proves frustrating.

Even as adults, we never completely leave behind this longing for the oneness we once knew with our mothers. As Judith Viorst writes,

> *Although we do not remember it, we also never forget it. We acknowledge it in religion and myth and fairy tales and our conscious and unconscious fantasies. We acknowledge it as reality or as dream. And while we fiercely protect the boundaries of self that clearly demark the you from the me, we also yearn to recapture the lost paradise of that ultimate connection. . . . Through sex, through religion, through nature, through art, through drugs, through meditation, even through jogging, we try to blur the boundaries that divide us. We try to escape the imprisonment of separateness. We sometimes succeed.*

Temporarily reexperiencing this "world-embracing oneness" can supply us with strength, an illusion of safety, and a sense of connection to the world. When this impulse becomes predominant—when it becomes a central, life-shaping ideal, when there is no joy in the return of personal boundaries and the ordinary life of a separate person who relates intimately with another individual—then the wish to merge is regressive, a yearning for the symbiosis of infancy. The connection implies safety and power. Though compelling, it does not make room for the two separate identities that are needed for a relationship. For Sophie, breaking out of her repeated episodes of drinking, romance, and disillusionment meant letting go of her fantasy of being fulfilled in someone else, and realizing that "growing up isn't something that just happens to you. You have to work for it. It's a choice you make." Now "a citizen of the world," she has an arena where she takes responsibility, and she no longer runs from the challenges that used to prompt her to take refuge in a drink or the arms of a man.

For Tamara, relationships were also largely a matter of power, but in different ways. When she was drinking, she got a further high from the hold she had over men, from the way she could get them to buy her drinks and do whatever she wanted. When she was sober, she would work out for three hours a day to keep her body perfect. She would walk into a room and know that everybody there was looking at her. At a gym or a swimming pool, all heads turned her way. "It didn't provide the action that drinking did, but it was exciting," she told me. She relied on this attention to make her feel real, since, like many others who struggle with lifelong feelings of inferiority, she believed she existed in the eyes of others. Underconfident, unaware of any other way she might achieve a sense of being worthy, she knew she could at least manipulate men with her beauty. She could get them into bed with her once, even if she couldn't make them come back. Her body was a tool to gain power and control, and sex, though it didn't interest her, still allowed moments of physical affection. In a sense, Tamara settled for being an object of desire and admiration as a substitute for genuine love and wholeness.

I am stressing the role that power plays in many people's drive for connection as a way of compensating for the current way of talking about women's needs in terms of their talent for relationships. For most women, the language of relationship is a comfortable way of framing their needs, because it is consistent with their socialization and describes a familiar feminine ideal. It's so comfortable, in fact, that it becomes an easy refuge, and it may push any impulse toward aggression, or any wish to exercise power, out of one's awareness. I recently came across an article on high-achieving women in recovery that exemplifies the danger of idealizing women's relationships. The authors, two practicing clinicians in New York, identify "the need to nurture and enable others" as the most authentic aspect of women's character, the part of themselves high-achieving women will uncover as they heal. They acknowledge that a recovering woman needs to be mirrored by others, and they suggest that AA fills this need. But, they caution, "power and success strivings are not consistent with the emphasis of self-actualization within the framework of a spiritual life." These authors tell stories of high-achieving clients who left their competitive occupations once they identified with being female and tapped into their own capacity for nurturance. This formulation sounds very much like the old prescriptive ideal of femininity that shut women out of "men's work."

Clearly, it is useful to point out how women's development is different from men's, and to see it in its own terms. It is also important to recognize that traditional male models of development, which focus on separation and autonomy, may lead to exaggerated ideals of independence and self-reliance. Women, because of their traditional nurturing roles, may be less likely than men to forget that human beings are mutually interdependent. They are well-situated to articulate a morality that emphasizes our need for one another. Yet to be fully themselves, women, like men, need to acknowledge their aggression and their need for power, accomplishment, and a sense of self, and to accept these needs as natural sources of energy. If they don't, they may have trouble arranging their lives in ways that address their own needs. They may look to relationships to satisfy needs that are better met through work and creativity.

Tamara spoke feelingly of the self-enclosed cycle in which she was trapped, setting her sights on a man, bringing him in, experiencing first elation, then despair, then anticipation of another romance. She spoke of how little sense of self she brought to any relationship. Even when she was in therapy and AA, this self-enclosed, self-perpetuating cycle persisted. I asked her how she broke out of it, and her answer was telling. "By doing things," she said. What things? "I went back to graduate school," she said. "I got a job."

Once Tamara had genuine accomplishments behind her, and a working community to mirror her strengths and weaknesses, she had less need to tell "self-esteem lies" to the men she dated. In her relationships, she took steps toward further intimacy and more mutual exchange. The rewards of love given and received gave her courage to reach further into herself and acknowledge feelings she had buried, which released more energy for love and work. As with all developmental progress, hers didn't take a linear course but rather was a spiral or a circle, with a bit of movement in one area allowing for movement in another. Her example illustrates how growth in personal development, relationships, and engagement with the world all grow in concert with one another.

THE FORCE THAT DRIVES ADDICTION

THE FORCE that drives addiction is powerful and doesn't disappear when drinking stops. Alcoholics often leave drinking behind only to find themselves in the grip of some other compulsive behavior. Many women shift from one addiction to another—from alcohol to another drug, or to compulsive sex, gambling, or spending, or to bingeing and purging, and back to alcohol again—each destructive behavior providing a temporary relief from unnamed inner cravings. All have in common an anticipatory high and some kind of release; then come shame and self-castigation and another search for relief.

Mary, who was a topless waitress when she was drinking, is now living a conventional life as the wife of a banker in London. Her compulsive behavior has been rechanneled into physical fitness and shopping. Two hours a day on the treadmill keep her body nearly perfect, even after two children, and daily shopping in exclusive boutiques yields fabulous clothing and jewelry. She no longer goes topless, but people still look up when she enters a room. "I guess I'm still an exhibitionist," said Mary, who keeps her sense of humor. Though her husband makes plenty of money, she shops so extravagantly—a Prada handbag for $900 is nothing—that they are always struggling to pay their bills. She still craves the high that comes from living in a danger zone. "My best friend in AA says I haven't made a dent in my alcoholism," said Mary, "even though I haven't had a drink in five years."

Alice, the lawyer whose story appears in Chapter 6, said that two months after her inpatient treatment, her craving for alcohol entirely disappeared; but the eating disorder she'd struggled with in college came back in triple force. The need that had driven her workaholism, her drinking, and her fear of relationships was transformed into literal hunger: "Once my eating disorder was triggered, obsessive thoughts were almost unbearable. They took up all of my mental space. It was awful. It was crippling." She described her obsessive planning of meals: the time she spent shopping for food, her intricate rituals of preparation, her reverence for a perfect place setting, the conditions that had to be met before she would eat. "I had a medical condition that kept me thin—I knew without doubt that I was not overweight—but that didn't matter. I was consumed by my diet."

Compulsions like these fall along a continuum that has to do with consumption. At one end, you have women working on their bodies, hoping they will feel better when they are showpieces, the object of men's desire, adornments that make men feel powerful. In a culture where women's bodies are used to sell everything from cigarettes to automobiles, women are led to assess their own value as a commodity. At the other end of this continuum, women themselves become consumers—buying designer handbags, bingeing on doughnuts, obsessing over a perfect meal, drinking a fifth of gin—in an effort to fill up their emptiness. Our culture encourages us to find solutions in the marketplace.

Often, as with Sophie's spiraling relationships, the compulsion that plagues a woman in sobriety operates alongside her drinking. Sometimes—as with Tamara and sex, or with Alice and food—it gains momentum when the drinking stops. Multiple addictions to drugs or behaviors can drain a woman so completely that she may be forced to give up and seek help. Many younger women turn to cocaine specifically to increase their tolerance for alcohol. Tamara took cocaine for this reason, and she believes that its devastating highs and lows brought her into treatment ten years sooner than alcohol alone would have done. Multiple addictions may also provide just enough relief from one another to widen the self-destructive circle and keep it going for a while longer. In her memoir, Caroline Knapp writes,

> *I am consistently amazed to hear women talk about their multiple relationships with addictions, the way they combine two or three, the way they shift from one to another, so naturally and gracefully you might think they were changing partners in a dance. Addictions segue into one another with such ease: a bout of compulsive overeating fills you with shame and sexual inferiority, which fills you with self-loathing and doubt, which leads you to a drink, which temporarily counters the self-hatred and fills you with chemical confidence, which leads you to sleep with a man you don't love, which leads you circling back to shame, and voilà: the dance can begin again. The dance will begin again, for the music is always there in women's minds, laced with undertones of fear and anger, urging us on into the same sad circles of restraint and abandon, courtship and flight.*

It is tremendously painful to live this way, but these cycles serve several purposes. They distract a woman from self-loathing, and they give her the punishment that she feels she deserves. They provide brief relief as well as excitement and drama. They create a comprehensible set of rules and this gives an illusion of relative safety, a familiar set of obsessions. They offer a strategy for shutting out a world that feels increasingly unmanageable and living within a world with a comprehensible shape and structure. In a healthier (but still misguided) sense, such repetitive behavior is impelled by a desire to get it right this time, to master impulses, grow up, get a handle on life. Isn't this drinking problem basically a lack of restraint? Isn't it time to seize the reins and take control of life? Isn't that what everybody around the drinker is *begging* her to do?

Contradictions, double binds, and paradoxes are at the heart of addiction and recovery. The drinker drinks to find love, but drinking chases love away. The drinker drinks to find relief, but after that initial release she finds only pain in the bottle. The drinker feels powerless and drinks to escape and to assert her power, but drinking renders her helpless. If she turns to a substitute addiction, it tightens the self-destructive cycle and delivers her back to drink. Her determination to get control of her addiction exacerbates her problem. It's a closed system, and she's in it by herself. The spiral keeps on tightening. There is no way out from within.

Even the wish to break out and get a larger perspective can lead to more drinking. Allison, a recovering alcoholic who has also been diagnosed with obsessive-compulsive disorder, described her desperation to break away from "the engine that drives me every day." "At the end of the day, I wanted to get outside myself. I wanted to reach that state where I wasn't like a cork, swept along by the ocean. I wanted a higher perspective, one foot in my life, and one foot out. When I drank, at first, I could finally let go of all the trivial things that bothered me and see myself, and my life, from a larger perspective. That's what I wanted; that's why I drank. But it was a lie. Alcohol doesn't transcend. It obliterates."

For all of us, our ordinary inner life—our subjectivity—is fairly chaotic and complex. Thoughts, feelings, and impulses come and go. We hide from our awareness of being alone. We struggle along, attempting to choose a path, but we find ourselves caught in conflicting desires. All of us are capable of sinking to a frightening level of unconsciousness, a point of primitive aggression, rage, and lust. We wish for some larger sense of purpose, but we find it hard to achieve or sustain. For an alcoholic in a tightening spiral, the desire to break out can be desperate.

In our secular society, many people have no way of understanding or talking about the basic human desire to transcend the self. We lack a cultural context for the ecstatic experience—that temporary state of pure focus, of inner and outer harmony, that can become a vehicle for personal transformation, as the memory of oneness with the world is gradually integrated into daily life. The oceanic feelings alcohol brings may be as near as we get to being in touch with the ineffable. When alcohol disinhibits us, and our inner censor and judge takes a holiday, our warm, loving feelings may be as close as we get to being in harmony with ourselves and all of life. One woman told me—sincerely and even passionately—that she was a better person when she drank.

For many women, the experience of oneness is what makes alcohol so compelling. Love, power, and alcohol are all related. To paraphrase Tamara, they represent attempts to get out of the self and make some connection with the world. To be sure, this pursuit is misguided. There is a difference between swelling the ego and transcending it, and alcohol betrays you in the end. Although compulsive behaviors arise in part from a shaky sense of self and feelings of despair and emptiness, the motivations for drinking often include health and striving for wholeness. It's just that alcoholics have chosen, as a Buddhist might say, "unskillful means" of achieving their goal.

In recovery, the alcoholic needs to learn "skillful means" of breaking through her isolation, repairing her connections to self and others, and discovering how to transcend the self in a way that can liberate her from a self-destructive cycle. Since alcoholism is, in part, a relational problem, genuine recovery must take place among people. More and more of the alcoholic's inner life, which often has been buried even from her own awareness, must be brought into her relationships. Telling her story—at recovery meetings, in therapy, among friends— becomes a crucial means of breaking down the boundaries that have separated a living soul from other living souls. As connections strengthen and life expands—including more experiences, more people, more feelings—she may learn to find strength in community, depend on other people, and let others depend on her.

Sometimes, said Tamara, when she calls her sponsor about something she has done that worries her, her sponsor says, "We're going to ignore that right now."

"She doesn't say *you* are going to ignore this," said Tamara. "She says *we*. That word means someone else is on my side. I have a connection to a human lifeline."

8

Springs of Sorrow:
Drinking at Times of Loss

Margaret, are you grieving
Over Goldengrove unleaving?
Leaves, like the things of man, you
With your fresh thoughts care for, can you?
Ah! as the heart grows older
It will come to such sights colder
By and by, nor spare a sigh
Though worlds of wanwood leafmeal lie;
And yet you will weep and know why.
Now no matter, child, the name:
Sorrow's springs are the same.
Nor mouth had, no nor mind, expressed
What heart heard of, ghost guessed:
It is the blight man was born for,
It is Margaret you mourn for.
—GERARD MANLEY HOPKINS,
"SPRING AND FALL"

LOSS REPEATS ITSELF THROUGHOUT OUR LIVES. THE EVO-
lution from infant to child to adolescent to adult involves a series of little deaths. A baby who develops separation anxiety has realized that she
and her mother are separate people, and her mother can go away. Not
without a struggle, she gives up the illusion of perfect safety and

harmony, of oneness with her mother. This is the first and primal renunciation in a life that will be conditioned by loss.

Women's biology and cultural roles entail particular losses. When a girl has her first period, sometimes as early as eight years old, the loss of childhood may seem particularly abrupt. Adolescence beckons, and though she may greet it with excitement, there is usually nostalgia for what is left behind. Bearing children involves many forms of loss. Miscarriages are common and can be emotionally devastating. Even abortions may require mourning. Infertile women must reconcile themselves to never being biological mothers. Raising children involves giving up aspects of the self. With menopause comes new freedom, but it also marks a loss of possibilities. If a woman's sense of usefulness has derived chiefly from her service to her children, when they leave home, not only will she miss them; she will have lost the meaning in her life.

For some women aging can bring a sense of doom. As her sexual power diminishes, a woman whose self-worth has been linked to youth and beauty may feel useless and unloved. She may fear that she will be discarded by her mate—no doubt, she knows men who have left their wives for younger women. Older age brings a loss of health and a loss of friends through death and illness. Since men die younger, and widows are less likely than widowers to remarry, many women end their days alone.

In *The Seasons of a Woman's Life*, the research psychologist Daniel Levinson estimates that we spend nearly half our adult lives in transition between periods of relative stability. During these transitional times, we challenge our operating definitions, question our values, explore our own wishes and motivations. We relinquish previous self-images. Although each metamorphosis brings new potential, we need to pause to mourn our losses before we go on.

At any point in the process, we may become stuck. Our crisis may be developmental, as we are suspended in transit between ending one life structure and beginning another; or we may be adapting to some highly stressful situation, such as illness or violence; or both of these crises may be happening at once. We feel shaken, scared, wrenched. The past—and sometimes even the future—collapses around us.

Even the most adaptable people are likely to struggle before they let go. Some hold on longer, becoming rigid, refusing to adapt. Some fight to stay young, or develop psychosomatic illnesses, or distract themselves—as Judith Viorst describes it in *Necessary Losses,* "running too fast to notice what they have lost." Some people develop compulsive behavior. One option is to drown one's awareness in drink.

LATE-ONSET ALCOHOLISM

WHILE NOT BLAMING their drinking on events or seeing themselves as victims, many of the women I interviewed dated their drinking problems from a major transition or loss. Stephie, whose husband had encouraged her drinking (Chapter 3), had been sober for five years when she was plunged into grief—and a relapse—by the death of her brother. Billie took to drinking when she lost her job as an administrative assistant and despaired of finding another. Jill, the woman whose mother told her, at age eight, never to touch her again and whose "second mother" killed herself, first got drunk after the suicide; her alcoholic drinking was triggered by her father's death.

Dale, the thirty-six-year-old computer programmer in Washington state, was happier than she'd ever been just before her world fell apart. She was working part-time as a legal transcriber, taking care of two small children, and actively involved in the Catholic church with her husband—they sang at mass each week and led retreats for married couples. Having been a lonely child, she now felt like a valued member of a community for the first time in her life. Neither she nor her husband drank more than an occasional glass of wine. Then one June, on her husband's last day of teaching for the school year, he came home distraught and told her he was "beginning to have feelings" for another teacher. In retrospect, Dale believes that he had begun an affair that day. This woman was going away for the summer, he said, to give them both time to think. "I want us to spend the summer as though there is nothing going on," he told Dale, "just you and me and the kids."

That night Dale and her husband got drunk on Black Russians, and their nightmarish summer began. She drove the kids around to the swimming pool, bought Burger King dinners for the family, stopped eating, and lost twenty-five pounds, all the while pretending that everything was okay. "If I'd known then what I know now, I wouldn't have gone along with it," Dale told me. "But I was terrified of losing him. This was the person I had fallen in love with the night I met him. He was everything I wanted in a husband. When I first saw him, I was twenty-one, and I knew right away that I was going to marry him."

Three years later, when they were finally divorced, Dale started drinking every night on her own. "I chose white wine because I had gone back to school, and if I spilled red wine on my homework, I'd have to copy it over." When she was offered a job in Seattle, she moved there with her children within a week. Desperately lonely, she escalated her drinking. Three months later, she was laid off, Seattle's rain kept coming down, and all she could do was worry that she'd run out of money and not be able to buy wine or Valium.

It is hard to assess how commonly or how directly women who develop drinking problems are reacting to situations. More often than men, they report that their heavy drinking followed such a crisis as miscarriage, a divorce, unemployment, or a child's leaving home. In some cases—especially when domestic violence is involved—it may be that drinking contributes to a crisis, as much as the other way around. Sometimes, alcoholic women may see a loss as an explanation that doesn't cause them shame. Men, on the other hand, may find it shameful—a sign of weakness—to attribute their drinking to grief.

As we have seen, researchers debate whether women's problems with alcohol may be more reactive and less genetic than men's. Some researchers believe that early-onset and late-onset alcoholism differ in their precipitating causes: people who develop problems in adolescence are genetically predisposed to addiction, whereas those whose problems develop in midlife or later are more likely to be responding to such stress and loss as death, retirement, and illness. Later onset of problems (defined differently by different studies) appears to be more common among women. Among elderly respondents in a general population study who reported alcohol-related problems within the last six months, fewer than one-third of the men but more than half of the women reported an onset after age forty. In another study of older women and men in treatment, the mean age of onset was twenty-seven for men but over forty-six for women.

Investigators have tried to distinguish different subtypes of alcoholism, looking at such factors as age of onset, family history, and the relative contribution of environmental and genetic factors. Cloninger's typology for men is probably most influential. He distinguishes between type 1 alcoholism, which begins later and includes a strong element of psychological dependence and a stronger contribution of environmental factors; and type 2 alcoholism, which starts early—usually in adolescence—and involves a stronger family history and more antisocial behavior. In 1995, the researcher Shirley Hill presented evidence for a premise that there are two types of alcoholism in women as well. Hill's "primary alcoholism" corresponds more or less to Cloninger's type 2, which is thought to be more influenced by genetics and more severe. Drinking tends to begin in adolescence, problems escalate, behavior is antisocial, and treatment is difficult. "Secondary alcoholism" is largely the result of environmental pressures. A woman with secondary alcoholism is less likely to have a family history of alcohol abuse. She probably began to drink regularly in her twenties or thirties, and her problem is likely to peak in her forties or later.

Several women I interviewed had been told that they were "primary" or "secondary" alcoholics, but scientists dispute whether there are genuinely distinct subtypes of alcoholism. As we have discussed, genetic and environmental influences interact, and there is no clear way to isolate their effects, though researchers do try.

Some research into the etiology of alcohol problems highlights individual responses to negative events. Edith Gomberg found a similar number of negative events in early life among 301 alcoholic women and a nonalcoholic control group, but the alcoholic women interpreted those events more negatively. Gomberg found that they felt more deprived, managed anger in self-destructive ways, felt more depressed, and experienced a higher degree of guilt and shame.

Why do some women respond to trauma, or to "ordinary losses," by adapting and building new life structures, while some become depressed or self-destructive? In psychology, research into resilience reflects a shift in attention from why some people succumb to fate to why others thrive in the face of adversity. We know, for instance, that a family history of alcoholism is one of the strongest predictors of alcohol problems, yet most people reared in an alcoholic home never develop an alcohol problem or a related behavioral disorder. What protects these people? According to one study, adolescents are protected by positive communication with their parents, parental support, and close monitoring. Another study showed that among adults, social support from friends is protective—more so than family support.

Very often, if a loss in adulthood sets us spinning in a downward spiral, we are recapitulating an earlier loss, when support was insufficient and mourning was never completed. When Dale was a little girl, her family moved every three years, and she didn't fit with any group of kids. Her mother favored her sister and shamed Dale for being "selfish, lazy, and disagreeable." The shaming took. At ten years old, Dale wet her bed at night and washed her hands so fiercely during the day that her wrists bled. She was her father's favorite, but he was usually overseas. She longed for him to return. Throughout her childhood, she said, it was as if she "lived in a glass phone booth, but nobody could see I was enclosed in there."

In adulthood, having a stable marriage, success as a mother and a worker, and perhaps most important, strong community support, Dale was able to grow, learn, and thrive. When her husband left and she suddenly moved to a new apartment in a new city, she reenacted the drama of her childhood, desperately grieving in a place she could not call home. Her isolation became intense, as did her shame and her sense of worthlessness. Alcohol and Valium replaced the support of her husband and friends.

Drinking and Depression

There is a high incidence of depression among alcoholics, and this complicates their problems. Depression can be reactive—a response to loss or trauma—or it can be a chronic underlying condition. Some would argue that this state of despair, with its stream of self-denigrating, self-flagellating thoughts, is purely biological, a disease of neurotransmitters. Others believe that underlying all depression is some kind of loss, whether current or long-buried. Most seem to take a middle road, believing that some individuals are predisposed to depression, and a loss can trigger it.

According to *DSM IV*, a diagnostic manual, such symptoms as insomnia, poor appetite, and weight loss in a grieving person should be diagnosed as "bereavement" for two months. After that—but who doesn't grieve longer than two months?—the diagnosis changes to "major depressive disorder." As this example makes clear, grief and depression are often intertwined; the boundaries between them are probably different for different people.

Assessing an alcoholic's depression is particularly complicated, because alcohol itself depresses the central nervous system. Even relatively small amounts can worsen depression and increase anger. Conversely, symptoms of depression—guilt, sleep disturbances, loss of appetite, and irritability—often diminish in periods of sobriety. In addition, the life circumstances of an alcoholic make sadness inevitable. Many have compromised their health, lost their jobs, and lost their spouses (this is true of women more often than men). In treatment, not only are they giving up alcohol, which dulled the grief of other losses, but if they have been drinking and using drugs with friends, they may be advised to give up their friends, too. If a woman has been clinging to an idealized image of herself, corresponding to her sense of what a woman *ought* to be, she must also recognize the gap between that image and reality—perhaps the hardest loss of all.

Since so much depression is induced by alcohol, twelve-step treatment has traditionally shunned antidepressant drugs. Until 1994, doctors at Hazelden, the most influential substance abuse treatment center in the country, recommended that depressed patients achieve two years of sobriety before considering drug treatment. Perhaps the most important shift in treatment is the recent recognition that untreated depression can sabotage sobriety and the acceptance of antidepressant drugs and other therapies. Since depression and alcoholism have a synergistic effect, treatment for both is critical.

Estimates of the prevalence of depression among alcoholics vary widely—from 15 percent to as high as 70 percent—depending on the source of subjects and the definition used. Studies comparing male and female alcoholics consistently find higher rates of depression among women. On the one hand, this is not surprising, since women's risk of depression generally exceeds men's by two to one. On the other hand, male alcoholics are depressed at about the same rate as male nonalcoholics, while female alcoholics are more frequently depressed than female nonalcoholics, suggesting that alcohol problems and depression are often closely related among women. In addition, women's depressive symptoms are more likely to persist into sobriety, and to have preceded their dependence on alcohol, whereas men's depression tends to follow drinking. It's not clear why this should be so. It may merely reflect the fact that men tend to become alcoholic at earlier ages than women, before clinical depression is likely to be diagnosed. Yet younger women alcoholics have even higher levels of depression than older women—a finding that would seem inconsistent with this argument. Scientific evidence seems to keep shifting, but it may well be that alcoholism is more reactive in women than in men.

Amy's Story:
Drinking, Loss, and the Life Cycle

DANIEL LEVINSON OUTLINES the developmental periods of women's adulthood and notes that although each new phase involves growth and dissolution—the building of new life structures and the falling away of structures we have outgrown—the balance changes as we age. In childhood, each step forward entails some loss, but we are moving toward our full potential. After forty, we begin a gradual biological decline. We will still grow psychologically and emotionally, but our losses multiply.

A sixty-three-year-old painter whose career has only recently taken off, Amy would seem to defy the usual arc of life. Yet she describes how, in later life, she sank under the weight of accumulated losses.

I met Amy through my friend Jonathan, who, when I told him about the interviews I was doing for this book, took me to see Amy, a woman with, he said, "a torrential sense of humor." A year before, at the age of sixty-two, she had gone to the Betty Ford Center in Rancho Mirage, California, for treatment of her alcoholism.

Her loft in Manhattan had a big central room, crowded with bookcases, paintings, and wood furniture. Brushes, paints, and supplies were laid out in front of the window. A half-finished painting was propped on an easel. Amy's mother was also a painter, and her father was a noted political cartoonist. The couple met in Paris in the 1920s, and Amy grew up in a social milieu that included Scott Fitzgerald, Hemingway, and H. L. Mencken, who was her godfather. She decided early on to stay away from painting even though she loved to draw and was well-schooled in it. "I didn't want to compete with my parents," she explained. She wrote instead but wasn't successful, she said, on her own terms or anybody else's. "Then I got married and had three babies, and I did that with a vengeance. I loved having children." When they were grown and Amy got divorced, she returned to writing for a while. Finally, in her late forties, she picked up watercolors and then oil paints. She had a successful exhibit, and since then, her paintings have sold so fast that she has to borrow them back to get a show together.

Amy wore big round glasses and looked up at us expectantly from her modest height. Her thick white hair was cropped around her face; she wore casual, loose clothing. Her parrot screeched, and Amy told us she was sad today, quite upset, in fact, because a friend had died after a long illness. She and Jonathan—who have known each other since both were very young—gossiped about old friends, several now dead. A neighbor knocked at the door and told Amy he was throwing out a footstool. Would it be useful to her? "Increasingly," she said. "You don't happen to be throwing out a walker too?"

Among the many photographs around the loft, one in particular held my attention, a large one pinned to the bookcase, of a little boy with a self-inflicted haircut. He was about six years old, sensitive-looking and elfin. This was Amy's grandson. In our private interview, Amy would tell me of his central place in the story of her alcoholism.

When the little boy, Luke, was eight months old, Amy's daughter returned to work and needed a baby-sitter. Amy volunteered. Three days a week, she cared for Luke from seven in the morning until seven at night. "I fell for him completely," she told me. She had three other grandchildren, but he was the one she took care of, and he was the one she understood. They took walks together, did errands, read books. When he was older, she took him to a nursery school for a couple of hours in the morning and was there to pick him up afterward. They loved to chat but were equally happy to be with each other in silence. "We were completely at home with each other," said Amy. Four days a week she painted; the other three days she devoted herself to her grandson. Amy's life was in balance, and the schedule suited her perfectly.

When Luke was four and a half, he moved away with his mother and father. Amy found she had no reason to go on. "I felt so bereft and alone and sad. . . . I was heartbroken. I couldn't work. I had a major breakdown. To me, when Luke left, it was like everybody leaving."

A pint of whiskey every day helped Amy cope with her depression. But she never kept it in her house. Instead, she made a daily trip to the liquor store, not drinking on Sunday, when it was closed—which proved to her that she didn't have a problem. Previously, Amy drank on social occasions. Now she shunned alcohol when she was with others, preferring to hide herself away with her drink. "I did it the way I would have taken heroin—all by myself."

Though Amy had a circle of friends and was in close touch with her daughters, she looked ahead and saw herself ending her life alone. Her work had been thriving, but she had always felt her deepest satisfaction in mothering someone. Now she felt less useful, less important.

The alcohol dissolved her loneliness. It also helped her avoid obsessing about her bills and her health, which worried her overwhelmingly, for no particular reason. "I was tied up with drinking, and I stopped worrying about money and about getting cancer. I also liked being unconscious and irresponsible, calling people and telling them to go to hell. It freed me up. It didn't ease my anxiety, but it moved me into a different room."

The afternoon of my visit to Amy's loft, she showed me her father's cartoons, her mother's wooden easel, and both of their faces in her paintings. I was highly aware of the prominence of the past in her imagination. Her enormous, bright parrot, which squawked from time to time, gave a figure to my thought. Thirty-six years old, he had been raised with Amy's daughters, and, said Amy, he still sometimes spoke in the voices of the girls when they were young. "It's eerie," she said. Especially because of her friend's death, voices from the past seemed to be the day's theme. Clearly, they enriched the present, giving context and meaning to each moment, but they also suggested a time that could not be recaptured. When Amy's grandson moved away, her intimate, daily care of him also belonged to the past. Ahead, with age, would come more losses: of people, health, memory, choices, status, and work.

When Older Women Drink Too Much

In older women, a drinking problem is often precipitated by the death of a spouse or friends, financial stress, depression, or illness. Among elderly women who seek treatment, there is a typical pattern: drinking first with a husband or significant other, then becoming a widow, then drinking more and more.

The number of women problem drinkers over sixty is generally thought to be quite small. In 1991, in a national survey, only about 3 percent of women aged sixty-one to seventy reported alcohol-related problems in the previous twelve months, compared with 26 percent of women aged twenty-one to thirty, 17 percent of women aged thirty-one to forty, 10 percent of women aged forty-one to fifty, and 7 percent of women aged fifty-one to sixty. Yet many experts believe that alcohol abuse by the elderly is widely underreported. At Johns Hopkins Hospital in Baltimore, doctors failed to diagnose alcohol dependence in 63 percent of the patients over sixty who met the criteria—and they missed *all* the elderly alcoholic women.

Released in June 1998, a report on substance abuse and the mature woman by the National Center on Addiction and Substance Abuse at Columbia University (CASA) declared, "By any standard of public health measurement, substance abuse and addiction has reached epidemic levels for American women over age fifty-nine," and noted that mature women are more likely to be hospitalized for ailments related to substance abuse (smoking, drinking, abuse of psychoactive prescription drugs) than for heart attacks. Smoking accounts for a high proportion of these ailments, yet CASA also found that more than 10 percent of mature women drink more than the limit of one drink per day recommended by the National Institute on Alcohol Abuse and Alcoholism. White women who were fairly affluent—with incomes of over $40,000—were particularly likely to abuse alcohol.

Even two drinks a day are a matter of concern among elderly women, because they get addicted faster, using smaller amounts, than any other group of adults. Tolerance for alcohol and prescription drugs falls with age. The two martinis a woman could handle in her forties are far over her limit at sixty-five. Also, one in four mature women is using at least one psychoactive drug—often inappropriately prescribed.

Amy is one of the lucky ones. Her daughters were alert to her drinking. Instead of rationalizing that their mother should be allowed to drink because she was lonely and had few pleasures—a common attitude that can condemn older women to ill health and early death—they persuaded her to get treatment. More often than not, a mature woman's addiction is swept under the rug by her physician, family, and friends. Relatives may notice symptoms—depression, memory loss, accidents, stomach trouble, and difficulty sleeping—but, according to CASA, they can't believe their grandmother or aunt is abusing alcohol or prescription drugs.

Echoes of an Early Loss

Amy's loss brought back painful early memories, but she did not refer to them until I asked detailed questions about her paintings. Her paintings now are often very large, oil on wood; but when she started fifteen years ago, she said, she did watercolors of little, empty, box-sized rooms, and eventually some people appeared in these rooms. They reminded her of the dollhouse that was her salvation when she was a small child. "It was a humdinger of a dollhouse," she said. "My mother made it. It had lights and running water. I played out my life in it."

Amy created an unusual floor plan. The dining room became a hospital waiting room, with tiny magazines, and the kitchen became an operating room—not surprisingly, perhaps, when you know that she had been hospitalized for a year at the age of five after suffering a burst appendix, before this modern age of drugs. At that time, there were rigid rules, restricting even parental visits. In addition, Amy's mother was terrified of pain and hospitals. During her year in the hospital, the five-year-old girl never once saw her parents.

It is hard to grasp the ramifications of such a separation. Dr. Sylvia Staub, a clinical psychologist in private practice in Cambridge, Massachusetts, says, "It's a profound and complete disconnection. Your parents are the people who reflect back to you who you are, that you exist and are worthwhile, that you are loved and lovable. When a child loses the parents on whom she depends for her very existence, it always feels like rejection and abandonment. She internalizes this and comes to feel there is something wrong with her, something bad, that caused her parents to leave her."

A child who experiences such a separation, who is not certain that she will see her parents again, is likely to become anxious. Her early, primitive terror of being alone and helpless in the world is likely to color her future attachments, making her particularly vulnerable to losses in adulthood. "There's a kind of echo chamber," says Sylvia Staub. "New losses set off echoes of previous losses. It's not necessarily conscious—we may not say, 'I'm feeling the way I did when I was five'—

but deep inside, in that echo chamber, there are resonances of the child-hood trauma that intensify our reaction to a current loss." Studies of the physiological response to loss of parents in childhood also suggest that basic mood-regulating mechanisms may be permanently altered.

Since children who suffer early loss are at higher risk of many problems, it isn't surprising that they are also more prone to alco-holism. Nonetheless, said Sharon Wilsnack, she was startled to dis-cover the strength of the correlation between early separation from a parent and problem drinking among women. As we have noted, Sharon and Richard Wilsnack followed the drinking habits of 696 representa-tive American women over a ten-year period. They found that women who had been separated from either parent before the age of six were five times more likely than other women to develop a drinking prob-lem, or to have an existing problem get worse.

When Luke left with his parents, Amy was hit at once with all the losses of her life. "It was like everybody leaving," she had said. Liv-ing in a heavy cloud of depression, she felt unloved and unwanted. Her anxieties about her health escalated—not surprisingly, since ill health had led to that first, most shattering separation. Ironically, the daily pint of whiskey that eased her mind was putting her health at risk.

Letting Go of Grief

Late-onset drinking can devastate lives, but thankfully, it is often quite responsive to treatment. This was certainly the case for Amy, who opened herself up to the healing power of the group of people in her inpatient treatment. As reported in Chapter 4, she said to me in awestruck tones, "I don't know why I was cured. There's a sense of mys-tery about it."

"Mind you," she added, "I'd already had ten years of Freudian analysis in early adulthood, and I did take care of a great deal of what was troubling me in my life before I went to Betty Ford."

Today some psychologists believe that the earlier mode of analy-sis—in which the analyst remained very neutral, very reserved—

retraumatized patients who were suffering from childhood disconnections. Amy's analysis had not protected her from being overwhelmed by feelings of abandonment, or from turning to alcohol for solace, but it had allowed her to let go of many problems, and it may have laid the groundwork for her healing experience at Betty Ford. There, among many struggling people and their families, in an atmosphere of acceptance and honesty, she felt a profound sense of connectedness. The image of herself as lost and abandoned dissolved as she experienced the reality of what she shared with other people.

The transcendent quality of this experience has changed Amy's life. Much of her anxiety has dropped away, and she no longer frets about her health. She still feels lonely at times, and the past may preside in her imagination, but she now experiences joy at least as frequently as pain, and she has no impulse to wash the pain away with drink.

Other women, too, speak of their recovery from alcohol as an opportunity to shed a grief that has dogged them through life.

Jill is working hard to grow beyond the legacy of her father's violence, her mother's abandonment of her, her "second mother's" suicide, her father's early death. After a relapse, she decided to get therapy: "I had to admit I needed more help. I was hanging on to hurts in ways I wasn't aware of." As her hidden fears come into her awareness, they have less power over her. Gradually, she is freeing herself from the grief, anger, and fear that have dominated her emotional life. Recently, she sent me an e-mail describing how she and a friend in AA—an older woman whom she thinks of as her "third mother"—enacted a ritual to help her let go of the past.

"I went to San Diego," the note began, "and finally put closure on my past." Before she left, she wrote letters to all the people she had loved and lost, describing her feelings, including her guilt, and exploring her own role in the sadness of her life. As her friend Nell watched, she placed the letters and some poems in a burlap bag and tied a rose to it. The two women walked to the cliffs not far from Nell's house. "I threw the bag, and together we watched it as it landed in the Pacific Ocean, and it got carried away. Eventually, we no longer saw the bag or the rose any longer. . . . The feeling of peace that I found as I walked away that morning was something I have no words to describe."

Eleven days later marked the tenth anniversary of Jill's mother's death. "This year I looked upon it in calm," wrote Jill, "with fond memories of my mother for the first time ever." She returned home "without the heavy burdens of things that are long gone," and she is enjoying her new freedom. She ended her letter on a note of quiet confidence: "More things will come my way when the time is right."

Though no one would recommend loss or addiction as a path toward spiritual fulfillment, many women have learned and grown from these struggles.

While telling me her story, Dale stopped talking when she got to the part where her husband announced that he was leaving. "This is different from telling my story in AA," she said quietly. "I'm feeling as sad now as I felt then. . . . But I don't regret anything. Everything that's happened in my life has led to where I am now. I'm in a good place."

Looking back, she saw how she had carried her childhood hunger into her marriage and relied on her husband to fill her up. "He was overwhelmed by my need for affirmation, direction, and stability. I was brainy, but I had no self-awareness. Inside, I felt blank. Not depressed, just blank."

As Dale described it, her new life was not as miraculous as Amy's. There were no sudden changes, and now, in her new marriage, she and her husband struggle with children who have problems with drugs. Yet, through hard work in AA, Al-Anon, and therapy, she has let go of old hurts and gained an inner freedom that she treasures. "I don't need to rely on one particular person anymore," she said. "I have enough inside myself." Importantly, Dale's "having enough" is not utter self-reliance. She also relies on her husband; on "good supportive friends" both in and outside AA; and her sponsor, whom she meets every Monday for lunch. "I'm still learning how to mind my own business and stop trying to control other people," she said. "I'm pretty well convinced that if everyone would do what I want, the world would be a better place!"

Coming to terms with her mother (her father is dead) isn't easy. Her mother still likes to taunt her daughters, both of whom recently received a telegram from out of the blue, which read: "Changing my will—Going to live it up—Guess who."

"When I see my mother," said Dale, "it's bizarre to think that I grew inside of her. I don't have any sense of connection to her at all except blood. She's let me down many, many times—not out of hostility, but just because that's all she knows. I have made the decision to call her once or twice a month and chat about inconsequential things—what the kids are doing, trips, recipes—because that's the level at which I can safely talk, and I don't have a need to go deeper. It would be a losing proposition. But I wouldn't want her to die in one of those periods where she wasn't communicating. I want to keep in touch, and I'm healthy enough to do that."

Where Dale can do more, she does. Four years ago, her ex-husband's mother had a stroke, and Dale helped nurse her during her convalescence. "People were flabbergasted that I would do this, because I hadn't been her daughter-in-law for ten years. But I had a fine relationship with her. She taught me to be a mom, and she really nurtured me. I was very lucky.

"It was my turn to help her, just as it's my turn to nurture my twenty-seven-year-old stepdaughter. Now I have money, and I can counsel. I have a great sense of the continuity of things." The child who never fit in has learned that she belongs to the circle of life.

9

Stealing Courage
from a Turtle's Heart:
Sexually Abused Women
Fighting Alcohol

"START ANYWHERE YOU LIKE," I SAID TO LINDSEY, A
mature-looking eighteen-year-old with pretty dark eyes and curled
eyelashes, brushed with mascara. At our second meeting, she would be
visibly more relaxed, tucking her legs beneath her and sipping a mug
of tea, but during this first conversation she held herself to attention.

"I have two brothers and two sisters," she began, "and my family
was always hanging on by the skin of our teeth. My dad was in and out
of work, and my mom ran the farm—we had a cow, calves, and a pig
for meat; chickens for eggs; and a huge garden. We did everything for
ourselves."

Lindsey's high school teacher, a friend of mine, had described her
as strong and gutsy, bright but underachieving, a girl who'd drunk her
way through her teenage years until she decided to get sober. She and
Lindsey became close, and that is why Lindsey agreed to talk to me. I
sensed now that she didn't want to be interrupted. There was pride in
her voice, even when she told me about getting forced out of her family's farmhouse when it was quarantined by the state because the owner
wouldn't fix it up. She made it clear that she didn't want pity.

"My father wanted to be a writer, and in his spare time he would write and otherwise fill in at a factory or do carpentry and mow lawns, anything he could find. My mother skipped meals so the kids could have enough food. She was always counting pennies, and that taught me how to save. The kids down the street had millions of toys, and they would go outside and break them. We might get one or two toys at Christmas, but we knew our parents had cut out something else to give us those toys, and we appreciated them.

"We grew up in an atmosphere of love and respect. My parents respected us and we respected them. Instead of punishing us when we did something wrong, they talked to us about their values. They taught us to take responsibility."

Perhaps this idealized family picture should have alerted me, but I was unprepared for what came next.

In the same deliberate voice, Lindsey continued, "When I was in ninth grade, my sisters and I turned my father in for sexually molesting us."

EARLY TRAUMA: STUDIES MAKE THE LINK

THIS WAS my first experience of what were to become familiar dynamics in my interviews with women about the place of alcohol in their lives. Somewhere along the line, they would drop information like a bomb, and everything they'd said up to that point would have to be looked at in a different light. This was most true of the younger women and those newest to sobriety, who were struggling to make sense of their personal stories. There's a saying in AA: "You're as sick as your secrets." These women were trying to dredge up their secrets without drowning in the pain. They needed to look calmly at their guilt, their shame, their sorrow and loss, and to integrate their experience into a larger narrative, which, if it didn't exactly redeem them, still offered them a future different from their past. Those who had come further told stories that seemed more continuous. They were conscious of building new lives—often full of ordinary joys—on the ground of the misery they'd lived through and helped to create.

Many women spoke of early experiences of violence, abuse, abandonment, and loss. I expected to hear such things—dysfunction may well be the norm for family life—but the degree of hardship they described was startling. It would be misleading and reductive to suggest that such trauma *causes* alcoholism. Of course, many women who suffer childhood trauma do *not* become problem drinkers. But studies have consistently shown that a disrupted early family life—a death, a divorce, a parent's absence or psychiatric illness—is a common experience among those who later develop problems with alcohol, and women report such experiences more frequently than men. Some researchers do posit that trauma precipitates women's problem drinking, but others, including Edith Gomberg, point out that among women who report similar painful early life events, the problem drinkers are more likely to respond negatively, and to view their childhoods as unhappy and lacking in love. These women may, for reasons of temperament and circumstance, have less capacity to cope with major stress.

In the case of sexual abuse, the trauma seems to be so overwhelming that even resilient children can suffer such long-term consequences as anxiety, depression, poor self-esteem, difficulty trusting others, emotional reactivity, and rapid shifts in mental and physical abilities, as well as addictive disorders. Primarily, girls are affected. Not only are they three to four times more likely to be sexually abused, but the abuse is typically longer in duration, and the perpetrator is more often a parent, so that they have no safe retreat.

In the late 1980s and early 1990s, when researchers began trying to quantify how sexual abuse is implicated in women's alcohol problems, the numbers were startling. Studies of women in substance abuse treatment centers found that up to 75 percent reported a history of physical or sexual abuse. In a study reported in 1993, data were collected from in-depth interviews of forty-seven women between the ages of eighteen and forty-five. Forty-five percent of women seeking treatment for alcohol-related problems said they had been sexually and physically abused by their parents in childhood, compared with 11 percent of first-time drinking and driving offenders, and 14 percent of women in randomly selected households. Even compared with female psychiatric patients who were not abused, women who were sexually abused in childhood have higher rates of alcohol and drug abuse; this suggests an actual association between childhood victimization and problems with alcohol—not simply a greater tendency by abused women to seek help. There is greater long-term harm when abuse occurs before puberty, and when it involves vaginal penetration. Childhood rape doubles the number of alcoholic symptoms in women.

Some of these studies have been criticized for using too small a sample or for being poorly designed, and indeed, this kind of research presents many challenges. First, definitions of abuse and alcohol-related problems must be very specific. Findings vary broadly depending on the researchers' definitions and the methods they use to collect data. For instance, if women are asked a broad question about whether they were "abused" before a certain age, they are more likely to say no than if they are asked a list of questions about specific sexual interactions. When definitions vary, it is difficult to compare results among studies.

Second, most of these studies focus on women in treatment, and it's not clear if these women are representative. A theory called Berkson's selection bias suggests that people with multiple problems—whether related to abuse or alcohol—are more likely to seek treatment than people with only one problem. It's possible, then, that studies of women in treatment overestimate the association between sexual abuse and alcohol-related problems. Only 14 percent of alcoholic women get treatment. Do the 86 percent of women who don't get treatment have similar histories of sexual abuse? And what of women with a drinking problem who aren't necessarily addicted? Does sexual abuse also play a role in their drinking?

Finally, most studies rely on retrospective reports of abuse, and it is possible that some alcoholic women, in great distress, are straining to find an explanation for their problems. Would they have identified themselves as victims of abuse *before* they started drinking? Also, not only may alcoholic or psychiatric patients be more apt to report sexual or physical abuse; the control groups may include "false negatives"— that is, women who are in denial about abuse. This too would distort the comparison. (There are not enough data to confirm a link between childhood abuse and alcohol problems in men, because no studies of males in treatment have compared them with control groups of males without alcohol problems.)

Some recent longitudinal studies have found ways to minimize the bias of retrospective reports and a focus on women in treatment. In Norway, a population sample of adolescents was followed over six years; 17 percent of the girls, but only 1 percent of the boys, reported having been sexually assaulted at some time. Researchers gathered data five times. They found that the female victims reported a dramatic increase in alcohol-related problems by the time of their late teens.

In May 1997, Sharon and Richard Wilsnack published the results of a landmark study of the general population, the largest one of its kind, in which they conducted ninety-minute personal interviews of a nationally representative sample of nearly 1,100 women, including 354 who had been followed since 1981. They asked questions to ascertain the women's level of drinking and the number of ensuing problems. Instead of asking a general question about sexual abuse, they asked about specific sexual activities, including exposure of the woman's own genitals, exhibitionism (by the perpetrator), touching or fondling, sexual kissing, oral-genital activity, anal intercourse, and vaginal intercourse. These activities did not count as abuse unless they occurred before age thirteen with a family member who was five or more years older, or before eighteen and were unwanted, also with a perpetrator five or more years older.

When they analyzed the data, the Wilsnacks found that controlling for age, childhood sexual abuse predicted the onset of problem drinking over a five-year follow-up period: 51 percent of the women who were not problem drinkers in 1981, but who reported sexual abuse, had *become* problem drinkers five years later, compared with 19 percent of those who had not been abused. Women abused in childhood were three times more likely to report such symptoms as blackouts and the inability to control themselves while drinking, and were more than twice as likely to report drinking-related problems in the last year. Some 50 percent of the women who had alcohol problems reported sexual abuse in their childhood. Says Sharon Wilsnack, "When you find the same thing in treatment centers and in the general population, you know you're on to something real."

Wilsnack said that in this study, "Childhood sexual abuse is the single strongest predictor of alcohol dependency in women, even stronger than a family history of drinking."

LINDSEY'S STORY

SOME OF LINDSEY'S fondest memories are of fixing up their family farmhouse in Vermont with her father, Mark. "I'd run home from school, drop my book bag, change my clothes, and go outside to work with him," she recalled. "Whenever he had a project, I was beside him, and he taught me everything—electrical wiring, plumbing, Sheetrock. It was fun working together.

"We talked about everything under the sun. For breaks, I'd sit beside him and tell him everything I'd learned in school. He was always so understanding.

"Then as soon as the sun set, he was the abuser. He would sneak into my room and touch me. . . . My mother worked nights at a center for the elderly, and my father always said he had the nights to himself. When he came into my room, I didn't remember the day or how nice it had been. The next morning, when he looked at me as if nothing had happened, I blocked out the abuser. I saw my father as two different people."

She whispered, "I loved my dad so much. I didn't want him to go away."

I had the impression that Lindsey was referring not to a literal abandonment, but to a fear that she would no longer be able to connect to the loving part of her father if she allowed herself to see the whole truth. Seeing her father as "two different people" enabled her to compartmentalize her perceptions, switching from one perspective to the other without ever putting the two together. Lindsey defended her "good father" by keeping the "bad" one in another part of her mind. She also wrapped up her anger and kept it in a separate box, afraid it would demolish the father she desperately needed.

This kind of "splitting" is thought to be universal in early childhood. In *Necessary Losses*, Judith Viorst explains, "In our immature state we cannot hold in our head the strange notion that those who are good can sometimes also be bad. And so our inner images—of mother and of self—are split in two." At age two or three, we may typically see a parent as two people—one is an all-nurturing mommy or daddy, and the other is all-frustrating. Our image of ourselves is also divided: there's a lovable self and a rotten one. Gradually we learn to mend these splits, to understand that the loving mother who soothes us and the hateful mother who goes away are really one mother, toward whom we have both positive and negative feelings. We also unite the good girl and the bad one in a single image of the self. Viorst writes, "Instead of parts of people we begin to see the whole—the merely but magnificently human. And we come to know a self in which feelings of hate can intermingle with feelings of love."

The task of uniting these inner images is never complete. As we continue to develop, our images of self and other become increasingly complex. From time to time, most of us slip back into black-and-white thinking, and some adults continue to vacillate between grandiosity and self-hatred, between idealizing and demonizing their loved ones.

In Lindsey's case, her father's abuse forced her back into a primitive kind of perception. It was intolerable to her that the man she needed so badly and loved so much could be the same one who caused her so much pain. In many ways, it is astonishing that today she can talk about this process and grasp it so well—astonishing because, as she revealed to me later, she cannot remember a time when her father did not fondle her genitals. In his court-ordered therapy, he confessed that it began when she was still in diapers. If a nonabusive father can seem like a monster to a child, imagine the monstrous proportions of the abusive father in the child's mind, and how hard it would be to reconcile this figure with the father who nourishes.

"You can't overestimate how important it is for a child to have a good view of her parents," says Rita Teusch, Ph.D., a psychologist who works with sexually abused women in therapy in Cambridge and Wellesley, Massachusetts, and has written on the connection between sexual abuse and chemical dependency. "She will see them as good at all costs, even if the cost is distorting reality.

"To hold your daddy in your mind as good and bad both, you have to have a reasonably safe childhood. You have to be able to think, 'Well, he's sometimes good and sometimes bad, but I can tolerate both.' When there's abuse going on, the child can't tolerate it. The experience gets split off, denied, dissociated."

Dissociation is commonly used as a coping strategy among girls who are abused. In its mildest form, familiar to us all, it simply means doing one thing while thinking about something else. Dissociation may also involve feeling detached from one's own mind and body—many girls describe a sensation of hovering over the scene of their own abuse. While the body is being punished for being bad, the mind is "good" and safe and far away. In this sense, dissociation and splitting are related. In daily life, dissociation allows a victim to confine her awareness of the abuse to a realm outside her normal perceptions. So that she does not have to contend with overwhelming anxiety, fear, and anger, the traumatic events are split off. These events don't figure in the story she tells herself about her life. When the trauma is happening, or when it is recalled, she may enter an altered state of consciousness, like a trance, in which she is less susceptible to pain. A more extreme form of dissociation occurs in dissociative identity disorder, where self and memory are broken into fragments.

Dissociation allowed Lindsey to have breakfast with her father in the morning as if nothing had happened the night before. It allowed her to rush home from school, drop her book bag, change her clothes, and run out to work with him. It allowed her to view her mother as a self-sacrificing saint, and never to blame her for being weak or for failing to protect her daughters.

"Our father wasn't affectionate with our mother," Lindsey told me. "She would cry." Lindsey believed she must sacrifice herself for her mother's sake. "I thought, if I do this with my father, maybe it will help my mom."

Keyed into Lindsey's psychology, her father told her, "If you don't love me, then I can't love your mother. Mommy needs love. If I give it to you, then I can give it to her."

Sitting on my sofa, Lindsey blew her nose and looked around for a wastebasket. "He didn't need to threaten violence," she said.

Lindsey tried to protect herself in practical ways. She learned to take a three-minute shower, including the time it took to shave her legs and dry herself off, so she was out of the bathroom before he could invite himself in. Finding safety in numbers, she became best friends with her little sister Heidi, stayed with her whenever she could, and shared a bedroom with her. "He wouldn't touch you if you were with someone else," she explained. Still, he found other ways. He'd invite her to his band practice, for instance, and pull off the road on the way home. Her constant anxiety about when he might approach her was nearly as traumatic as the episodes themselves.

By the time she was in ninth grade, she was conscious that her father's actions were abusive.

I asked her how she got from the state of mind in which she submitted to his fondling for her mother's sake to the point at which she said to herself, "This is wrong."

"I think it was just hormonal changes," she told me. "I was attracted to boys—instead of to my father—and that made me think differently."

Indeed, says Dr. Teusch, many girls who have blocked out memories of early abuse remember it when adolescence hits, and their hormones are going haywire. Also, adolescence brings a whole new level of comprehension. Teenagers know which rules are universal. They know the difference between, as the developmental psychologist David Elkind describes it, "rules that hold for the one and rules that hold for the many." Specifically, though Lindsey had once believed her father when he said, "People will laugh at you if you complain about what I'm doing, because *all* daddies do this with their daughters," she now came to know that he was breaking a taboo.

"I stood up to him," she told me. "I was taking a bath, and he came in and said, 'Let me look at you.' When I said no, he said, 'I promise I won't touch.' I said, 'What's your problem? You have a wife you're supposed to do that with. Get out of here or I'll tell.'"

She said proudly, "This was two whole months before my mother found out he was molesting us, but after this incident, he never attempted it with me again."

As it happened, Lindsey's older sister Emily was reaching her own limit at just about the same time. One morning at breakfast, in the presence of her mother, she asked him for a ride to her boyfriend's house, and he said no. She nearly spat at him, and he said, "What's wrong? Why are you so pissed at me?"

"I have a good reason to be pissed at you," she snarled, and stormed up to her bedroom.

Something cued her mother in. She followed Emily to her room and said, "Has he been touching you?" Emily began to moan. She hugged herself and fell to the floor.

Her screaming woke Lindsey up. When Lindsey ran into Emily's bedroom, her mother turned to her, white-faced. "Has he been touching you, too?" she asked.

Lindsey couldn't find a voice, but the tears streaming from her eyes were answer enough.

For two intolerable months they continued to live as a family, on the condition that Lindsey's father, Mark, didn't touch the girls again. When Lindsey's mother broke down at work, a colleague persuaded her to turn in her husband. She and her daughters went to the authorities. There was a trial, and the judge sentenced Mark to fifteen months in jail.

When he left, Lindsey felt "a thousand times lighter. I could take a shower without worrying; I could be alone without fear." At the same time, she told me, she felt tremendously sad.

"What was the sadness?" I asked softly.

Lindsey's eyes filled up with tears. I thought about the loss of her childhood, her guilty feelings about her father, her family in pieces, but Lindsey was not thinking of herself.

"It upset my mom," she whispered. "She was living with this turmoil inside."

The Aftermath

Lindsey is early in the process of coming to terms with her abuse and still needs to protect herself from the force of her experience. She is able to talk with understanding, but emotionally, it needs time to sink in. She's apt to deliver contradictory statements about her parents without seeing any problem. At one moment in our interview, she described her father as inspiring and two sentences later commented on his selfishness, saying that while her mother was skipping meals so the children could eat, her father was "buying candy for himself and hiding it in his room." He was, she said, "overall not abusive," but then she noted that he had "a flaring temper" and "if something went wrong he might throw a hammer across the room." But typically, she said, "no one would get hurt."

Her mother, her "most important teacher," taught her that "you have to love yourself before you can love other people"—this being the same mother who cried for years because her husband didn't love her and put up with hammers being hurled. Lindsey described her mother as consistently overwhelmed, then called her "a very strong person." Still unconscious of any anger toward her mother, still protecting her, Lindsey needs to see her mother as a wonderful parent.

Most painfully, Lindsey expressed the split in her own frame of mind, at one moment describing herself as "feeling better—myself again," and at another saying, "I can't concentrate on anything because I'm so unhappy." She works hard to keep any guilt and anger invisible to herself. She wants to be loving and giving, and indeed, by the end of our second meeting, when she gave me a warm hug, I was under her spell. I remembered that my friend, Lindsey's teacher, had told me that boys fall all over her, not because she is seductive, but because "she's warm and cuddly, and they want to lay their heads on her chest and cry." Lindsey's voice grew affectionate when she talked about "looking out for her mother," who gets lonely and needs more social life.

Lindsey, like many survivors of incest, grew up taking care of her parents' emotional needs. In a way, this made her feel powerful and special. She may have imagined that she could appease them with her care and make them feel so loved that they would become capable of taking care of her. To maintain her sympathy for them, she focuses on their suffering. Not surprisingly—abuse is often an intergenerational problem—Lindsey's mother was also abused as a child. Her father's father despised him, and his mother was schizophrenic.

Her role as caretaker has, of course, been severely challenged, but she's doing her best to maintain it. When her father—whom she took to calling "Mark" when his abuse was uncovered—was sentenced to fifteen months in jail, she said, "Everybody else was pissed off that it wasn't longer, but I didn't really care. I'm not the kind of person to hold grudges." Her mother was upset after learning about the abuse because "she thought we blamed her because she didn't notice it earlier"; but "we never felt anything bad toward her. It wasn't her fault."

Lindsey's anger flares up when the stakes are not so high. Her tone changed to genuine scorn when, in our first talk, I asked how she was doing in her freshman year at college. "I hate this college," she said. "I don't like it—my work has shown that. I don't like my professors. The rooms are like prison rooms. . . . I'm not coming back for sure, no way." She also got angry with her older sister, noting, "She hates Mark now, but she always wanted her own room, and I wonder if perhaps she wanted the extra attention." Apparently, the girls found it safer to express their anger at each other than at their father. Lindsey noted that when they were younger they were "vicious." "We pulled each other's hair, and Emily scratched me till I bled." Now, they enjoy a closer relationship.

In our conversation, Lindsey saved her most intense rage for the counselors who worked with her after her father's arrest. "I hated my first counselor, so—stupid them—they put me in group counseling with my sister Emily! I couldn't say a word because she'd use anything I said against me, and everything I said she contradicted. So I said, I'm not doing counseling, I hate it. Fuck it! I can get through this by myself. They were drilling stuff into my head that I didn't feel was true or right, and that pissed me off. They were telling me things about myself that weren't true, and I said, 'Why are you filling my head with this shit?'"

I asked Lindsey what they were telling her.

"That I should be angry and upset!" she answered. "That I should not want anything to do with my dad, and I wanted to see him again and be friends with him. They tried to tell me that that's not what I wanted, and I was like, no, I'm not that angry person, you're not going to tell me who I am. I was really peeved. They kept telling me that it wasn't my fault, and I'm like, I know that."

I was especially struck by the formulation, "I'm not that angry person; you're not going to tell me who I am." To Lindsey, love and anger were not just feelings common to all of us; they were the basis for two incompatible identities. There were people who love, and there were people who hate and are angry. With her maternal air and solicitous manner, her dream of working with children and handicapped people, Lindsey intended to be someone who loves.

Lindsey did like the counselor at her high school, who was more sensitive and took a comforting but neutral stance. She did not try to force Lindsey into territory she wasn't ready to navigate. But Lindsey was not ready to depend on anyone else. Their meetings were only sporadic, and Lindsey did not confide in this counselor when her life went from bad to worse.

In tenth grade, with her father in jail and her mother divorced, remarried within days, and divorced again, Lindsey began her first experiments with alcohol. She was in a school play, and before the cast party, she and a friend drank five shots of rum. "Whoa," she thought, "this is nothing—like drinking a cup of water." At the party she got sick, and a friend had to drive her home.

Lindsey was not particularly young by national standards—in the Monitoring the Future survey, 40 percent of tenth-graders reported drinking within the previous month. There was no heavy drinking in her nuclear or extended family, so presumably she wasn't genetically predisposed to alcohol dependence. At first, Lindsey was cautious about drinking too much, not for her own sake, but because she wanted to be sober if anything happened to her friends. "I was with a wild crowd," she explained. "I was worried about alcohol poisoning, or someone falling into the river. . . . One night a friend broke his ankle, and another night someone passed out in the snow and came in blue-lipped and pretty much in hypothermia. I was sober enough to take care of them."

Girls who are sexually molested are significantly more likely to have early consensual sexual intercourse. By the age of fifteen, if Lindsey liked a boy, she slept with him. "It was drilled into my head for so long that sex is a must for someone to love you, and so I was always really free about sex—always, always, always. I thought, That's what he wants, that's what will make him happy." During her junior year, she hooked up with a steady boyfriend, Freddie. "I had this hollowness from Mark being gone," she said. "Freddie filled the spot." He was a big drinker, and over time she began to keep pace with him, often staying drunk from Friday afternoon until Sunday night. She took care of him as if he were a child: making him breakfast, doing his laundry, and cleaning up after him when, drunk out of his mind, he vomited and peed all over himself.

Lindsey's behavior, says Dr. Teusch, probably had several unconscious motivations. Tending to Freddie and that whole gang of boys—"I was like a mother to them," said Lindsey—she became the caretaker and protector that her own mother wasn't, allowing her to be less

helpless than she was as a young child. The sex and the caretaking
could also be unconscious ways of trying to appease an abuser. If you
give a boy what he wants, perhaps he will not hurt you. Also, Lindsey
might have been trying to assuage the guilt she would naturally feel as
the result of her father's imprisonment. "I knew it wasn't my fault,"
Lindsey maintained at first, but later she said, "In some ways I feel
guilty for letting the abuse happen. . . . I didn't say anything right
away."

I said, "Right. When you were in diapers, you didn't say anything."

She replied, "That's so true, but it doesn't click in my head."

In spite of all her efforts, Freddie eventually left Lindsey for his
first love, and she fell apart completely. It's not that she loved him so
much—"We were just used to each other," she said—but her feeling of
helplessness redoubled. Neither sex nor her fanatical attention to her
boyfriend had kept her in control. Panicky and desperate, unable to
cope with her life, she started stealing brandy from her mother. When
that ran out—her mother never noticed—she got a friend to bring her
more. She hid it under her bed so she could take a few chugs in the
morning. She kept another bottle in her locker at school. At the end of
the day, she and her buddies, "my guy friends," as she still calls them,
would go out "and drink and drink and drink till we were passed out
all over the place." At times, she stayed home from school and took a
bottle to bed with her.

When she drank, Lindsey said, "It was like I was in a bubble.
Nothing could touch me. Nothing could harm me." When there was
no alcohol to be found, "I'd be like, AAAh!" said Lindsey, mimicking a
scream. At these times, she turned on herself. With a dull knife, she
would saw at her arm "until it was just like shredded." She had done
this once before, just after her father left their home, during that time
when she was "a thousand times lighter . . . and tremendously sad."
The cuts were always shallow; she never went to the emergency room,
and she never told anyone. She cared for her own wounds and wore long
sleeves throughout the summer to hide the scabbing. The cutting gave

her a feeling of being high, and it eased her tension. The physical pain covered over the far worse pain of her anger and fear.

It is estimated that close to 2 million Americans injure themselves by such means as cutting, burning, bone-breaking, and rubbing glass into the skin. In an essay in the *New York Times Magazine*, Jennifer Egan describes the typical profile of a self-injurer, and it fits Lindsey. She is likely to be white and female and to have been sexually abused. She probably suffers from other compulsive disorders, like alcoholism, has a powerful need to be in control, and may be driven by a "mix of toughness and a hypervigilant desire to please." Terrified of expressing rage and sadness for fear of chasing people away, she turns her feelings on herself. "In a sense," writes Egan, "self-injury becomes a perverse ritual of self-caretaking in which the injurer assumes all roles of an abusive relationship: the abuser, the victim and the comforting presence who soothes her afterward." By enacting a drama in which she played all the parts, Lindsey tried to gain control.

Although the typical self-injurer is likely to continue into her late twenties, often with increasing severity, for Lindsey, "it seemed like it just stopped." Alcohol remained her favorite release, and her favorite way to punish herself. Consuming little but alcohol, she lost twenty pounds in a month and found herself contemplating suicide. She was stumbling on the ugly truth about alcohol: though it may "work" at first to lighten your mood and ease your pain, it stops working after a while. You have to drink more, and then more again, to achieve the same high. You go on chasing elusive feelings, though they seem to get farther from view. Meanwhile, you suffer the hangovers, illness, alienation from yourself and your loved ones. The pain you were seeking to escape intensifies. But you go on drinking, because by now you have to drink—your body craves it, your hands tremble in the morning, and you feel like jumping out of your skin until you do. In Lindsey's pithy words: "Alcohol knocked everything out, but in the long run, it kicked my ass."

Lindsey never had treatment for her alcohol dependence. At some point, it dawned on her that drinking made her feel worse, and she was able to cut back. She began to feel moderately better, and then a little better than that. She started eating again and catching up at school.

When I first spoke with Lindsey, during the spring of her freshman year in college, I was under the impression that she was committed to staying sober, but it soon became clear that she is not out of the woods. Indeed, she hasn't fully acknowledged that she has a problem with alcohol. I had to put this together from contradictory bits of information she revealed to me—at one point referring to her recovery when she was a senior in high school, and later describing the summer that followed, when she moved in with her gang of "guy friends" and got drunk every night, even experimenting with LSD and mescaline. But now, she said, she wasn't into the drug scene and never had more than one or two beers. When I asked, she said she never worried about drinking.

The summer passed. We met again in the fall, and Lindsey said she had decided to take a year off from college to work and think about her goals. More open with me now—and perhaps with herself—she acknowledged that her attitude toward drinking was inconsistent. One day, she said, she'll be on the wagon, and the next she'll ask her mother to get her a six-pack, because she needs to relax. She'd gotten drunk with her new boyfriend the night before. It's not uncommon for her to down five shots of hard liquor. She got a little worried, she said, when she realized that over the summer, hardly a day went by when she didn't have a beer at lunch and another at dinner.

Lindsey's evasiveness alternates with piercing honesty—a pattern familiar to many alcoholics and their families. It sometimes seems that the honesty is a cunning way for the drinker to convince herself and others that she's got a handle on the situation. In the meantime, she goes home and has another drink. Denial is far more complicated than an outright refusal to acknowledge a drinking problem.

The way Lindsey revealed her struggles with alcohol reminded me of the way she revealed the abuse: contradictions, a combination of openness and secretiveness, emotional distance with dips into real feeling. For her, denial is not something that developed with dependence on alcohol; it is part of the mental world she constructed when she had to pretend that she had a loving, respectful father.

There are parts of that story she still can't say out loud. She first led me to believe that her father's abuse had stopped with fondling her genitals, but she must have wanted to correct that impression, because she sent me a poem in the mail, called "What a Great Daddy." It describes her father putting his fingers inside her. When she complains that it hurts, he kisses her "down there"—to make her feel better, she decides, the way he kisses the scrapes on her elbows and knees. The next visit, he slides his penis in. She cries. He gets off, hugs her, and says he's sorry. She feels blessed to have such a wonderful daddy, who's "always thinking of others." Lindsey told me that she sent this poem to her father to let him know how much he'd hurt her.

Denial is still protecting Lindsey from the full horror of her childhood, which is connected to her use of alcohol; thus denial of her drinking problem is another loop in an already complicated system of defense. Says Dr. Teusch, "The feeling that you are actually out of control, as an alcoholic really is, is intolerable to abuse survivors. It complicates the recovery. They have a real reason to fear being out of control." She adds that, even more than other alcoholics, survivors of abuse need to believe that they can cut back and can take care of any problems on their own.

Lindsey communicates fierce independence. When I saw that she was struggling, I tried to think of ways to broach the subject. I went so far as to get the names of some therapists who had worked successfully with girls who have alcohol problems and were sexually abused, hoping I'd be able to say, "Look, if you do want help . . ." I'm still hoping for that moment, but so far, Lindsey has made it clear that she doesn't want suggestions. She was telling me how hard sex is for her, how as a child she trained herself not to feel any pleasure, and now she has to fight her own repulsion to have an orgasm. She described some difficult sex to me. She had suddenly got frightened, had yelled at her boyfriend, and had curled up into a little ball "to deal with it on my own." I commented, "You're so *much* on your own." She answered,

"If I'm going to do something, I'm going to do it on my own, and I don't want any help." To illustrate her point, she told me about getting a fever of 105 and hallucinating, but refusing to go to the hospital and refusing medication. She was determined to get better by herself.

This anecdote points up a paradox: Lindsey's need to be entirely self-sufficient undermines her ability to take care of herself. Until she learns to rely on other people, she'll have a hard time relying on herself, and she'll be vulnerable to self-destructive impulses. To ask for help, she'll have to make two leaps—believing that someone can help, and believing that she deserves help.

She has several things going for her. Cognitively, she understands her history, and she can talk about it. That, says Rita Teusch, is the big first step. It always takes time to integrate knowledge. And then, she's taking certain healthy steps. She's made a rule that she won't have sex unless she really wants it. Instead of going out with friends every night, she finds herself "becoming quieter and more self-oriented"—because, she says, "it's something my body is asking for." When she and I went to lunch, she wanted to talk about an *Oprah* show in which a guest claimed that when women lose themselves in caring for their families, their bodies grow fat as a way of saying, "Pay some attention to me." Lindsey is learning that she needs to pay attention to her own needs— her needs, not her boyfriend's. Not her mother's. Not her father's.

And then, there's the warmth and concern she has for others. Though it still has a desperate edge, it will be there for her to return to, if—as I trust she will—she dares to walk through the mess of her rage and shame into a place of greater freedom.

Why Do Sexually Abused Women So Often Turn to Drink?

First of all, many don't. In the Wilsnacks' survey, 24 percent of abused women in the general population developed alcohol-related problems. Note that this is different from the percentage of alcoholic women who were sexually abused—that figure is at least 50 percent. This means that over 75 percent of sexually abused women did not develop alcohol problems. The effects of childhood sexual abuse are wide-ranging and vary from one individual to the next. Some therapists note that their abused clients avoid alcohol because they associate it with losing control, the last thing they want to do.

In Lindsey's story, we've seen how alcohol covers up her pain and allows her to stay in partial denial about her abuse, continuing—with one part of her brain—to believe that she grew up in an atmosphere of love and respect. Alcohol numbs and soothes her temporarily; it makes it easier to have sex. When she was at her lowest, cutting herself, convinced of her own guilt and unworthiness, alcohol was a way of harming herself, and it may still be. For some women, alcohol keeps them from remembering. The addictive cycle is so preoccupying—the craving for a drink, the drinking itself, the hangover, the depression, the new craving—that there's simply no psychological space for anything else. If they suffer from severe dissociation due to the sexual abuse—including frightening gaps in their memory—they may prefer to blame it on alcohol, which also causes blackouts. And extreme instances of dissociation can be frightening in themselves—when you blank out for periods of time, you can't rely on your own mind. This impairs your ability to work or interact with people. Alcohol can be an escape from this problem, and it can also exacerbate it. Abused women also often drink to be able to tolerate adult sexual relationships and to numb themselves against abuse from their current partners.

Some of the newest research explores how severe trauma in childhood, especially when the central nervous system is still developing, can cause lasting neurological damage. "The shock absorbers of the brain are shot," explains Dr. Bessel van der Kolk, a professor of psychiatry at Boston University who specializes in trauma. "If everything is running smoothly, if it crawls along just fine—as it does in nobody's life—you're fine. But the moment you get hurt, jealous, upset, fall in love, fall out of love, your reaction becomes much stronger."

Women who were severely and chronically traumatized as children may fit the diagnosis of posttraumatic stress disorder (PTSD), which used to be called "shell shock," because veterans of war so often develop it. It involves frightening hallucinations and flashbacks, irritability and angry outbursts, difficulty concentrating, hyperarousal, insomnia, and an exaggerated startle response.

Corinna Stewart, a psychologist with the Counseling Service of Addison County in Middlebury, Vermont, works with teenagers who abuse drugs and alcohol and also have PTSD. "Imagine what they're dealing with," she says. "They have all the usual difficulties of recovering, plus they have to learn how to detach from their bodies' own responses. When you or I step out into the crosswalk and hear a siren, we have a moment of fear, and we jump back onto the sidewalk. These young women might hear a door shut and experience that same fear: the adrenaline rush, the sweating, a sense of doom. They feel like they can't get out of the way. To deal with it, they may need medication, and they need—through long training—to learn to experience the body's panic without taking it too seriously, without having to act on the impulses of the body, which may never change."

Women with PTSD may feel that they absolutely *need* to drink, to relieve their symptoms. This was the case with Louise, a forty-two-year-old African American who made a conscious decision to start drinking at fifteen "to have the numbness. To bear the agony and pain." An attractive woman with a mass of cornrows, she described herself as "very sad," and indeed, throughout our interview, she stared at the floor and looked disconsolate. She had a way of raising her eyebrows in two slanting lines, as if she were perplexed. By the time she was fourteen, Louise had been raped three times—first by her mother's boyfriend, then by an uncle, and then date raped at gunpoint by her own "boyfriend." She developed a terror of men. In school, if she was assigned a male teacher, she would sit in the back of the class and sob until she was moved to another room. She had two marriages to abusive men and has never in her life had sex without being drunk. She has twice tried to kill herself, and she spent years hiding in her dark house. "I couldn't stand the sunlight," she told me. "I was like Dracula."

At the time of our interview, she had been sober for seven months, and many of the memories and feelings she'd kept at bay with alcohol had started to come back. "I'm having nightmares," she said. "Waking up, cold sweat. My hands, my nails—I'm going to have to cut them because I sleep with my fists balled up and my fingers constantly ache, ache, ache. I'm getting headaches, because there's too much going on. I told my counselor, the stuff coming back to me, I want it to stay buried. I tried to get out of seeing her, but she told me I needed to."

Louise has a hard time leaving her house, because, as she says, "I'm paranoid about men. I was walking, I dropped something, and this man said, 'Miss,' and he talked to me. I'm telling you, I ran two miles. It freaked me out."

Louise's addiction to alcohol has cost her enormously—when she sees her children hurting because of the years she was lost in a fog, it's "the saddest sight I ever saw in my life." But she still says, "I'm glad I had the alcohol. I just couldn't cope. I couldn't. I told my counselor, I'm glad I had the alcohol. It helped."

For Louise, seven months of sobriety is a magnificent achievement. She still has a long road ahead of her. Although medication will help, she'll probably always have to contend with anxiety and panic. In time, these should become less distressing, as she comes to see that she is not in genuine danger. She has people to help her: her children and sister are devoted to her, and now she has a counselor she's come to trust. She understands her vulnerability; now she's trying to learn about her strength.

WHAT DOES IT TAKE TO RECOVER?

FOR A LONG time experts in treating alcoholism insisted that getting sober must come first; only then could other problems be addressed. Fortunately, in recent years many have changed their tune—now women and men are also advised to get treatment for coexisting disorders. For women like Louise, whose alcohol abuse is intricately bound up with a history of sexual abuse, whose trauma-related emotions come flooding back when they stop drinking, it simply isn't possible to set aside their feelings while they work on getting sober. They need help in understanding how substance abuse and their history of sexual abuse are interrelated and mutually reinforcing.

It is becoming clear that insisting on sobriety as a prerequisite for exploring a history of incest sets some women up for failure. Their half-hearted commitment to getting sober often reflects their fear of reliving their traumatic past. Clinicians who treat survivors of trauma say it works best to encourage such clients to express or contain their fears without resorting to alcohol or drugs, and to set goals appropriate to their stage of recovery—all the while making safety the first priority. This difficult transitional period challenges the therapist, who may be reduced to such stopgap measures as getting the client to agree not to drink and drive, or to stay away from dangerous neighborhoods. "The clinical task," writes Joan Ellen Zweben, Ph.D., executive director of the 14th Street Clinic and Medical Group and East Bay Community Recovery Project in Oakland, California, "is to fine-tune one's sense of timing, to maintain clear goals when deciding how much to explore painful experiences, and to devise ways to secure cooperation with safety measures despite turmoil and distress."

Zweben adds that much treatment for addiction relies heavily on group counseling, and in some settings there is a bias against individual therapy. Yet survivors of trauma are often ashamed of their history; they need private attention. Zweben refers to a study in 1994, in which 70 percent of clients who were substance abusers and had a history of incest preferred individual counseling. This study did not surprise me, since of the six women I interviewed who discussed sexual abuse, all but Lindsey—who is at the beginning of her journey—referred frequently and gratefully to their therapists. One woman said simply, "A therapist is the best gift a woman can give to herself."

In her chapter "Substance-Abusing Women and Sexual Abuse" in *Gender and Addictions*, Rita Teusch outlines common issues in the treatment and recovery of sexually abused women who abuse substances, from the period of initial stabilization through longer-term goals:

Developing a Therapeutic Alliance

Women who were chronically abused as children will not trust anyone easily and may try to sabotage their relationship with a therapist, because they are frightened of becoming dependent and thus vulnerable to being traumatized again. "Even to accept a suggestion and follow it may be associated with unbearable fear," writes Teusch, adding that in such cases it can take a year or more to develop an alliance.

Maintaining Safety

A woman who is suicidal or can't control her use of alcohol or drugs might need to be hospitalized, sometimes repeatedly. Many women reenact their childhood abuse by getting involved with an abusive partner. They may need the therapist's help to leave.

A woman usually feels safer in therapy if she works with another woman, especially if her abuser was a man, but sometimes she feels so betrayed by a mother who failed to protect her that she may work better with a man. Survivors of incest often test their therapists to see if they care by relapsing or otherwise hurting themselves. They need a therapist to notice and address even subtle danger signs.

Educating About the Impact of Sexual Trauma and Substance Abuse

Many survivors feel hopeless and overwhelmed and cannot imagine recovering. It helps to learn about physiological reactions to alcohol and drugs, depression, flashbacks, and dissociation. It helps to know that hyperarousal, mistrust, and self-destructive impulses are common among women who have been abused, and that recovery takes a lot of time and work. Such reassurance needs to be ongoing.

Separating Recovery from Substance Abuse and Sexual Abuse

A major task for the recovering woman is separating out and articulating her feelings. Nightmares and flashbacks can be described in words, tolerated, and worked through. Negative feelings not directly related to the trauma—fear of being isolated, fear of making changes—need to be identified and connected to the urge to relapse. When triggers of relapse are discussed and understood, there is less need to act on impulse. Instead, rage, disappointment, and hurt can be tolerated and expressed.

Shifting Addictions

Sexually abused women commonly shift addictions during recovery. A woman who has used alcohol to soothe herself may achieve the same effect when sober by turning to other drugs or developing addictive behaviors: shoplifting, compulsive eating, cutting herself, or compulsive sex. Early recognition of the tendency may be enough to prevent its escalation. In more severe cases, the new problem may need specific treatment. Many women feel like failures when they develop new addictions. They need to be reminded that recovery is always complicated.

Difficulties Using Twelve-Step Programs

Many sexually abused women do not want to show their vulnerability or rely on others for support. Sometimes they need to develop trust in one person first, perhaps a therapist, before they can trust other people. A woman who suffers from flashbacks and panic attacks may hesitate to join a group, but joining becomes easier when she understands her triggers and has options for dealing with them. A woman with dissociative identity disorder—what used to be called multiple personality disorder—may have child personalities that need to be reassured. She may need to take "baby steps" in her recovery, perhaps standing for five minutes at the door of the room where the group is meeting, rather than trying to stay the whole hour. She may find a support group less stressful if it has a leader. Finally, some women feel uncomfortable about discussing their abuse at twelve-step meetings. Such women can find a smaller group or an all-women's group. As Louise said to me, "I've been to some meetings, but when I walk in and see a lot of men, I'm gone." Some women do well with AA when they accept that it's meant specifically to help them stay sober, and that they'll need another format to discuss their abuse issues.

Use of Medication

Many sexually abused women need medication to relieve overwhelming anxiety, depression, sleep problems, and hearing voices from dissociated parts of themselves. A woman in this situation needs a physician or psychiatrist who is sensitive to clients' potential to abuse a medication and who can help clients work through any anxiety they have about depending on medication.

Reenactment of Abusive Situations

A woman who has been sexually abused will commonly experience a crisis with her therapist over issues of control. If the therapist fails to understand what's happening, it can escalate into an adversarial relationship, in which the therapist is experienced as another abuser. Such a scenario stirs up painful feelings for both client and therapist, and the work can be long and slow.

A woman who has been sexually abused may associate caring and nurturing with sexual contact and may long for a sexual relationship with her therapist. She may have trouble setting her own limits. She may have trouble saying no when she doesn't want sex. She may want to please her therapist and may see sex as the best way. Since she was taught that sex can equal power, she may see sex as a way of taking control of the therapy. A sensitive therapist makes it clear that all the client's feelings, including sexual feelings, can be talked about and sorted out, and that none of them will be acted on. Obviously, it is critical that a sexually abused woman find a reputable, well-trained, morally sound therapist who is comfortable with all of these dynamics and is easily able to recognize and discuss them.

Longer-Term Treatment Goals

Even when an abused client feels completely secure with her therapist, treatment can be a rocky road. Regression is inevitable, because each time a woman feels strong enough to explore her painful feelings, her anxiety mounts, and she becomes vulnerable to relapse. Gradually, as she becomes familiar with the range of her feelings, she can learn to get some distance from them, to recognize that she doesn't have to act on self-destructive impulses, that she can choose healthier behaviors.

SAMANTHA: SHE'S COME THROUGH

HAVING INTERVIEWED several women who were struggling through the early stages of recovering from sexual abuse and alcohol problems, I was alert to the awesome challenges they faced. I was especially glad to meet Samantha, age forty, who had been sober for twelve years and whose curiosity, liveliness, ease, and mischievous manner suggested a woman at peace with herself and engaged in the world around her. Samantha—an Ojibwa woman with long, black hair down to her thighs, suggested that we enjoy the spring sunshine by sitting on the lawn of the Minnesota Indian Women's Resource Center, where she works as a chemical dependency counselor. She amused both of us by quizzing me about my other interviewees with a slightly competitive edge—she wanted to be sure she was going to make it into this book.

We sat down beneath a shade tree, and she began her story. "My family lived on a reservation in a little one-room shack. No electricity or running water. My dad was an alcoholic, and there was a lot of violence. Now, you hear some women say, 'He made me drink.' I always think that's BS, because everybody has a choice. But I think my mom was one of the people who actually are made to drink. My dad used to pull her hair and jam the bottle down her throat. He'd hold her head back and pour it down her throat, and if she moved he'd slug her.

"There are a lot of stories about abuse, but I always think it wasn't anything compared with what my mom went through and what we went through."

At this point, Samantha gave me a searching look and a half-smile. "Are you sure you want to know all this?"

I nodded, and she proceeded with a story of such violence and pain that it seemed surreal. In one incident, when Samantha was five or six, she watched her father go after her mother with an ax. She now suspects that her father suffered posttraumatic stress disorder. He had been in the Marine Corps in Korea and engaged in hand-to-hand combat. When he was sober, he was loving to his wife and six children, but when they heard him coming home singing "exactly like Hank Williams," they knew that he was drunk, and they would throw blankets and pillows out the window, jump out on top of them, and run into the woods to spend the night.

Samantha's grandparents lived in a wigwam village built for tourists. They dressed in buckskin, and her grandmother would sit under a birch bark awning weaving baskets. When Samantha was eight, they made a "jingle dress" for her, and she and her cousins would dance for the tourists. Samantha liked the chance to get paid, to leave the reservation, and to be with her grandmother, who loved her passionately. She loved to watch her grandmother tan deer hide, and to help her cook. Wrinkling up her nose, she told me, "One time when we were really little, my grandfather caught a great big turtle. I watched him. He tipped it over on a table and the head came out, and then he chopped it off. It stunk. My grandmother's house—sometimes it would stink. She cooked all this stuff they caught. We could see the turtle floating around, bubbling in the water. After they cut it up, they cut the turtle's heart up. The turtle has courage and perseverence. They cut the heart right up when it was beating, and they made us eat it."

I asked, "To give you courage and perseverence?"

She nodded. "Raw. We were really little, and they lined us all up, and my grandma took it on a spoon, and made us eat it."

There were no turtles at the tourist village. Though she loved to see her grandmother, the worst memories of Samantha's life are also from this period. Every afternoon when the village closed, Samantha's grandfather got her alone and raped her.

Some researchers point out that the strong link between childhood sexual abuse and later alcohol problems does not establish causality. Both substance abuse and such traumatic events as child abuse, they argue, might share a deeper cause, rising out of a disturbed family environment that fails to nurture and protect a child. When Samantha looks back at all the violence and physical abuse in her life, what she experienced and what she witnessed, including the times when she was taken from her mother and placed in foster homes, her grandfather's abuse, which began when she was eight, is what hurts and enrages her the most. One detail in particular still overwhelms her. Every time he raped her, he bought her a hamburger afterward. This was a child who was used to eating raw oatmeal sandwiches, who would take a sheet of paper and roll it up into a cone, fill it with a dab of government peanut butter, and if there was sugar, sprinkle some on top, so she could pretend it was an ice cream cone. Samantha scowled as she told me, "It got to where I let him rape me so I could get that hamburger. . . . And he knew. He knew we were poor. He knew how old I was. He knew how it was at our house. He knew. He knew. God."

She shook her head. "What else could I have become but an alcoholic?"

Samantha and all of her siblings started drinking early, keeping their parents company. All had their own children young, and, said Samantha, "We were all the time getting drunk, beating each other up, going to detox, going to jail—just the same stuff we grew up with." All but Samantha and one sister are still drinking.

Samantha first got sober in an effort to win back custody of her children. After a period of sobriety, she shifted addictions—as Rita Teusch points out, this is a common pitfall—and began to shoot cocaine. Her memories were deeply traumatic, but harder to cope with was her overwhelming guilt. Her son was born with fetal alcohol syndrome and became an alcoholic before he was twelve years old. Chronically drunk, she had neglected her son and her daughter until they were taken away by the state. Furthermore, she had seduced countless men for the pleasure of walking out on them. And then there were all the losses: the drug-addicted friends who had died, and the recent death from cancer of Bruce, the father of her children. She had loved Bruce since the age of thirteen, though when he made her choose between alcohol and him, she chose alcohol. When Bruce lay dying in the hospital, he asked her what would make her happy in her life, and she answered, "Being your wife." They were married ten days before he died.

Shortly after his death, after speaking to her son on the phone—he was in a treatment center—Samantha lay down on Bruce's bed and cried. She was living in his old house, but the landlord had called and was coming to kick her out. Bruce's brothers were coming to pick up his belongings, and she had nowhere to go. She had three bottles of Bruce's pain pills. She thought that if she sold them she could buy enough cocaine to kill herself. She could hardly bear the thought of leaving her kids, but she told herself that Bruce's parents would take care of them. When she heard a far-off sound, she sat up and looked around, wondering what it was. On a dresser stacked with jeans, she found a little radio, one she'd never seen before. It must have belonged to Bruce. The radio was on. She turned it louder, and listening to the words, she felt the hair stand up on the back of her neck. The song, by Corey Hart, was called "Never Surrender." She realized that she wasn't going to kill herself. She would go on, no matter what.

Samantha did get sober, and she regained custody of her children. Her son is still in and out of treatment. When her daughter started experimenting with marijuana in high school, Samantha immediately noticed the slide in her grades and had her in therapy and a support group before any serious problems developed. Samantha went back to school and began her work as a counselor.

Six years after her last high, Samantha was beseiged by night-mares and overwhelming memories and was diagnosed with delayed PTSD. She was placed on medication. She went back to therapy for four more years. She had to work through much of her fear, her sadness, and her rage—but, said Samantha, she didn't exactly follow the thera-peutic prescription. "They say, oh, you need to forgive the ones who abused you, but when I was in therapy I made a decision: I was never going to forgive my grandfather. I don't care who did what to him, that was no reason for him to do it to me. I'll die not forgiving him, and can I live with that? Yes, I can. And not only that. In therapy, I decided that I would not go all the way into my rage. I went maybe halfway, a little less than halfway, and then I decided, I'm keeping the rest of it for me. Because some day I may be in a situation where that rage is going to save my life."

I wondered if rage had kept Samantha alive through so much sor-row, and if that's why she wanted to hang on to it. Sitting there in the shade as a gang of kids played ball nearby, I was in awe of her achieve-ment. By turns fierce, passionate, tender, and funny, she all the while communicated a peaceful sense of having come to terms with herself. She was open about her shortcomings, but not judgmental. Much of her story she told me with wry amusement, and sometimes with comic flair. She still worries about her mother—"she's probably drunk with my son right now," she laughed—but she seems to know the limits to how she can and cannot help. She's excited about her future, having applied for a further year of schooling with some hope of a scholarship.

I asked where she got her strength. She said, first of all, that she had been loved by many people: her grandmother; a social worker she met in seventh grade; a foster mother who hugged her, encouraged her, and told her that the white girls who taunted her, calling her a "savage," were jealous of her straight A's. Then there was the therapist who saw her through her flashbacks, encouraging her to call his emer-gency number when she was at the hardest stage. Perhaps all that love helped her develop her faith in the Creator—"or God or Allah," she said. "He knows I'm talking about him." She cautions that her faith is not about believing life can get easy, because "Life isn't like that. Things happen. People die. Your whole sky could fall down, and it does. But it passes. And the pain passes too. As long as you allow yourself to grieve, it will pass."

In her work as a counselor, Samantha sometimes has to guard against a sense that she's been through worse than her clients. As soon as she listens to their stories, she understands that they share pain. "Life hurts," she said. "Not only for Native Americans. I do evaluations, and I see it's the same for whites, for blacks. I'd say that 99 percent of my clients are sexually abused."

"That many?" I asked. Though sexual abuse cuts across lines of class and race, it can be endemic in impoverished, embattled communities.

"That's right. I think about how hard it was for me to go through therapy, and I always tell my clients, 'You can, you really can, you can get sober. I know it.'

"I don't know what part of me is the part that stays sober, but whatever it is I wish I could cut it out, and cut it into little bitty tiny pieces, and feed it to all my clients."

I asked her, "Like a turtle's heart?"

She rewarded me with a winsome smile. "Whatever God gave me he gave to everybody. I try to help my clients find what he gave them to go on. He didn't discriminate. He said, 'Oh, you're going to earth—here, have this. You're going to need this on your way.' He didn't give anybody less than what he gave me."

Part Four

Women's Paths
in Recovery

10

Doctors Still
Don't Get It

MORE AND MORE, THE ALCOHOL TREATMENT COMMUNITY is focused on early intervention to try to help people change their drinking habits and divert them from "end-stage alcoholism," which wastes so many lives and is so very difficult to treat. Yet the major components of this new emphasis are drunk driving programs, in which women are underrepresented (because they more often drink at home, and because, when they go out with a man, the man more often drives), and employee assistance programs, which may reach men more effectively.

Though women who are problem drinkers are less likely than men to run up against the law and less likely to be referred to treatment by their employers, they are apt to visit physicians and mental health professionals much more frequently. Women seek medical attention more often than men, and among women who see physicians—family doctors, gynecologists, obstetricians, pediatricians—or other health care professionals, the prevalence of alcohol-related disorders is at least double that in the general population. Men seeking help with alcoholism are more likely to go to a substance abuse treatment center, and women are more likely to see a personal physician or a psychiatrist. Unfortunately, the stereotypical perceptions of what it means to be female—especially a female with a drinking problem—go with a woman into the doctor's office and work against objective assessment.

Like Daphne, whose story was told in Chapter 3, many women who are dependent on alcohol are in denial, and they go to their doctors to seek relief from a concurrent disorder, such as depression. They also go to seek relief from symptoms directly attributable to alcohol: fatigue, sleeplessness, anxiety, irritability, weight loss, chronic heartburn. Such symptoms, taken together, should alert doctors to potential substance abuse, particularly when other risk factors are present— including depression, a family history of alcoholism, and a history of sexual abuse—but doctors frequently fail to make the diagnosis. Many initial assessment forms ask the patient about alcohol and drugs; but although these forms may protect a physician from a lawsuit, they are all but useless when an alcoholic is intent on hiding her problem. Across the country, thousands of doctors and mental health professionals are missing the signs of drinking problems in women.

Of course, it is hard to work around a patient's and her family's denial. When Daphne went to the doctor with complaints about depression, clumsiness, sleeplessness, fatigue, heartburn, and irritability, she did not consciously attribute her symptoms to the effects of alcohol. Nor did she make the connection when antidepressants failed to take effect. Though her husband, Paul, never saw her with her tall glass of vodka, he must have sensed she was drinking—he told his friend she *seemed* drunk. That he never put two and two together over a period of ten years might seem bizarre and extreme, but such denial and despair are familiar in alcoholic families and are not at all surprising to workers in the field.

Recovering women tell of being discouraged by their doctors even when they actively sought help. One woman said, "When I told my gynecologist I might have a problem, he said to me, 'You're too smart to be an alcoholic.'" Another woman went into a hospital for gall bladder tests and suffered withdrawal symptoms under the doctor's nose. He pretended not to notice. In one study, physicians were given hypothetical patients in a computer simulation and asked to elicit additional information and arrive at a diagnosis. Two-thirds of these well-trained clinicians missed the diagnosis of alcoholism in cases that were considered obvious by others. Although this is a problem for both men and women patients, a range of studies have found that physicians are particularly blind about alcohol problems in women. In one study, hospital doctors were three times more likely to fail to diagnose a female alcoholic than a male alcoholic. Another study found that even when physicians did recognize signs of alcohol abuse in their patients, they addressed the problem in only 24 percent of cases.

The stories proliferate. I interviewed a man who, like Paul, had missed his wife Diana's alcoholism over a period of many years. When, still clueless, he accompanied her on a visit to her psychiatrist—a well-known clinical diagnostician—the doctor announced that he was referring them to somebody else for treatment, because Diana reminded him painfully of a personal case, and he could not treat her objectively. After the session, this husband wondered aloud what this could possibly mean. "He told me I remind him of his wife," said Diana. "She was a closet drinker for years, and he never figured it out. His children had to tell him. Isn't it sad?" For the first time, the lights went on in this husband's head.

Alcoholism nearly always refuses to see itself. The tragedy deepens when suffering people place their trust in a health establishment that shares in their own denial.

Physicians have a real opportunity to help. A range of studies and clinical experience suggest that even brief counseling by a physician can reduce drinking and decrease the costs of health care for alcohol-related problems. A recent community-based study found evidence that should encourage any physician about the usefulness of careful screening. Among men who consumed more than fourteen drinks per week and women who consumed more than eleven drinks per week, brief intervention by a physician—two short counseling sessions and follow-up telephone interviews—resulted twelve months later in a 14 percent reduction in alcohol use in men—and a 31 percent reduction in women. As noted previously, a single motivational session offering feedback to heavy-drinking freshmen resulted in fewer alcohol-related problems over the first two years of college. Among the women I interviewed, one—Dale—was confronted by her physician after a fairly brief period of dependence on alcohol. She left his office, joined AA, and never had another drink.

In May 1997, a committee of the American Medical Association presented a report addressing the poor record of physicians in identifying alcohol-related problems in their patients, particularly women. The report recommended that the AMA urge physicians to be alert for alcohol-related problems, to screen patients more thoroughly for alcohol abuse and dependence, and to educate women of all ages about their increased risk of liver and heart disease from alcohol and about the effect of alcohol on the developing fetus. It included advice on how to counsel patients with problems, and screening instruments that might be more effective than those currently in place.

This is an important first step—and one hopes that the AMA will follow through. If a survey of 400 physicians done in late 1997 by the National Center on Addiction and Substance Abuse at Columbia University (CASA) is any indication, this issue had not yet penetrated many physicians' awareness. When asked how many drinks per day would constitute problem drinking, their answers (from 2.3 to 2.5 drinks per day) were virtually equal for patients of both sexes and all ages. They did not take into account women's lower tolerance for alcohol, or the changes that age brings. The survey found that only one in seventeen physicians asks patients to complete an alcohol assessment form at every visit. Only one in five uses the sensitive CAGE questionnaire. (CAGE is an acronym for four brief questions: Have you ever felt you should *cut* down on your drinking? Have people *annoyed* you by criticizing your drinking? Have you ever felt *guilty* about your drinking? Have you ever had a drink first thing in the morning (*eye-opener*) to steady your nerves or get rid of a hangover? One doctor in thirty-three uses the TWEAK, a version of CAGE modified for women (see Appendix A). And when presented with a hypothetical patient who presented a full array of symptoms consistent with alcohol problems, only 1 to 2 percent considered the possibility of substance abuse. The results of this survey are clear. Too many physicians do not have substance abuse on their diagnostic radar screen.

On the other hand, 82 percent of these physicians suggested depression—the most common diagnosis. Twenty percent suggested anxiety, stress, or psychological problems other than depression. These are reasonable diagnoses, but if substance abuse is not screened for, the stage is set for such inappropriate medication as antianxiety drugs, sedatives, and certain antidepressants that complicate and exacerbate addiction, which goes untreated. Doctors who miss the signs of alcoholism often send a woman away with a prescription for tranquilizers tucked into her purse, setting her up for a dual addiction. Female alcoholics like Daphne and Dale, who abused Valium along with alcohol, often combine alcohol and prescription drugs.

Similarly, doctors confuse the signs of drinking in older women with side effects of medications and senility. When an old woman trips and falls, her doctor often doesn't consider that the two martinis she could handle twenty years ago now have an increased effect on her body and may be causing her clumsiness.

What is the problem here?

Physicians, like the rest of us, may have stereotyped ideas of what an alcoholic looks like.

Unfortunately, the stereotypes of the alcoholic hooker and the alcoholic bag lady persists. In the study at Johns Hopkins University Hospital, doctors were even less likely to consider alcohol as a potential problem if the women had private insurance or higher incomes and education. It boils down to this: If a woman doesn't fit the stereotype of an alcoholic, she cannot be a problem drinker.

Physicians may wink at a woman's heavy drinking, believing she needs alcohol to cope.

In CASA's survey of 400 physicians, more than one-third agreed with the statement, "Many physicians fail to address problem drinking among mature patients because they believe drinking is one of the last few pleasures left for the elderly." Thus, they overlook or wink at early signs of trouble.

While this attitude may be most exaggerated in relation to elderly women, it may pertain to women patients of all ages. In *Substance and Shadow: Women and Addiction in the United States*, Stephen R. Kandall describes the long history of women being excessively medicated by physicians. This, along with women's own self-medication, has been a significant factor in addiction. Women have been thought to need special protection, to be less able than men to deal with physical or psychic pain. During the Victorian era, doctors medicated "women's diseases" and "nervous weakness" excessively, contributing to addiction. By the end of the nineteenth century, two-thirds of the nation's opium and morphine addicts were women. Today we have different pressures and different ways of conceiving them—for example, competing in a male-dominated workplace, or coping with an empty nest. Yet today, if a woman is anxious or lonely, a doctor is still apt to prescribe tranquilizers and sedatives, making her less likely to adapt creatively and more vulnerable to addiction.

Physicians are not properly educated about substance abuse.

A national panel of doctors, representatives of insurance companies, public officials, business executives, and leaders in medical education concluded that physicians are being inadequately trained. Doctors may not know that most of their alcoholic patients will come to the office sober with no trace of liver disease and no obvious signs of withdrawal, and that these patients may have periods of abstinence lasting for days, for months, or even longer. They're often unaware that such other conditions as a modest elevation of blood pressure and an increase in triglycerides are likely to be observed with heavy drinking. When a patient complains about insomnia and mood swings, doctors may not know enough to ask about alcohol. They're often unaware of clues that might help identify "hidden" alcoholics.

Questionnaires and indices of alcohol consumption are geared toward men.

In taking a medical history, doctors may ask about alcohol and may even use a questionnaire intended to help diagnose drinking problems. But many of the screening techniques used on women to measure the quantity and frequency of drinking were developed for men. These techniques don't take women's different metabolism into account. What's more, they ask about issues more common among male problem drinkers—legal troubles and trouble at work, for instance—and neglect to ask about family conflict, domestic violence, sexual abuse, and reproductive dysfunction, which are more common markers of heavy drinking in women. Since so many problem drinkers underreport their consumption—even modest drinkers do that—it is critical to gather a careful history of alcohol-related life problems. New screening tests geared toward women sometimes approach the problem by asking, for instance, "Do you ever carry alcohol in your purse?"

Physicians don't think it's their job to identify alcoholics.

When an oral surgeon treats a woman for broken teeth, he may know she broke them by falling down steps when she was drunk, but alcohol problems, he reasons, are not within the realm of his practice. Even internists often hesitate to accept responsibility, though this seems hard to understand, given the serious health risks to alcoholic patients.

Physicians are not trained in intervention.

Even when doctors recognize that a patient has a drinking problem and feel responsibility, they still may not know what to say or do. Especially if they associate women's alcoholism with promiscuity, they may have trouble discussing drinking problems in a nonthreatening, non-judgmental way. They may not even know where to send their patients for help. They may be pessimistic about treatment.

When physicians intervene, they are not supported by the health care establishment.

Many insurance companies, as well as managed care and Medicare, do not pay doctors for time spent on efforts to prevent or intervene in an alcohol or drug abuse problem.

Physicians have too little time.

In the CASA survey, physicians reported lack of time as a crucial barrier to screening for substance abuse. Importantly, neither managed care, many health insurers, nor Medicare will pay doctors for the time they spend on efforts to prevent or intervene in a case of substance abuse. The average visit to a primary care physician is less than eight minutes—hardly enough time to address sensitive issues such as substance use, especially if the appointment has been scheduled to address other problems. Says CASA: "We must pay physicians to talk to patients, not just to treat them with needles, pills, and surgery."

There is a high rate of alcohol abuse in the medical profession.

Indirect measures of alcohol abuse suggest that members of the medical profession are more likely than other highly educated men and women to develop a drinking problem. The rate of hospitalization for alcohol-related difficulties among physicians, for instance, is three times that of other highly educated, high-income groups. A study in Britain found that 23 percent of male medical students consumed an average of thirty-five or more drinks per week. A survey of medical students in the United States revealed that almost 20 percent had experienced an alcoholic blackout. These figures are not markedly higher than those for the general college population, but even if members of the medical profession have rates of alcohol abuse that are the same as in the population at large, 10 percent of our doctors would be affected at some point. Doctors in denial about their own condition aren't as likely to see it in others.

Mental health professionals are also missing the boat.

Women like Daphne often have problems to deal with apart from their alcoholism. Daphne's depression predated her drinking, and her life circumstances needed attention. None of her psychiatrists, clinical psychologists, and therapists ever asked about her drinking habits. I heard many versions of this story as I was writing this book, including reports of mental health professionals who knew how much a client was drinking but didn't see the problem or minimized it when the client brought it up. I was relieved when, finally, Alice (the lawyer in Chapter 6) told me that her therapist had helped her confront her drinking problem, and another woman, Kim, said that her therapist had ended the treatment because she did not want to collude with Kim's pretense that she could do the work of therapy and change her life while she was still actively drinking.

Of course, it can be hard to diagnose a problem if a client hides all the signs. A Jungian analyst told me that she has sometimes been clued in by a patient's dreams. In *Many Roads, One Journey: Moving Beyond the Twelve Steps*, Charlotte Davis Kasl says she begins to suspect substance abuse

- When a client never seems to push through problems.
- When significant progress one week seems forgotten the next.
- When each week brings a new topic, with little follow-through.
- When a person reports behavior that seems out of character.
- When a person seems immature, like an adolescent who has never grown up.

Kasl urges therapists to ask clients directly about alcohol and drugs—"when, where, how much, and about all the effects." She suggests a period of abstinence from mind-altering drugs as a way of closing "the back door on their emotional escape hatches," in order to make progress in therapy. Often, this suggestion stimulates important discussions, from which the therapist can learn a lot.

Traditionally, providers of twelve-step-based treatment have been biased against psychotherapy, especially in the early stages of recovery. They point out that it is hard to disentangle the effects of alcohol from ongoing emotional problems, hard to know which problems will persist and which will fall away when the patient becomes sober. They object when alcoholism is seen as a symptom of underlying problems instead of the chief cause of problems in and of itself. In addition, they argue, someone who is newly sober does not have the mental resources for analytical work and responds best to the simplest kind of encouragement and advice. In speaking with families of alcoholics, I heard angry stories of psychotherapists who helped alcoholics trace the intricate roots of personal problems but were helpless in diagnosing or treating a disease in which the immediate stakes were life and death. Some therapists in effect collude with the alcoholic, reinforcing her feelings of victimhood and getting in the way of her taking responsibility for recovery. Some have little understanding of AA and do not fully support their patients' involvement.

Though studies suggest that mental health professionals frequently recommend AA, many have negative feelings about it. Some of the objections of therapists are discussed elsewhere in this book: they see women and men for whom the emphasis on powerlessness and disease has not been liberating; who are involved in more rigid AA groups that adopt an isolating "we versus the world" stance and are suspicious of any display of feeling; and who, when they begin a healthy questioning of what they believe and what they want, are frightened by friends in AA who insist that they will start drinking again if they stop looking to the group for answers. While the procedures and practices of AA groups are remarkably consistent around the world, individual meetings do tend to develop a kind of personality. Naturally enough, just as there are good and bad therapists, there are AA groups that range from rigid and literal-minded to warm, supportive, and deeply growth-enhancing.

Recently, addiction specialists have made an attempt to move beyond this mutual suspicion, arguing for the benefits of simultaneous involvement in AA and psychotherapy. At the most basic level, AA helps people stay sober, and therapy provides a place for people to work through their feelings about AA sponsors and group dynamics, and to come to terms with unconscious impulses which thwart their recovery efforts. More broadly, AA and psychotherapy can work together to facilitate emotional and spiritual growth, with insights achieved in one context enhanced and reinforced in the other.

WE CAN DO BETTER

IN DAPHNE'S CASE, it took years of mistakes by important health professionals before the truth of her condition could no longer be ignored. By then, her addiction was firmly established, her disease was well advanced, and her personal life was in chaos.

Although no solution will be perfect, many such tragedies could be averted by early detection of alcohol-related problems. Evaluations of alcohol treatment suggest that, particularly for women, the earlier a patient enters treatment, the better the outcome. Physicians and mental health professionals need to be better educated about substance abuse, and we need to call on insurance companies and Medicare to cover prevention and early interventions. In a guide to substance abuse services for primary care clinicians, five critical components of brief early interventions are established:

- Explain how a patient's level of alcohol use may create impairment and health risks.
- Inform the patient about safe consumption limits and, where appropriate, offer advice about change.
- Assess the patient's readiness to change.
- Negotiate goals and strategies for change.
- Arrange for follow-up treatment.

In an overview of drinking problems in women, Nancy Vogeltanz and Sharon Wilsnack also suggest ways we can do a better job of prevention:

- Health professionals and other practitioners should have a high "index of suspicion" regarding drinking problems among both women and men. About 10 to 15 percent of American women report some type of alcohol-related problem, and about 4 percent, or 4 million women, meet diagnostic criteria for alcohol abuse or dependence.
- Familiarity with risk factors—biological, genetic, demographic, social, psychological, and environmental—should prompt special attention to high-risk subgroups.
- For women, many physical, psychological, and environmental problems are associated with alcohol abuse—as antecedents, consequences, or both. Research findings can be used to educate a large variety of practitioners about the links between women's alcohol problems and their own speciality. Gynecologists, for instance, can be made aware of the link between alcohol and sexual dysfunction. Doctors and other health professionals; mental health practitioners, including marriage and sex therapists; workplace professionals; personnel in the legal and criminal justice system; educators; child service specialists; and other personnel in social service agencies can all be trained to detect problems and intervene.

Vogeltanz and Wilsnack suggest that knowledge about risk factors may eventually lead to such effective prevention strategies as skills training for women with heavy-drinking partners; early intervention for sexually abused girls; and alcohol education and prevention for women in transition (due to unemployment, divorce, children leaving home, or rapid acculturation), women in male-dominated workplaces, and women with mood or anxiety disorders.

Until things change, too many women with alcohol problems will be slipping through the cracks. We need to press our doctors and mental health professionals to accept responsibility as the first-line response to women with drinking problems. We need to support their efforts to intervene and reimburse them for time spent on prevention. Medical schools, health centers, and psychology departments need to teach practitioners how to screen for early and advanced drinking problems in ways that help get around a patient's denial, and educate them in the many faces of alcoholism and drug abuse, so that stereotypes of bag ladies and prostitutes stop interfering with objective diagnosis. Doctors must be alerted to the indirect ways a drinking problem can present itself. They must learn to intervene effectively, or refer the patient to other services.

For this to happen, the first step must be taken. Doctors and therapists must acknowledge their crucial role and recognize the active harm that they can do when they ignore a woman's symptoms of drinking problems. Looking the problem in the face is the crucial first step to recovery. A clear diagnosis by a doctor or a therapist can help a woman see the demon she's been hiding from. Even if she is in active denial—lying about how much she drinks, even leaving in anger—the practitioner's questions and concern can bring her closer to acknowledging her problem before precious years slip by.

11

Working with Difference:
Minnesota Indian Women's Resource Center and African-American Family Services

THE TREATMENT INDUSTRY IN AMERICA HAS ALMOST entirely accepted the concept of alcoholism and drug abuse as a disease. Patients are taught that alcoholism is a medical condition that can happen to anyone, regardless of class, race, or gender. Counselors stress what alcoholics have in common with one another because of their disease. At AA meetings—usually strongly recommended by treatment providers—I have myself witnessed mutual respect among crowds that can be quite diverse. At the beginning of each meeting, someone reads the rules, which emphasize the importance of anonymity and state that the only requirement for belonging is a desire to be clean and sober. An alcoholic is an alcoholic, and no one is excluded because of race, sex, class, creed, or sexual preference. Why then, one might wonder, are minority groups across the country creating their own treatment programs and support groups?

The Minnesota Indian Women's Resource Center (MIWRC) and African-American Family Services (AAFS), both in Minneapolis, offer culturally specific outpatient treatment for substance abuse. The stories of Samantha and Rachel, Ojibwa women in recovery, appear in other chapters. The stories of Victoria, Ruth, and Pat, African Americans who say they owe their lives to AAFS, follow. But first, here's what staff members and other recovering women said about the advantages of culturally specific treatment.

You have sober role models of your own race.

The women with whom I spoke agreed that role models are vital. Having counselors who are female, who had been addicted and now are sober, who have faced many of the same obstacles, who look like them, who have professional credentials, and who are operating successfully in the world—this validates the education being offered and gives a message of hope. Clients at both facilities see the staff as a kind of buffer zone between themselves and the white establishment, which may have ordered them into treatment because of child neglect or some other violation of the law.

It's comforting to be with a group of people who understand you and accept you in the context of your background.

Some minority women may hesitate to discuss problems that exist in their communities, for fear that they will be misperceived and reinforce negative stereotypes. In addition, cultural misunderstandings can get in the way of true sharing.

Denise Bond, director of MIWRC, explained why some Native Americans have trouble talking at twelve-step meetings: "We have longer pauses in our speech. Growing up, we were socialized to wait for our elders to get done talking before we jumped in. Sometimes their pauses seemed like minutes or hours! But we learned to wait. For us that's simple respect, but other people have different communication patterns. I met a man who told me that in the part of New York where he comes from, if you breathe in, somebody else jumps into the conversation. In Minnesota, we have this 'Minnesota nice' thing—we wait for people to finish talking. When he came here he kept talking and talking and couldn't figure out why no one was jumping in! Native Americans take 'Minnesota Nice' a further step.

"We have Talking Circle every week in our treatment program, and the women pass around a fan of eagle feathers; the woman holding the fan speaks. It's a good thing to incorporate any time a group includes Native people."

Bond added that many Native tribes see the eagle as the creature closest to the Creator. Holding the feather is symbolic—it takes your words to God.

Leslie Ann Sparks, the women's program coordinator at AAFS, used to work in a predominantly white treatment center. She said that the white staff there had little frame of reference for understanding African-American clients, and misunderstandings could be problematic. "For example," said Sparks, "when an African-American woman is angry, she uses her hands a lot and gets very animated, and from the tone and loudness of her voice, you know she's angry. You might also hear more cursing—it's the language of the class she's from. It doesn't mean that the next thing she's going to do is hit you! But you'll see the white staff backing off, saying, 'This woman needs anger management,' instead of understanding that people communicate in different ways."

Even among well-educated, middle-class people, said Sparks, there are often misunderstandings: "If you're in a town meeting, say, of educated people, half white and half black, and someone's talking or making a presentation that has little content, really blowing his own horn, the black people will say, 'Next! Get on down, be quiet!' We'll move them along! Whereas in white culture everyone gets a certain amount of time. When we say, 'Next,' the whites will see us as being threatening and disrespectful.

"This happens in treatment, too, when you have two different populations, or a white staff and a black group. It blows the staff away, because they don't understand that kind of dialogue."

In culturally specific treatment, such misunderstandings do not arise.

Since most alcoholics have suffered from feeling isolated and unique, the sense of belonging that comes from connecting to their ethnic or racial roots can help women gather their strength. At MIWRC, a number of clients were adopted as children into white homes, and they know little about their culture, even though they may look Native American. The agency has a library of videos and books, and elders from the Ojibwa and Lakota tribes give talks on traditional ways.

Confrontational approaches and "bottoming out" may not work when you need a message of hope.

Alcohol and other addictive substances hijack the brain, including natural systems of learning and memory, and steer it toward another fix. This is why addicts will lie and manipulate people—sometimes consciously, sometimes not. Basically, alcohol has fooled the brain into thinking it needs the substance to survive. At times, alcohol may seem more vital than food and water. Since addicted people are often caught in a web of deceit that allows them to continue their habit, counselors at treatment centers—usually recovering addicts themselves—will try to cut through the cobwebs and strip away the client's defenses, so the client is forced, again and again, to face the naked truth about where alcohol has brought her. A single counselor may be "fooled" by a client who believes she is utterly sincere in her intention to quit; that is why group therapy is so important. A roomful of fifteen other addicts can often spot the mental thread by which someone is clinging to her habit. The approach tends to be confrontational. Counselors walk a fine line between ripping away the defenses that a client needs to function and leading her to self-knowledge that can save her life. After treatment, in AA groups, recovering alcoholics continue to confront one another with their weaknesses and justifications in various aspects of their lives, with the idea that honesty and assumption of responsibility are critical for continuing sobriety.

Another prominent idea is that an alcoholic has to "hit bottom" before she can recover, that to become motivated she must sink to a level of behavior and feeling she can't tolerate. Thus others almost seem to wash their hands of an alcoholic who goes back to the bottle. I don't mean to imply a lack of caring and concern—that is certainly not the case. But there is a sad recognition that no one but the alcoholic can choose to get well, and a belief that if she hasn't yet reached bottom, interfering with her habit may only delay the day of reckoning.

Such approaches probably work best for people who have a certain amount of ego strength; who can tolerate confrontation; who have resources of their own to fall back on; who, even if filled with self-loathing, believe that their life is worth saving; and who have faith that counselors, staffers, and fellow alcoholics understand them and accept them on a very basic level. Those who fit this description and have been helped in this way are, naturally, attached to the method, but it may not work for everyone.

At AAFS, the male counselors say that after the first half of treatment, when the focus is on education and applying new knowledge to everyday life, they do get confrontational. George Lewis, lead counselor for a program called Male Oppression and Violence Elimination (MOVE), challenges his clients about their ideas of manhood and appropriate behavior, and it can get heated. "People raise their voices, vent, and curse you out," he told me. "There's only one rule: never leave your seat when you're angry. If you do, you're immediately terminated. But you can curse me out and attack my mom—those words come out when you get pissed."

It's different with women, according to Leslie Ann Sparks. When I asked her if she, too, became more confrontational during the second half of treatment, she said, "These women have been beat around enough!" Direct confrontation can be destructive, since it triggers their fears and defenses and reminds them of the abuse they've experienced, sometimes all their lives. You can't use confrontation to get through to women with a very shaky sense of themselves. Instead, said Sparks, "When a woman hears someone else repeat what she's been through, someone who understands it, it's the most healing thing that can happen. I had a woman come in recently who's been with an abusive, alcoholic partner for twenty-two years. She met him at thirteen, and they have five children. He keeps her isolated and confined, but she has all sorts of reasons for putting up with this. Instead of challenging her, I said, 'Aren't you tired of living like this?' She looked at me and started crying. Someone else had told her what her life looks like, and now she could see it too."

At conventional treatment centers, when someone doesn't show up for two or three meetings, he or she is kicked out. AAFS also sets clear limits, but before taking such action, Sparks and her colleagues ask a lot of questions. They may find that a woman has been ordered into treatment by a court for three different issues—say domestic violence, child neglect, and substance abuse—and two of them are scheduled too close together. The client may want to do her best but may not have the communication skills to let you know your expectations are not realistic. Sparks explained that she has to stay alert and walk a fine line between understanding and being duped—"My clients do know how to work the system," she laughed, referring to a woman who had recently sold her bus pass and used this as an excuse for not coming to treatment.

At MIWRC and AAFS, the counselors try to be flexible. They get clients from all walks of life, and each client responds differently. Still, 80 percent of their clients have been ordered into treatment by a court.

Sparks's observations were affirmed by Maya Hennessey, who works for the Illinois Department of Human Services and helped to develop Project Safe, which offers innovative treatment for substance abuse at locations across Illinois. Project Safe sends outreach workers to coax women into treatment who otherwise would never go—often minority women, many of them pregnant and with children, who have lived amid poverty and violence since they were born and who have never believed that a good life was possible. Usually the women have been identified by the child welfare system as needing screening for substance abuse. Sometimes they are open to treatment, but often, when outreach workers knock at the door, they find that the woman has moved, or she is hiding. "The outreach workers don't give up," Hennessey told me. "They'll be aggressive in tracking her down. They'll find a way to convince her there might be a better way." Again, such tactics contradict the theory that, for treatment to be successful, a person has to "hit bottom" first. These women live at the bottom, and as one counselor commented, "If we wait for them to bottom out, they'll die." When asked how they came to treatment, they are likely to say: "That woman—I couldn't get rid of her!"

Project Safe tolerates some infringement of the rules. A woman may come in high, shout profanities, and then call later to see if she can come back. "It used to be that if you broke the rules or relapsed, you got thrown out," said Hennessey. "But we saw that as people became part of this community of recovering women, they would relapse less, and the relapses would be less severe." Now the policy might be summed up as, "There's no failure; there's just feedback." Hennessey explained that experienced staffers at Project Safe have learned how to take a relapse and assist a woman in making it therapeutic. "Sometimes, as a result of a crisis, a woman will come back with greater gusto and more determination, more commitment to recovery. She drops her denial and is prepared to face painful issues." Hennessey added, "We don't get sudden conversions. We get destructive and healthy behaviors side by side. Over time, the one gets weaker, the other stronger." A woman may say four or five times that her partner is abusive and she needs to get out. Instead of confronting her about being all talk and no action, the staff at Project Safe understands that each time she says it, she's getting a little bit more strength to do something about it.

For women at MIWRC, AAFS, and Project Safe, the most powerful motivator for getting sober is seeing other women like themselves who have been in the same boat—addiction, domestic violence, a life on welfare, single motherhood—but who have managed to get out and make real lives for themselves. Fear won't work as motivation—these clients have lived with fear for a long time. Instead, they need to be surprised by hope.

The centers offer a holistic approach.

Minority women who develop addictions often have particular environmental vulnerabilities. A review of 172 treatment record charts of American Indian and Alaska Native women showed that their life conditions were extreme.

- Sixty-three percent had been separated from at least one parent as a child.
- A large percentage were physically, emotionally, or sexually abused as children.
- Seventy-eight percent had been abused as adults.
- Forty-nine percent reported an underlying health condition.
- Their partners were frequently unsupportive of treatment.
- After treatment, they returned to communities where substance abuse was widespread.

There are tribal differences in drinking patterns and in the consequences of drinking, but taken as a whole, American Indian women are more likely to die at a younger age from alcohol-related causes than American Indian men and white or black men and women.

When treatment providers stress the similarities between racial and ethnic groups, they commonly say, "We all have feelings," "I look at each person on an individual basis," "I see no color," "We're here to treat substance abuse, not to deal with differences," "An addict is an addict." They may mean well, but in essence they trivialize the conditions of their clients' lives. When they focus narrowly on the need to change as an individual, they imply that minority women must adapt to a sexist and racist society.

At AAFS and MIWRC, addiction is understood as one piece of a larger picture. At intake meetings, the staffers interview the clients extensively and try to ferret out the factors in their addiction. These factors may include domestic abuse; medical and legal problems; lack of job skills, housing, social support, and education; parenting problems; and destructive, misunderstood values and beliefs. All of these problems are within the purview of the agencies. If they can't address a problem directly, they make other arrangements. Child care is provided for women in treatment. At AAFS, if a woman has an abusive partner, they ask her permission to contact him as well. Abusive men, instead of being seen solely as perpetrators of violence, are understood in terms of a larger, unhealthy system, and are offered treatment and a chance to change. There is anger management for children who are acting out. Instead of viewing addiction as a relationship between a drug and a person, they see it as part of the fabric of a whole social world.

Since most of their clients have been through treatment elsewhere, it's important to discover what was missing at those other places. Along with the problems inherent in programs that aren't culturally specific, there's the problem of the quick treatment encouraged by insurance companies and HMOs. "When women have multiple issues, these programs can't provide the services," said Leslie Ann Sparks.

The programs at AAFS and MIWRC maintain many aspects of twelve-step-based treatment, including counseling by recovering addicts, an emphasis on complete abstinence, and ongoing support groups. AA or Women for Sobriety is strongly recommended, though many women find their chief sustenance in reconnecting with their church. Education and talk therapy—one-on-one and in groups—is a large part of the work of these agencies, but they emphasize that their talking is different. "The teaching at most centers is impersonal," said George Lewis of AAFS. "Here, we never give information without putting it in the context of someone's life. Before every lesson, each member of the group tells you about her week. If a woman says, 'I had an argument with my partner, and I felt like smacking him in the face, but I remembered the program and walked away,' we say, 'That's good; that's a great beginning. Now, suppose he blocked your way, suppose he stood in the door. What would you do then?' We use their personal experience to teach them something else."

Denise Bond at MIWRC told me that many women who can't be reached by talk will begin to trust when they're engaged in other ways.

"We offer massage and aromatherapy, and once a month, there's an option of going to a traditional sweat lodge, either Ojibwa or Lakota." MIWRC also offers a class in Native arts and crafts. Some women, while making dreamcatchers or moccasins, will open up in ways they haven't dared before. Their treatment takes another step forward. At the beginning of each week, the counselors burn sage, sweetgrass, and cedar. The women entering the building recognize the symbol of cleansing and purification. It's a small gesture, but it evokes pride in a common heritage, and it challenges the women's hidden feeling of shame and worthlessness regarding both themselves and their culture.

It is a place to come to terms with "cultural pain."

Many members of minorities consider a narrow focus on keeping sober appropriate to treatment, but others feel that not talking about race removes addiction from the context of actual life. It can even make them feel as if they have to sacrifice their racial identity in order to get sober. When treatment ignores social and cultural implications, it is unwittingly assuming a political perspective. This idea may be puzzling and annoying to, say, a white man who believes, quite rightly, that if he reforms himself and tends to his own ills, he will have access to a world of options. On the other hand, an alcoholic Native American woman who grew up on a reservation, whose ancestors were conquered by alcohol as surely as by gunfire, may bridle when she's told that her addiction is a purely personal problem. More important, such an approach may not give her the tools she needs to recover. Her dependence on alcohol may be so embedded in her culture that an understanding of that culture and her role in it is essential to her recovery.

It is understandable that counselors at treatment centers may want to avoid the topic of race. They may not feel competent to deal with it, or they may worry about their ignorance of a client's culture. They may not have dealt fully with their own prejudices and may fear that the treatment will get sidetracked from the real issue—the client's

addiction. They may worry that the client will use racism and prejudice as an excuse for her behavior, and won't "own" her own part in her
troubles. They may think they don't have the right to challenge the
client on the subject of race. Also, there is a long tradition of emphasizing what's common in the experience of alcoholics, and a belief that
accepting this commonality is a prerequisite to healing. But when a
recovering person has painful feelings about race and racism, those feelings need to be talked about and sorted through. Clients need help
sorting out realistic obstacles from a "victim posture" that may be used
to avoid taking responsibility for their behavior. Without such help,
their painful feelings are likely to continue to cause trouble, and to be
a factor in relapse.

In *Cultural Pain and African Americans: Unspoken Issues in Early
Recovery*, Peter Bell describes cultural pain as feeling "insecure, embarrassed, angry, confused, torn, apologetic, uncertain, or inadequate
because of conflicting expectations of and pressures from being a
minority and an African American," and he notes that all recovering
African Americans must learn to deal with the challenge of this pain,
or their ability to stay sober will be threatened.

I asked two counselors—one male and one female—at AAFS
about how they deal with the subject of racism and cultural pain in
treatment. As on the issue of confrontation, they had quite different
answers. The male counselor emphasized, "We don't have to approach
the subject of racism. The clients will. We don't, because we don't want
to give them excuses. If they feel racism is a serious piece of why they
feel the way they do, they will vent, and we will take it and use it to
help them. If a man rants and raves about not having the right opportunities, because white people stop him from doing this, that, and the
other, our question to that person is: What are you going to do about
that? We turn the responsibility back to him. We say, you may be
right, but that still doesn't tell me what you're going to do about it.
Are you going to use it as an excuse to keep on the way you are? Or are
you going to find a solution, and succeed in spite of it, instead of failing because of it?"

On the other hand, Leslie Ann Sparks said that the women rarely use race as an excuse. She emphasized educating women about their rights: "A lot of times, what the women talk about as racist is illegal! But they're terrified of challenging the system. So we educate them about their legal rights; we'll explain, for instance, that they don't have to take a complaint to their supervisor, they can go to the employee assistance program. We also help them process their feelings. They need to learn not to personalize the pain they feel, and not to let it jeopardize what they are trying to do for themselves."

African Americans may feel cultural pain in many situations— not just when they face overt or covert racism. They may also feel it when another African American seems to be denying her blackness, or when a white person expects them to explain or defend questionable behavior by other African Americans, or when they or other African Americans have two different sets of mannerisms, speech, and humor: one for blacks and one for whites. Peter Bell writes, "As African Americans in treatment or in aftercare, we usually feel great relief when we begin to look at the cultural pain in our lives. We realize we are not alone; we are not abnormal. As we share our feelings and experiences with other African Americans, we begin to rid ourselves of bottled-up secrets, and as a result develop more positive attitudes and new coping skills. When we share our problems, we also share solutions."

African-American Family Services

IN 1975, a group of African Americans in recovery saw that they were the exception to a rule—most African Americans were not getting clean and sober. These recovering addicts founded the Metropolitan Institute on Black Chemical Abuse, which later became African-American Family Services. They started up in the back of a barbershop and began reaching out to addicted inner-city blacks; and they were so successful that the community began requesting other services.

Today, AAFS has three offices in Minneapolis and Saint Paul, Minnesota, and more than twenty programs addressing such issues as

domestic violence, parenting skills, juvenile delinquency, and substance abuse. These programs are funded by a range of grants—some
national, though mostly from within the community—but the programs for male perpetrators of violence are hard to support. "The men
have been dismissed as just criminals, and nothing more," George
Lewis told me. "But they have their own stressors and their own pain,
and if things are going to change in our community, they need treatment too. Here, we're committed to the whole picture." AAFS works
closely with the child protection agency and the courts, which may
refer clients to them for assessment, and which sometimes make treatment and education a condition of probation. If their insurance or the
county will pay, some of the clients begin with inpatient treatment for
substance abuse at a local facility, but guidelines are getting much
stiffer. Many clients are not getting the inpatient treatment that would
give them time to assimilate new attitudes and behaviors before they
return to their lives, where all the old triggers of substance abuse are
waiting. This puts even more of a burden on the outpatient work done
at AAFS, which can last from twelve weeks to a year or longer and
includes preventing relapses. In an average year, more than 2,000
recovering alcoholics and drug addicts are actively involved in AAFS's
long-term aftercare support services. Because of their success with a
population that had been considered resistant to treatment, AAFS
counselors are often courted by other treatment centers with African-
American populations. For agencies from Russia to Belize, AAFS has
become a resource for information on culturally specific treatment.

A counselor in the women's program, Victoria, had arranged for me to
speak with herself and two other women, so that I could hear firsthand
the stories of women who were transforming their lives with the help
of African-American Family Services, and for whom addiction was one
piece of a large, complex picture. We agreed to meet at the headquar-
ters of AAFS, an imposing stone building that used to be the Franklin
Avenue Bank in Minneapolis. I walked up the massive front steps in
the bright sunshine and entered a large front hall paneled with dark

wood; it had a twenty-foot ceiling and a central reception desk like an island in a sea, with a grand central stairway behind it. The atmosphere was cheerful in spite of the dim stateliness. Clients and staff members chatted amicably with one another. Announcements of meetings and opportunities were pinned to the walls.

I was directed to a cavernous seminar room where Ruth, Victoria, and Pat waited for me at a table that must have been twelve feet long. The night before, I'd met Ruth, Victoria, and other women at the Saint Paul site of AAFS, in a cozy office in the somewhat shabby building, where I had explained my project and answered their questions. They had laughed and spoken freely, teasing one another and launching into their stories. Ruth came in late—she'd been walking her boss through a computer problem over the telephone—and announced that for her, and for most alcohol- or drug-dependent women that she knew, sexual abuse was the beginning of the path to addiction. The other women murmured. "I still remember what I was wearing the first time," Ruth said. "It was a beautiful fall day, and I had on a red-and-black-check flannel dress."

"That's what I remember too!" a woman named Jenny had said. "For my fifth birthday, my mother had got me a yellow-and-white-check pinafore dress. I was playing in the basement, and my uncle came down. He raped me in the coal bin. The dress got all dirty, and I threw it away. For years my mother asked me: 'Whatever happened to that dress?'"

I was struck by the matter-of-factness with which the women referred to childhood rape (an objectivity achieved through years of support groups and therapy), their easiness with one another, their mutual sympathy, and their jocularity. When the talk turned to prostitution, Ruth—who had now been clean for four years after drinking every day from age six to thirty-nine—said that until she quit, only three things made sense to her: money, sex, and drugs. "And it was easier to stop drinking than to stop doing tricks. Sober and *broke?*" She laughed. "Now *that's* a bummer."

This afternoon—perhaps because of the somber paneling in this

oversized room, or the ghosts of bankers looking over our shoulders, or
the tape recorder ticking on the table—the mood was tentative and
quiet.

RUTH

WE STARTED and ended with Ruth's story. She sat across from me; her
long straight hair was neatly combed, and she was wearing an embroi-
dered beige-on-beige blouse and a loose skirt. I reminded her of that
red-and-black dress—I'd woken in the night with those little girls'
dresses on my mind.

"I remember the dress because I liked it," she began. "I was
proud of it. It was one of those beautiful fall afternoons—sunny and
fresh—and I was walking home from kindergarten. As I approached
the corner of my block, I saw my godfather sitting on his porch. He
said, 'How was school today?' I always rode my bike around the block,
and he and his wife were friends of the family, so I stopped to talk on
the porch, and from there . . . We talked on the porch for a minute,
and then we went inside. He closed the door. I can't remember . . . he
might have given me candy. I was getting ready to leave and he stood
me up on a chair and started to kiss me and fondle me. I knew it was a
bad thing. I felt it was a bad thing. Right after, he said, 'Now don't go
home and tell your mom, 'cause you'll get in trouble,' and he picked
me up and set me down off the chair. I went home and it was really
scary. I walked into my mom's kitchen through the back door, and I
must have had a funny look on my face, because my mom asked me,
'What's wrong with you?' I was looking at her like she should be able
to *tell* that something's wrong, and she should be able to tell what it *is*.
And even though I'm saying nothing, I felt really hurt that she
couldn't tell."

I asked Ruth if she continued to be upset with her mother, and
she answered softly, "Real disappointed. Real abandoned."

For a while, she was able to avoid her godfather. One day he had
his wife call her parents and say, "What's wrong with Ruthie? We

haven't seen her for a while." The girl felt trapped. She went to see them, and the pattern of abuse began. He took her to an empty apartment—he owned two duplexes, and he always kept one apartment vacant except for a mattress on the floor. Their meetings continued every weekend and two or three times a week.

I wondered aloud how long the child Ruth had tried to avoid her godfather, and she looked a little upset, saying, "A lot of that is fuzzy . . ." and added, with a brave effort, "From the beginning he gave me an allowance. And he was giving me alcohol." I felt the presence of Victoria and Pat, as all three of us flushed with sympathy, sensing the shame Ruth still battles for having been—at the age of five!—seduced by attention, treats, money, and the numbing relief provided by a swig of bourbon. Shame is always inherent in sexual abuse, but it can triple in the girls and women who, in self-preservation, take what nurturing they can from their relationship with the abuser, and whose bodies—in spite of themselves—feel pleasure. The night before, Ruth had told me that the hardest thing for her to deal with when she became sober was the fact that her body had responded to her godfather.

I asked her about this now. "To me the term 'sexual abuse' meant bruises or being beaten," she replied. "It didn't mean a gentle sexual touch. How could I call him an abuser when he didn't harm me in that way? It didn't feel *painful,* though it was scary and painful in its own way. It was hard to admit that as I grew older, it wasn't so scary or painful anymore. . . . I never came out with all of this until I was in a sexual abuse survivors' group in my second treatment—the treatment I'm still clean from."

Ruth was a beneficiary of Minnesota's generous social services: the state paid for her first inpatient treatment of twenty-eight days, and six months later for another thirty days, followed by ninety days in a halfway house. She was then able to get a job—"a legitimate one," she jokes—and pay for four more months at a three-quarters house in Saint Cloud. Today, Minnesota still offers unusually liberal support, but in keeping with a national trend, its guidelines for treatment are much stiffer. A patient like Ruth would probably be allowed only ten days of inpatient care. Because of her relapse after six months, she would not qualify for time in a halfway house. Ruth feels certain that under these new rules, she would never have gotten sober.

I asked her if there were good things in her relationship with her godfather, and she told us about fishing trips, and how he taught her to use a 12-14-gauge shotgun. When she was just a little older, he took her along with him and his wife as they flew on jets to visit other cities.

"Wow, pretty seductive," I said, and Ruth laughed.

"Yeah, there were times, you know . . . A lot of the younger stuff is jumbled in my mind. There are specific times I remember, like when we were down at his mother's house in Kansas, and I was sleeping between him and his wife, and he was, you know . . . having a sexual relationship with me. He was entering me while I was in the bed facing toward his wife, and my back was toward him."

We were quiet for a while.

"I was about nine," said Ruth, "and that is the only recurring dream that I have. When I dream it, it's like watching me watch me get abused. So there are three of me. . . . His wife at one time slit both of her wrists, and I was told I shouldn't go down there for a while. I believe she knew what was going on."

"Your mother never knew?" I asked.

"My aunt has told me that my grandfather suspected, and he kept telling my parents, 'Don't let her go down there, something's going on.' My parents, I guess . . . being that my godfather had a lot of money, he used to buy my school clothes. There were ten of us, so that was a big help to them."

Silently, I tried to fill in the gaps. What did her parents have in mind when they handed their daughter over to her godfather, in exchange for a little support? After Ruth had been prostituted for the family at the age of five, her eventual career should have surprised no one. Nor should her long addiction. By the age of six, she was drinking nearly every day. She remembers stealing a little plastic bottle from her mother's suitcase—the kind that's meant for lotion or perfume—and filling it with liquor to take to school.

It has been theorized that the most devastating aspect of abuse is the child's isolation and abandonment. If the abuser is your parent, then the very person who is supposed to be nurturing you is hurting you instead—imagine the emotional complexity of running to your abuser for comfort. But even when a more peripheral adult is the abuser, the parents' failure to protect the child leaves her alone in the world.

Ruth recalled how lonely she felt when her parents failed to follow through on their suspicions—the time her mother questioned her about her dirty underpants, or the day her father put her in the car and said, "Show me where your godfather takes you." Ruth, in a panic, led her father to a place where she had never been.

Her godfather promised that the abuse would stop when she had her first boyfriend. "So I created one at the age of thirteen," said Ruth. He kept his word. Two years later, at the age of fifteen, Ruth ran away with a twenty-eight-year-old man; soon afterward she began working as a prostitute. At eighteen, she wrote her parents a letter detailing her godfather's abuse and the fact that she had drunk throughout her childhood. They didn't respond. At twenty, just before she added crack cocaine to her alcohol addiction, she visited her home and confronted them about those years of abuse. "Abuse?" they asked her. "We must have skipped over that part of the letter." They claimed, when pressed, that they didn't believe such things could have happened without their knowing. Ruth left their house and did not speak to them for twenty years.

"If your parents didn't nurture you, who did?" I asked her. She had such directness about her, such a way of connecting, it struck me that someone must have cared for her. Later, she would tell me about her brother, seven years older and a minister of the Nation of Islam. When she was brought home from the hospital, he named her Ruth, and he fed her and diapered her. She's still very close to him.

"Your godfather taught you to fish," I said. "He talked to you— did he nurture you in some ways, too?"

Ruth shook her head no. "He treated me like a woman," she said. "An adult woman."

"So you didn't get any nurturing from him."

"I remember the day my godfather actually entered me," she answered. "My school had gone on a tour of the Ramsey House—it used to be the governor's mansion—and I was so happy, so impressed with the nursery, where they had a big dollhouse and the grandchildren's original dolls. I kept talking about it, and my godfather said he'd take me back there on Saturday. So we went on the tour, and of course, like always, we stopped by one of his apartments. That was the day he actually entered me. I remember him panicking and saying, 'Okay, now, I'm going to have to get you a douche. You're going to have to take care of this so you don't get pregnant.' It was all on me. He made out like it was my fault."

I asked, "Were you old enough to get pregnant?"

"I was in third grade. I didn't have my period, but I bled from him entering me. So he got me a douche and made me take it, and then he showed me how to use a belt and put on the pad."

"Did he serve as a kind of mother to you?"

"No."

"He didn't tell you nice things, and make you feel . . ."

"He treated me like a woman. An adult woman."

"Did you ever feel abandoned by *him*?"

Ruth's face twitched a little. "It was so easy to cut off our relationship. I said, 'I have a boyfriend,' and he was like, 'Okay.' And that was it."

Sitting next to her, Victoria put her head in her hands.

"Plus"—Ruth's voice went up as if she were asking a question— "he adopted two little daughters, who were five and six at the time?"

With a sinking feeling, I asked the obvious question: "Did he abuse them?"

"That's what I hear," she said.

The women I interviewed have often told me it is therapeutic to revisit their traumas in the presence of sympathetic listeners, but I felt the devastation of Ruth's early life threatening to take us over. I reminded myself that this was a story of victory, since Ruth, somehow, had become the gracious woman sitting across from me. I asked her, "What was your motivation for getting sober?"

"I didn't want to live anymore," she said.

"So you had to choose . . ."

"Between life, being sober, or death. And that was it."

"And that was clear to you?"

"Very clear. I did not ever really have a very strong will to live. I never really cared. And I lived very carelessly, running crack houses, prostituting . . . I prostituted for about fifteen years . . ."

I said, "Last night you mentioned it was harder to give that up than the drink."

"Definitely," and laughing, she repeated the phrase of the evening before: "Being sober and broke was a bummer. Some of my clientele I had for fifteen years, so any time I called for money I could get it. And if I called for money and said, 'I'm in treatment getting sober,' I *really* could get it. I knew I couldn't do that. I knew if I did, I'd eventually use again. But it was real difficult not to call for money when you needed a cigarette. And still I'll run into ex-clients and"— she shrugged—"say no."

I wondered how she looked in the days when she was doing tricks, high on alcohol and crack, and what these ex-clients made of her now, this modest and sober woman, no makeup, a competent demeanor. They say in Alcoholics Anonymous that if you want to stay sober *everything* must change—your habits, your friends, your thinking, and sometimes even the clothes on your back. Ruth was a case in point.

"How long did you say you've been sober?"

"I have been sober . . . 1,407 days. It will be four years on June 16, and I'll be forty-one this month."

All of us smiled hugely, and when I asked what she was up to now, she told us that she was working as a chemical dependency assessor, going to school to get her certification for chemical dependency counseling, and working for a program that helps prostitutes find a better way of life. I remembered the banter of the night before, when the other women complained that they had no opportunity to bitch about being overworked, because Ruth—until recently working at three jobs and going to school—was busy around the clock. She explained that in therapy, she'd figured out that exhausting herself was an unconscious effort to deal with her shame. She hadn't believed she deserved a clean sober life: it had to hurt if she were to stay sober. In an effort to let up on herself, she let go of a job at another treatment center.

Referring to this, she said, "They gave me a party when I left. That was real different." Smiling, she added, "Usually I get shown the door."

VICTORIA

VICTORIA DESCRIBED HER MOTHER as an overprotective, competent, stay-at-home housewife, and she translated the plus side of that persona to the workplace, where, at AAFS, she had her hands on all the ropes, and, with a warm yet professional manner, encouraged her staff and her clients.

When I turned to her, she announced that she'd soon have been clean for five years, but then she became too distraught to speak. Recovering herself, she said, "My heart is still aching about Ruth's story! You know, I don't know how my own addiction got so out of control. I could be one of those where it's hereditary: my father was an alcoholic, and 90 percent of my relatives are, so alcohol was always in my life. I knew I liked the taste when I was about eight years old. My dad used to keep beer in the refrigerator and I used to pop the caps a little and suck a little out of each one. I thought he didn't notice!"

Victoria told us she never got along with her college-educated mother. "We were *never* close. I couldn't talk to her about anything." Her mother lorded it over her father, who had only an eighth-grade education and worked as a maintenance man at International Harvester. Victoria saw her mother as passive-aggressive and simply mean. Trained as a history teacher, she chose not to work, but she appeared downtrodden by the family's poverty, implicitly accusing her husband of being a bad provider. She disapproved of socializing in any way—she thought it was a waste of precious pennies—and wouldn't accompany her husband anywhere. Victoria remembers her father begging her mother to come with him to a banquet where he was to be honored for his volunteer work, and her mother saying she couldn't afford the clothes, and forbidding her husband to buy her any. "It looked like some kind of game to me," said Victoria. "You can be poor and still treat yourself!"

She sided with her father. "I was the only girl, the baby"—she has a brother six years older—"and my dad and I were real tight." Upset by the way her father begged and was rebuffed—and no stranger to her mother's sharp tongue—Victoria blamed her mother when her father skipped out for days at a time, and when he had girlfriends. Though they lived in the same house, her parents didn't have "a real marriage." Her father moved into a basement bedroom, and when he got drunk he came upstairs to her mother's room. "I'd wake up and they'd be arguing, and my daddy would go back downstairs. I was real resentful of my mother, because I thought she was just so square, and that was why my daddy stayed out, because she refused him in bed and she didn't drink."

Her voice warmed up, and she said emphatically, "I loved my dad; he could do no wrong. No matter how many times he didn't show up, no matter how many times he broke his promises, it was okay." Looking back, she can see that her mother's anger was largely because of her father's drinking, and she acknowledges that there were aspects of the marriage she never understood. Just a year ago, her mother revealed that her father—now long dead—had hit her a couple of times. "And I thought he was a perfect guy," Victoria mused. In the last few years, she had made an effort to repair her relationship with her mother, yet it's easy to see that for her, her father's warmth compensated for years of bad behavior, whereas the wounds from her mother's cold self-righteousness are still painful.

Early on, Victoria gave up on her mother, who, consumed by her

problematic marriage—and a little jealous of her daughter's relationship with her husband—tried to control her daughter's life but never
focused on her feelings or granted her respect, sympathy, or understanding.

Solidarity with Dad: "That's My Baby"

Victoria identified with her father, and this made her curious about
alcohol. "I loved my daddy, he wanted to drink, and I wanted to see
what it was about." At nine years old, she would sneak down in the
basement and taste his vodka. "It burned, but you know, I got the little buzz." At thirteen, she drank wine and smoked marijuana with her
friends. Her mother was on top of her at home—"she was on my every
move"—so she did most of her using with her church youth group. She
laughed now at the irony. "We'd all get together at the youth program
and go out in the back and get high. We'd go on retreats and take red
devils and yellow jackets, and this was the Christian youth retreat! And
we were falling all up and *down* the stairs. That's how my addiction
began, and it was *fun* then."

She recalled coming home from these retreats and, still high, staring up at the ceiling in her bedroom, while her mother, clueless, made
dinner. By the time Victoria was seventeen, she had tried "pretty much
everything except heroin and mushrooms," but her drug of choice—
just like her daddy's—remained alcohol.

In retrospect, it's heartbreaking to see the pattern developing—
with Victoria going away to be with her friends and coming back high,
deceiving her mother, angry, her needs unmet, just like her father. Imi-
tation, as they say, is the sincerest form of flattery. Her mother didn't
approve of her father, but Victoria approved of him. She, like so many
children of alcoholics, may have thought that if only she loved the
drinker enough, she could heal his wounds and make him feel good
about himself. Healthy and whole, he would turn to his daughter and
give her what she needed. She may also have wished he would act as a
buffer between her and her mother.

When a child believes she can control a parent by behaving in a particular way, her development gets stuck. She can't let go of the normal childish belief in her own omnipotence, because she needs it to feel safe. This desire for control is often noted in children of alcoholics, who are desperate to manage their chaotic environment. They are bound to fail. Sadly, this sword is double-edged. The child who tries to manage a parent's emotions does so because she can't feel good unless the parent is happy. Unable to identify her own subjective feelings, she doesn't learn that she can regulate them. Her emotional state depends on the moods of other people.

Moments of satisfaction reinforce a child's sense of mission. When Victoria recalled her father's pride in her, the occasion was her drinking. "My dad died when I was twenty-two, but before that I would see him in the bars, the local pubs, and he'd say, 'Oh, there's my baby!' I had this little air about me. I was real proper. He had taught me to drink top shelf, so when I ordered it was something fancy. He'd say, 'You gonna buy *my* girl a drink, gotta spend some money. That's my baby!' Being an alcoholic himself, he didn't recognize that I was in trouble."

Her father disapproved of drugs, however. When Victoria was fourteen, he caught her smoking marijuana in the bathroom. It was winter, and she was trying to blow the smoke out the window. He grabbed her by the collar, put her up on the windowframe, and yelled, "You think I'm so stupid I don't know what that stuff smells like?" It was the only time he raised his voice at his daughter.

Ever protective, Victoria said quietly, "He died before things got really bad for me, so he didn't have to see that."

Add Sex to the Picture

Victoria described her early sexual experimentation and her first taste of alcohol in similar terms: just what was this thing that her daddy liked so much? She told us an amusing story about an older girlfriend who decided she wanted to have intercourse with her boyfriend and took Victoria along to get birth control pills at the health department. Afterward, on the appointed day, Victoria tagged along with the girl, the girl's boyfriend, and the boyfriend's little brother. They went to an apartment building under construction and, said Victoria, the older kids went down in the basement "to do the wild thing."

"The little brother and I were supposed to be security, and then we decided that, well, why didn't we try it? And that's how I had my first sexual experience."

"Curiosity again," I said.

"Curiosity, and wanting to be grown up. In the community that I lived in, over in Saint Paul, it was real busy. And in the seventies there were all the black exploitation films, and there was a lot of prostitution in the area. I wanted to grow up and find out what everybody was doing. But those experiences were kind of devastating for me, because once I got my clothes off and I let the little brother play around and do what he thought he was going to do, then the older guys came and showed me what it was *really* about."

No one was laughing now, but Victoria said dramatically and comically, "Oh, yeah, I can *feel* that."

I asked if she had been free to refuse these older boys, and she said yes—there was an element of peer pressure, but mostly, she was curious about sex. The next day at the church program, all the kids were talking about her. Ashamed and confused, she stayed away from boys for about a year. When she got involved again, sex was definitely part of the plan. "I wanted to get attached to somebody and stay with him, and I thought that having sex was going to keep him. Because, you see, my mom and dad did not have sex—he was downstairs, she was upstairs—so I didn't blame my dad for having girlfriends. I thought, Well, I'm going to get a man and we're going to stay together, and I'm not going to deny him. I got into this mentality that if you want to keep the man, you have to do this."

I asked her, "But you also felt ashamed of it?"

"There was shame, and there was fear."

The fear was of being seen naked, and of being considered "loose" or "experienced." She explained, "A nice girl was a girl who made a man wait, date her for a long time, and who didn't really like sex, only just did it because the man wanted it. There were nice girls and party girls, and I didn't want to be a party girl."

Virgins and Sexual Slaves

Nice girls and party girls: an updated version of virgins and whores, women idealized as spiritual or scapegoated as sexually degenerate. In either case, they appear as men's objects, to worship and marry or screw and discard. When women buy into this age-old dichotomy, and think they have to choose, they're left disowning either their desires or their spiritual selves. Either way, they are depleted. As Audre Lorde argued in 1984, in her groundbreaking essay "Uses of the Erotic: The Erotic as Power," a woman's sexuality is deeply interwoven with her femininity and her spirituality. When it is corrupted or distorted by exploitation, the result is "a suppression of the erotic as a considered source of power and information in our lives."

Women of many cultures have been colonized by the dichotomy between virgin and whore, but black feminist historians such as Patricia Hill Collins have suggested that African-American women may be especially susceptible, in part because of the strong Baptist influence in the African-American community, and also because of the dichotomy that developed during slavery, between the image of the pure, passionless white woman and the primitively sexual slave. A black woman who accepts these images tries hard not to notice her own sexuality. Victoria, who very much wanted social acceptance, was humiliated by the knowledge that she actually liked sex, and not just the missionary position. Her struggle to mold herself into a good, pure woman further estranged her from her own body, and therefore from a sense of her own power.

Schooled in a family that ignored her needs, and in a culture that teaches girls to respond to the needs of men, she never thought of asking herself what she was feeling or what she wanted. She didn't know she had the power to manage her own emotions—except indirectly, by making a man feel good. If she made him feel good, then he might love her, and she would feel good too.

The stress that develops around such inner conflict would be hard for an adult to cope with—and not surprisingly, Victoria said, "it was easier when we were intoxicated. That stuff just went hand in hand. You have to drink and smoke a little weed, and then you have sex, and that's how you keep a man." It was during this time, her early teens, that her alcohol habit became entrenched.

The first man she "kept" was her high school boyfriend; their relationship lasted four years. "Once involved in a relationship, I was just real clingy. You just weren't going to get rid of me. No matter what he did, I'd be saying, 'It's all right, I'll be here for you, because I know you're a man and you've got to do what you've got to do.'"

That usually meant one-night stands. "If I was a man's main woman, I'd get to come out for a few hours early in the night, use my share of the drugs, and then the old boy was supposed to take me home, and then he'd go back and hang out with the big boys and the party girls. It was peer pressure—he wouldn't want to be a punk or look like he was whupped, so he'd drop me off and hang out with the players."

I teased Victoria, saying, "Couldn't you be a player?"

"A player? No no no no! You're either the good girl at home or the party girl. My boyfriend's family, his uncle and dad, were players, and he was intrigued by fancy cars and money and prestige and nightlife."

She laughed at my naïveté when I asked what "players" do. "There's players and hustlers. Hustlers usually do the illegal activities—after-hours gambling, drugs. Players just look good and work the ladies. Players were the kind of guys I was attracted to. Johnny Campus walks up and asks me out, I'd say *Oh, no*—too square."

Hypermasculine Culture

In their book *Cool Pose*, two black scholars, Richard Majors and Janet Mancini Billson, describe the hypermasculine culture Victoria refers to, outlining the ways young black men in the inner city establish a "rep" or reputation: by acting "loco"; adopting distinctive clothing, hand-shakes, hairstyles, hand signals, and nicknames; speaking in slurred obscenities; and engaging in heavy use of alcohol and drugs. As the rapper Ice T says, "You've got this walk, this attitude, that says: 'Don't fuck with me.'"

When Victoria described this world, she laughed and made us laugh—you could see her sense of fun, her appreciation of the show-manship of those "players" whose coolness is part of their public pose, who boast of criminal records, who love "fancy cars and money and prestige and nightlife." While it creates obvious problems, cool may have its roots in the African-American tradition of celebrating the "trickster," the wily, heroic predecessor of the "bad nigger," both of them resisters of white oppression—and in this sense, appealing to a community that has historically been exploited. This world, in which "bitch" and "ho" are generic terms for women, in which not being "whupped" is a prerequisite for manhood, and in which every woman needs "a main man," is a treacherous one for a woman to navigate in.

Victoria's illusion of control—her belief in her own power to make a man give her what she needed by being both a submissive, stay-at-home, good girl and a woman who gave her man some fun—was bound to be shattered.

Tricks Without a Pimp

When Victoria and her high school boyfriend broke up, her mood spi-raled downward and a big gap opened inside her. She tried to fill it with other men. She got pregnant, but the father of her child was see-ing another woman, who was also pregnant by him. Humiliated, she married someone else; she divorced soon afterward, vowing never to experience such emotional pain again. Since she didn't know how to be with a man "without going sticky on him," she would avoid relation-ships altogether.

Twenty-five and single, she tried to take care of herself and her baby by means of welfare and occasional jobs, but the problem was that "I liked living above my means." She liked nice things—clothes and jewelry and eating out—and she missed the buzz and excitement of criminal activities that she'd gotten used to from being with her boyfriend's family. Looking back, she thinks she was as addicted to the "lifestyle" as she was to alcohol. The problem as she saw it at that time was how to keep up that lifestyle without being dependent on a man, in a community where "business" and power were in the hands of men. In a series of psychological maneuvers designed to keep her self-respect—and true lovers at bay—Victoria took on a handful of older men who paid her to have sex: "more like sugar daddies," she said. The point was getting paid without having a pimp—a fairly subversive thing in itself—and furthermore, to work when she wanted to, for whatever she thought she needed.

In an ideal world—which is not where Victoria was living—she would have discovered better options, like education and a vocation. Yet I found myself deeply impressed by her resilience and her inventive adaptation to a difficult environment. Sex for money is hardly empowering, yet in her own way she was creating a space for herself. She was beginning a long struggle for autonomy and independence.

In conversation, Victoria, quite rightly, focused on her confusion and the alcoholic thinking that allowed her to live in such denial. "I considered those men to be my relationships, and today I know they were my *tricks*. I considered them my relationships! Because I didn't want to say the truth. Not until I got clean did I really face that and say, 'Yeah, that's what that was: it was *prostitution*!' No matter how I wanted to look at it."

A Female Supplier

This was only the beginning. In a culture where addicted women sell their bodies and addicted men sell drugs, Victoria broke the rules again when she became an equal partner with a supplier of crack cocaine—a man who was dating one of her friends. It started one afternoon when she was watching him weigh packages; she said: "I know enough people—I could sell some of that. No strings attached." Her supply went so fast that he tried her out with more, and it became clear that she had a knack for the business. "I never put any cut on my stuff—I served it like I got it, and it was stronger and straighter than most in the city. That's why my business was so good." Her partner soon trusted her to weigh the packages and count the money, and, ready himself to take a backseat—"He didn't want to be bothered with folks"—he essentially handed the business to Victoria. "He made me like the district manager and distributor," she said. "Anybody who wanted something had to come see me." Before long Victoria was making $4,000 a day—half went to her partner, half to herself.

Curious about the degree to which Victoria saw herself as playing a man's role and reversing the usual balance of power, I asked her if she had stopped tricking when she started selling crack—a stupid question, really—and her response was emphatic: "I was making $2,000 a day—no reason for me to trick! I didn't even want men in my life, because they wanted to get next to me and get my drugs and my money. If I felt like having some sex, *I'd* pick somebody. Take him to a hotel, wine him and dine him and then kick him to the curb!"

Meanwhile, Victoria was seeing how addicted women were treated by men in the business. Men made women do "nasty things" for drugs, and she was getting sick and angry as she got to know the wives and mistresses of her "colleagues." "Don't let this happen to you," they told her, and she told them, "You don't have to do that stuff with me." In solidarity, she found herself making loans and selling her stuff cheap to women.

Though her behavior was self-destructive and her well-being illusory, Victoria had respect among her peers, power, and financial independence. For the time being, she was at no one's mercy.

The Downhill Slide

Eventually, Victoria started using crack. Her customers taught her how, though she didn't see their motive at first. "I found out, boy, in the end," she told us. She made her voice go spacy, as if she were high,

and said, "Oh, yeah, here you go. You can have that, and I'll cook some
up, and I'll take this, and you want to buy this. . . . But they smoked
up more than they paid for before they left."

She began to take too much property instead of cash—something
she'd often done in a small way—and to overextend her credit. She lost
her apartment. When she got another one in the same building, somebody told her supplier that she had been busted and kicked out, and
now she was back in the same building because the police had set her
up, and she was snitching. Her supplier became alarmed. He trusted
her not to snitch, but he suspected that she was using. To test her, he
sent her to pick up a package and pay $900 out of her own money—
knowing she ought to have "large loot." Victoria, however, had smoked
her money up. She scrambled and managed to pay the $900 in one-
dollar bills, which she kept in shoe boxes in rubber bands. This cued
her partner in—she was in trouble.

Victoria shook her head, moved and troubled even now. Her relationship with her supplier had been a source of pride. He was a man,
but he wasn't her man, which meant that she was not under his control;
she was an equal partner. It was a rare achievement, one she clearly is
still proud of. "There was no physical relationship. It was strictly business. He had a lot of faith and trust in me. But a couple of weeks later
he said to me, 'Vicki, you're *sick*. You're getting sick now. This was
supposed to be about money, but I care too much about you. I know
you need some help, and the only thing I can do for you is not give you
anything else.'"

She tried to stay in business by getting another supplier, but
"they didn't like a woman out there trying to buy, and she's got no man.
Everywhere I went they always told me I needed a man, because they
didn't want me weighing their shit and telling them what's not right."

She found herself buying "lines" from the men she used to serve.
"They, you know, they made me . . ." Her voice trailed off and disappeared. When she spoke again, it was quietly. "They tried to make me
pay, and then it got to the point where sometimes I didn't have any
more money. I went from buying an ounce to a half-ounce to a quarter,

to trying to get an eight-ball, maybe three dollars short. And they start treating you bad! I got myself in a few ugly situations where I had to go into a room with my shirt off and wait for somebody to come with the package . . . even when I had money. But it wasn't a lot of money, so they treated me like the rest." By "the rest," Victoria means the rest of the women—the ones whose condition she had pitied, the ones who had warned her not to let this happen to her.

For a while, she stopped selling and stopped using crack. "When I stopped making money, I stopped using, and that's why I thought I wasn't an addict." She was still drinking, though, and still caught up in a criminal life.

"I got so tired of hearing I needed a man. I went to this gang moll, and she also said I needed a man, so she found me one. He had just got out of Stillwater—"

Ruth and Pat started laughing. They saw that I was confused.

Ruth said, "That's a prison."

"He'd come out of prison," said Victoria, "and she hooked me up."

I said, "And that was the solution, right?"

"Right!"

"The man came and saved you, right?"

"No," said Victoria. "The man came and he broke both my legs—"

"Oh, God," I said.

"—and I stabbed him and spent a night in jail, and"—her tone became facetious—"we were just using alcohol, because he didn't want that other stuff around, because it was nothing but trouble."

Having avoided men to preserve her independence, she now entered the most dependent, abusive relationship of her life. "I was thirty-five years old," she said, "and I had never been physically abused like that by anyone. This man was so controlling and domineering. . . ." Terrified, she drank whenever she was with him, and, never knowing when he might snap, she kept a knife in every room—on the window ledges, under the bed, in her underwear drawer. She wore her hair in spiral braids and stuck steak knives up into her hairdo. When he came at her one day—both her legs already in casts from his abuse—she grabbed a Boy Scout knife from the cushion on her chair and stuck it into his neck.

After a night in jail, Victoria got a restraining order on her boyfriend, but as soon as she got him out of her house, somebody else came and gave her a big package of dope, saying, "We know you can do this." Tempted—and frightened now of being on her own—Victoria accepted the offer. "Three months later," she said, "I was sprung and broke. I let that man back, because I didn't know how *not* to use crack, and I thought I needed him to keep it out of my life and keep the people away."

Predictably, the violence escalated once again, and Victoria decided that either this man was going to kill her or she would kill him. "In my mind I said, 'I'm going to kill him next time. The next time he raises his hand on me, I'm just going to kill him, and then, because of our history with the police, maybe I'll do six or seven years in Chockapee, and then—then maybe I can finally go to school. I'll get my degree in Chockapee, and then, you know, I can have . . .'"

At this moment, the extremity of Victoria's situation seemed to dawn on all of us. That little seed of hope inside the horror of her life—the thought of going to school in prison—was somehow devastating.

Finally I spoke. "You thought you had to kill him to go to school?"

"Yeah, because I didn't . . . That was really what was on my mind. In prison I could finally focus and be out from under this man, because I just was real twisted! I was twisted."

Getting Treatment, and Easing Him Out of Her Life

Instead of killing her lover, Victoria had inpatient treatment for alcoholism for ten days and then went to a halfway house, paid for by the county, for ninety days. She told her lover that he could come and see her only when he wasn't drunk. He tried to change her mind for about three months, but Victoria also had work and recovery meetings at AAFS, and she didn't waver. "He was going to have to find time between me being busy and his being drunk," said Victoria, "and he couldn't do it.

"This agency saved me. When I got out of the halfway house, I came to group meetings here every night of the week, because I was scared to be home. I worked at my little job in the daytime, took care of my son, was home for him when he got home from school. I cooked him some dinner, stayed with my kid, and then I would go to the agency. I might see my old man if he could manage not to be drunk between two and four, and then it was like, 'Oh, I've got to go to my meeting,' and that would save me, because I didn't have enough strength in myself to tell him to leave me alone.

"And he wasn't taking that—he wasn't going, you know? And he would get so violent. Those were times I thought I would relapse: when he called me, ranting and raving. I'd get that rumbling inside me, and I'd be looking around in my house, because I remembered where I used to keep the bottles. It would be automatic: look at those cupboards. Because that's what I would do. Carry a drink and a knife when I was with him.

"But instead I came to groups at AAFS every night. I'd tell him, 'I'll be back at ten o'clock, but you know you can't come over here if you're drunk.' He just couldn't do it, but he respected that, because we did, in a sick way, *love* each other.

"But he could not choose me over the chemicals, so eventually he eased on out of my life. Because I was busy."

I recalled the time sheets Victoria had showed me the night before—she gave them to her clients to make a plan for every half-hour of the day, so they don't find themselves at loose ends for an hour or two, and be tempted to use.

"No wonder you pass out those time sheets to people," I said. "They saved you."

"They saved me. I had to stick to it, no matter what was going on. I couldn't falter. Friends call, family call, I'd say, 'Well, you can stop by if you want to but I'm only going to be here for forty-five more minutes.' And some of them would come by and think they could dissuade me, but I said, 'Nope, van's coming, got to go.'"

"The van from the treatment center?"

"From here. It would come to get me every night, and I'd be *waiting*. And that would save me. I'd get home around ten o'clock; my baby and I would go straight to bed; then I'd get up and go to work. I did that until I got every certificate they had, two or three times, and they told me, 'Well, dang, make some coffee, set up some chairs, act like you're getting better.'"

We broke into laughter, and Victoria added, "I said *whatever*, just don't tell me I can't come back."

Flipping Between Two Poles

How did such an energetic, competent woman allow herself to be virtually imprisoned by an abusive man? For that matter, how did a woman who describes herself as "dependent" and "clingy" have the gumption to compete with hustlers selling crack cocaine? And when a woman has lived a life of risk and danger, has made thousands of dollars a day in illegal activities and wound up in jail for stabbing her lover, has navigated in a dangerous world, has been addicted, has committed herself to recovery, and has taken responsibility at work and at home, how can she still see her history as passive? "I lived vicariously," she told me. "I can't really say I did a whole lot, but I was always in the mix." If, as in some old assessment scales, you were to divide personality traits into those that are traditionally considered feminine or masculine, with submissiveness, dependency, passivity, warmth, and expressiveness at the one end, and aggression, self-reliance, and stoicism at the other, Victoria would be an interesting case. She'd have high scores on both ends of the spectrum, depending on the context. What she hasn't had—and today struggles to attain—is an integrated sense of her own potential, a choice about when to act out of one side of herself and when to act out of the other.

Her conflict about personal power and powerlessness was echoed by Ruth and Pat, and a woman named Louise I'd interviewed the night before—but it was played out in different ways. Ruth, traumatized and powerless the first half of her life, was left with a serious case of post-traumatic stress disorder, which a new study has found is more frequent and more severe among prostitutes than among Vietnam veterans. Yet she had begun to discover her own resources. By means of therapy, medication, school, a new vocation, and a commitment to helping other women, she embraced the work of mastering her own life.

Powerlessness, victimhood, and fear have seemed the only possibilities to Louise, who by age fourteen had been raped three times and as an adult spent seven months in a depression so deep that she had to be bathed and fed by her sister. Sober now for some time, her potential for anger was threatening to break through. "I can't stand it if somebody says something to me I don't like. I'm on them. This is not me. I don't like this person." Her psychiatrist told her anger is good and wanted her to check into a hospital and work it through, but Louise said she wouldn't go through that. "One time I started to get angry, and I think they almost had to put the oxygen on me. I started crying. I couldn't stop. I couldn't deal with it." At this point, Louise disowned her anger, saying it was part of some other "evil person." Her doctor wanted her to harness that rage to energize and motivate herself.

At the other extreme was Pat, who was with us that afternoon. Forty-three years old and sober for thirty days, Pat had a habit of getting into fights; she'd been jailed several times and was in treatment now because she didn't want to go back to jail. Where Louise shunned the experience of anger, Pat would do anything to keep from feeling vulnerable. She told us about watching her alcoholic grandfather abuse her sisters as she was growing up, and seeing those sisters become prostitutes. Early on, she determined to avoid their fate. A lesbian, she left little doubt about which end of the masculinity-femininity scale she wanted to emphasize. She was dressed in leather and chains, wearing tight black shorts, black ankle boots with white socks and chains around the ankles, a black leather choker an inch wide tight around her neck, and two metal links dangling down. Her necklace bore a silver cannonball.

USED BY ALCOHOL AND DRUGS

IT MAKES SENSE that Victoria, Ruth, Louise, and Pat would have inner conflicts about power and vulnerability, when you think of the outer conflict they've had with men, with their original families, and, as minority women, with the culture at large.

In the last twenty years, black feminist historians have analyzed how sexual oppression in their community is linked to, and hard to separate from, racial and class oppression. Though not excusing black men for their abuse of black women, they place this violence in the historical context of the lynching of black men, which was justified by the stereotype of the black rapist. The activist Angela Davis has suggested that one reason black women keep silent about rape and violence is that they are so alert to "the frame up rape charge as an incitement to racist aggression." At AAFS, George Lewis confirmed that this attitude persists: "A black woman might be in a bad situation for a while before she picks up the phone to get help. She knows the history of how black men are treated by police. She's not willing to expose her man to that. She convinces herself that it's an isolated experience and it won't happen again."

Alice Walker asserts:

> *At the root of the denial of easily observable and heavily documented sexist brutality in the black community—the assertion that black men don't act like Mister, and if they do, they're justified by the pressure they're under as black men in a white society—is our deep, painful refusal to accept the fact that we are not only descendants of slaves, but we are also descendants of slave owners. And that just as we have had to struggle to rid ourselves of slavish behaviors we must as ruthlessly eradicate any desire to be mistress or "master."*

When life presents a series of either-or options—slave or master, weak or strong—and when the image of the brutal slave master is the internalized alternative to slavery, black men who wish to be strong and free have a dangerous model.

Similarly, as Patricia Hill Collins argues in her book *Black Feminist Thought*, poor black prostitutes today cannot be understood without taking into account the historical legacy of their forced prostitution. Black women, from their arrival in this country, were sexual hostages. Naked on auction blocks, they were objects of voyeurs. As slaves, they were used as breeders and routinely raped by their masters. Rape was not just an expression of lust but a political tool used to demoralize slave women and their men, to weaken their will to resist, and as an aspect of economic exploitation, since mulatto slaves brought a higher price. Used in this way, black women soon came to stand for illicit and wicked sexuality in the imagination of white people. White men blamed them for their own carnal desires, and white women concurred—this protected them from having to confront their husbands' behavior and allowed them to share in the profits of slavery.

No matter that they had been bought and sold against their will, treated and imagined as animals, the idea of African-American women's illicit sexuality consolidated during the antebellum period and followed them through the great migrations of the first decades of the twentieth century. To this day, poor African-American women must deal with the image of themselves as sexually promiscuous and potential prostitutes.

When such historians as Patricia Hill Collins explore how race, gender, and class oppression have invaded the private lives of individual women and men, they illuminate the mechanisms that, when internalized, lead people into violence. Once the dynamics are clearly seen, alternatives become possible. In recent years, popular conservative critics have insisted that problems within black communities are a natural outcome of detrimental values and attitudes, and that the cry of "racism" is being used to excuse "black pathologies," which should rightly be blamed on the negative aspects of black culture. Such a simplistic account ignores not only a range of contributing factors, but also the fact that understanding the forces of racism and how they become internalized is a crucial step in taking responsibility for one's own attitudes. By naming the external sources of oppression, African Americans can more clearly recognize their own collusion. Far from claiming the privileges of victimhood, they undertake an exercise in empowerment, which can lead to the very hard work that Alice Walker refers to as the struggle not only "to rid ourselves of slavish behaviors" but to "ruthlessly eradicate any desire to be mistress or master."

And what does all this mean to an individual African American who picks up a bottle or gets high on heroin or crack cocaine? At AAFS, a poster offered a provocative interpretation. Above a strong black wrist bound in white cloth, used syringes in the palm of the hand, the caption read, "Yo, Slave!" It may be that drugs are as potent a master as any white man ever was—as destructive to health and happiness and as far-reaching in consequence, the damage cycling through generations, and as difficult to throw off. Like slave masters, drugs and alcohol divide families, separating children from their mothers as the state places them in foster homes. Worse, an addict believes she needs this particular master. At first, anyway, the pleasures it offers are in proportion to the pain. Alcohol and drugs seductively trick you into thinking you are in control. By offering a predictable high, they give you an illusion of managing your own feelings. Interestingly, in a study of African-American college students, women more than men reported that alcohol was useful for "feeling in charge" and "relieving emotional distress."

"I used it to cope," said Louise. At first, you think you are using alcohol or drugs. Only later do you realize that they are using you.

THE SCOPE OF THE PROBLEM

STUDIES OF AFRICAN-AMERICAN women and alcohol come up with contradictory findings. According to a few researchers, African-American women are less accepting than men of using alcohol to have fun: they disapprove of drunkenness generally, and more so if the drunk is a woman. But there is also research suggesting more tolerance of women's drinking among blacks. Blacks, both women and men, are more likely than whites to abstain from drinking altogether (46 percent of black women compared with 34 percent of white women; and 29 percent of black men compared with 24 percent of white men); but if they do drink, they may be somewhat more likely to drink heavily.

Trying to make sense of why black women's habits and attitudes are clustered at the two extremes, some analysts note opposing historical influences. On the one hand, the antislavery and temperance movements of the 1800s were closely linked, and fundamentalist religions, which forbid drinking, have shaped African-American values. On the other hand, prohibitionists often expressed white supremacist views, which, along with migration of African Americans to Northern cities in the 1920s and 1930s, helped to erode temperance. During this time, urban black nightclubs began to flourish in Harlem, Chicago, and San Francisco, and for both women and men, alcohol became associated with "sophistication and the good life."

A study based on a national survey of 1,947 black and 1,777 white men and women found that a given rate of heavy drinking created fewer problems (in health and daily life) for black women than for black men or whites of either sex. The author speculates that the black women could be protected by higher body weight. These results are hard to reconcile with disturbing statistics. Death from cirrhosis of the liver is 73 percent higher among black women than white women, and black alcoholic women die at nearly twice the rate of white alcoholic women. Furthermore, the incidence of fetal alcohol syndrome is about seven times higher among blacks than among whites. Black women are less likely to drink than white women, but when they do, the consequences to their health can be more extreme. It is not clear why.

You can't get the full picture by looking at alcohol alone. AAFS finds that the primary drug of most of its clients is crack cocaine, with alcohol often in the background. The National Client Data System, which collects information from substance abuse treatment programs that receive public funds, reported that in 1991, 72 percent of black women listed "other drugs" besides alcohol as primary, compared with 39 percent of white women; and only 12 percent of black women listed alcohol as their primary drug, compared with 38 percent of white women. (Sixteen percent of black women were equally addicted to alcohol and other drugs, compared with 23 percent of white women.) Smaller studies in various parts of the country show a similar pattern. In a study of sixty-three women in recovery from alcohol and other drug addiction on the Texas Gulf Coast, for instance, 76 percent of the Anglo women listed alcohol as their primary drug, whereas 72 percent of the ethnic minority women (almost all African American) cited cocaine-crack as primary. Their burgeoning AIDS rate—it is sixteen times higher among black women than white women—is partly due to sharing needles, having unprotected sex while using drugs, and trading drugs for sex. The overwhelming majority of HIV babies were infected by their mothers.

It is misleading to think of race as the primary factor accounting for variations in drug use. In 1991 the National Household Survey on Drug Abuse found that overall, blacks are four times more likely than whites to use crack cocaine, but when researchers separated out a range of other factors—including socioeconomic status, region, gender, and age—they discovered that the differences between the races were no longer significant. This is very important information, as it suggests that poverty and other variables—and black women are more likely than white women to live in poverty—may be more important than race in influencing drug use. In total, 2.2 million white women use drugs regularly, outnumbering all minority women combined (846,000).

It remains true that African-American women who drink or use drugs are suffering inordinately. Not only do they face more extreme health consequences, they are also more likely to be criminalized. When pregnant women who abuse alcohol or drugs are compared, black women are almost ten times more likely than white women to be reported to child abuse authorities. Since 1985, more than 200 pregnant and postpartum women in thirty states have been criminally charged for drug-related behavior—including delivering drugs to a fetus through the umbilical chord—and most of these women are black. They are caught in a bind: often sexually and physically abused as children, often victims of assault and rape, they face the wrath of society for being unable to protect their children. They are, in fact, links in a long chain, with plenty of blame to go around. Many want desperately to shake off their addictions, but they are frightened that if they reveal their histories of drug and alcohol abuse to professionals, they will meet with punishment instead of help.

PAT: EIGHT LITTLE PUPPIES IN A DOGHOUSE

PAT, WHO HAD been sober for only thirty days, began her story shyly, her eyes cast down, telling us she was in a bad state. Every day she wanted desperately to drink. She wasn't sure she was going to make it. She had a tendency to get into fights and wind up in jail. Her longtime "woman" had dumped her. She wanted her woman back and wanted to stay out of jail, and she figured she'd have to stay sober to achieve either goal.

Pat was raised by her Baptist grandparents, who were "real religious people, real strict people." She resented her grandmother for imposing so many household rules, for whipping her, and for making her come inside when the other neighborhood children were outside playing. The house had to stay perfectly clean and neat. The children had to dress and speak a certain way. In the background, Pat's grandfather was abusing her older sisters—which may have had something to do with the grandmother's furious attempt to impose control in some other arena. With dry humor, Pat described a picture of a doghouse with eight magnetic puppies that hung on the kitchen wall, each puppy bearing one of the children's names. "When my cousins came around, they'd go to the wall and say, 'Now, who's in the doghouse today?'" Pat felt ashamed when her little puppy was there, and begged her grandmother to take it out.

I noted the suggestion of sadomasochism in Pat's clothing—all the leather and chains—not to mention her big strong appearance, and I thought of all the shaming she described. Pat described her own belligerence and violence when she was drunk, but today, sober and shy, she was graceful and refined in her movements, and she spoke in a warm, low voice, with crisp pronunciation. I imagined that I could hear her grandmother's coaching in her precise consonants.

Pat grew up longing for her mother, whom she described as "a gypsy." "I always wanted to know why I didn't live with her," she said musingly, with a notable lack of anger. "She lived all over the place, and I didn't see her much, but when she did come around, I was really happy. I always hated to see her go."

Her relationship with her grandmother reached its lowest ebb when her grandmother found out that she was lesbian—"She sent me to a psychiatrist," exclaimed Pat, "and she told my preacher!" Victoria, Ruth, and I burst into laughter, and Pat gave us a wry smile. "Now she loves my woman," she told us. She recently made up with her grandmother, "Because she's just so old," said Pat with obvious affection. "She's teeny tiny and so weak, and I look at her and just can't believe how scary she used to be when I was little. I forgive her now. She *thought* she was doing right by me. She didn't know any better."

She got anxious when she told us her biggest problem. She had no job. She'd been working as a nurse's aide when her employer discovered her police record and fired her. This event had provoked the latest round of violence and bingeing. She had been so happy at her work and had been doing well. Now she had no money coming in. She was going for job assessment interviews and taking tests.

At this point Ruth broke in, with a big smile. She told Pat about a program through a division of rehabilitation services, which offers education and job training to minority women who want to get off, or stay off, welfare. "I just discovered it," said Ruth. "It's perfect for you." They made arrangements for Ruth to pass on information. I recalled what George Lewis told me: fully half of the jobs their clients get are found by other clients. They form a strong and supportive recovery network.

Pat didn't seem to want to talk much more, and it looked as if the interview was coming to an end. The four of us fell into a casual discussion about our parents' attitudes toward drinking, and how they were generally stricter with their girls than with their boys. Ruth seemed distracted. She kept glancing out the window. The evening before she had described how odd sounds and gestures could trigger panic, and how she was learning to ride out her body's experience of anxiety, while reminding herself that she was no longer in danger. Though she'd fought off taking medication for a year, she'd given in when she tried to go to school and simply couldn't concentrate. Her psychiatrist explained that her brain had been chemically damaged by her trauma and by alcohol and drugs. When he persuaded her to take 40 milligrams of Paxil and 300 of Wellbutrin, both antidepressants, her grades shot up. During this interview, both she and Victoria occasionally became trembly, and Ruth would get a kind of twitchiness around her face; but very quickly, they would be back in the room with us, totally focused and present. This was different. Ruth's agitation was rising. She played with her hands and blinked heavily.

Finally, she cut into our conversation. "The only thing I did want to add," she said, "as a piece of my story, and I guess I've been so much in denial about it, it's sometimes hard to talk about it . . . but that's about my sons. My kids. I do have children."

RUTH: WHAT TO DO WITH HER CHILDREN

ONCE AGAIN, the room fell silent.

"I'm a grandmother, actually," said Ruth. "I have a twenty-three-year-old daughter, a thirteen-year-old daughter, and two sons, five and six. And, uh, the twenty-three-year-old is an addict. She's lost three children to the system." Ruth described how she sent her thirteen-year-old to live with her father when she went into treatment for the first time, and called the county to have her two young sons put into foster care. When she got out, she lasted barely two weeks before she was drinking again. She got a job and tried to get clean so that she could get her sons back, but she found she couldn't do it. She became suicidal.

After her second treatment, when she'd been clean for about three months and was living in the halfway house, the county came to her and said, "It's time for you to get your sons back. They've been in the system a long time, and you're clean; you're doing well." She told them she wasn't ready. "I didn't want to find myself caught . . . in the system again, staying home on welfare with two sons and . . . *caught*." When she had been clean for six months, the county came to her again and told her she had to make a decision; she had to take her sons back or terminate her rights.

"I prayed and prayed on it," said Ruth. "I felt I had to give my sons the best chance at life, and give myself a chance. When I had been clean for nine months, I terminated my rights."

Deliberately, she repeated, "I terminated my rights to my sons. I was able to see them up until last April, when they were adopted. I won't be able to see them anymore."

I pushed away thoughts of my three-year-old son at home in Vermont.

Ruth said, "It was the most painful experience I've had clean. Letting them go. They had already gone through enough."

With her youngest son, she told us, she was three months pregnant before she knew it. She was working at a sauna, making about $1,500 a week. When she went to have an abortion at four months, she was already too far along. She kept on drinking and smoking crack cocaine daily. At six and a half months of pregnancy, her water broke, but she kept on smoking for two more days. "I was trying to kill myself," she said. A girlfriend came by and said that she was going to call the police if Ruth didn't get to the hospital. Ruth made a motion to go upstairs to get her suitcase. When she got up from the sofa, there was blood all over it. She smoked all the way to the hospital.

The baby weighed two pounds and three ounces, and Ruth was so ashamed that she couldn't bear to see him. "I wanted to die. I remember saying, let me die, die, die. My heart kept stopping, and I kept fighting them to leave me alone, and they kept bringing me back, and I prayed, *just let me go.*"

I asked if she was happy with where the boys are now, and she said, "Very. I don't know exactly where they are, but I know it's with a family where they have a chance." Her voice got livelier. "They're together. They're eleven months apart, and they're together. And they are very close. I'd always tell my son, Phineas, *take care your brother Reggie.*'" She laughed softly. "He'd hit him upside the head, and say, 'Okay, ma.' I told him he was doing a good job."

"Maybe he'll remember that," I said.

"Yeah. So, I've got a picture. Yeah, I'm very happy with my decision. Even with my thirteen-year-old being in Atlanta. I'm going to keep her there. I just, um, I'm scared. I'm not willing to take any chances."

"You don't trust yourself?"

"It's not myself so much as *being caught*. Not being able to keep accomplishing my goals. I know that going to school, going to work, helping others, going to meetings, getting up, knowing what I have to do and where I have to be . . . it's what's keeping me clean. I know that staying at home with my kids on welfare did not keep me clean. Okay? I can't distinguish. . . . I've never been clean in my entire life, my entire life of raising children and the drinking and the dope game and the prostitution—that's all I know. I don't know if I'm capable of being a mother, I don't know if I *am* one. I know that I gave birth."

I wondered how Ruth's godfather could have brought on so much destruction so thoughtlessly. What story would Ruth's children tell about the suffering in their early lives? And how would their children fare? So much misery tracing back to one man.

It was time to wind up the interview and walk out into the lobby of AAFS, where people take a larger view. No doubt, if Ruth's godfather were standing before us he would have a compelling story of his own. Though individuals needs to take responsibility for their own part, no one can change without a glimpse of his or her role in the larger machinery, and no larger change can happen without what is being done at AAFS—the patient, endless work of stopping the cycle. The work begins when people like Ruth and Victoria, and with luck

Pat and Louise, take a huge risk, leaving behind their old defenses and coping with shame and anxiety attacks and fear—not to mention violence and worries about money—without the help of their old friends alcohol and crack. Doing this, one of them said, feels like walking into gunfire without any armor. Especially in early sobriety, the world is a very frightening place.

"So you've got a whole new life," I said to Ruth.

She said, "I've got a whole new life."

Recovery:
Only Connect

THE RECOVERING WOMEN WHOSE STORIES APPEAR IN THIS book journeyed out of their addiction on paths nearly as various as their personal histories, but most of them had some kind of treatment and follow-up care. The good news is that women fare as well as men in alcoholism treatment, in spite of the fact that most treatment programs were designed for men, and women are expected to fit in.

WHAT TREATMENT IS

TREATMENT FOR WOMEN and men who are physically dependent on alcohol begins with detoxification. Withdrawal can be dangerous, even life-threatening. About 10 percent of alcohol-dependent patients need to be hospitalized for detoxification, and even in less severe cases, medication can ease withdrawal symptoms.

Inpatient treatment used to be considered the foundation of early recovery, but it is expensive. Some studies show inpatient treatment to be highly effective, but their results cannot be generalized because they do not include formal outpatient treatment groups for comparison. Studies that do compare inpatient and intensive outpatient treatment have found comparable long-term outcomes. Some people object that when researchers randomly assign patients to treatment modalities for purposes of comparison, they are not taking individual needs into account, which skews the results—because, for example, people who, if left to their own devices, would choose residential treatment may be the ones who would profit from it most. Nonetheless, many insurance companies have dropped coverage of inpatient treatment, except for detoxification.

Residential treatment is still preferred when a patient's life is especially chaotic, when her medical or mental health problems need close monitoring, or when outpatient treatment hasn't worked. It may be followed by a period in a halfway house, where patients live with other recovering alcoholics who can offer insight and support, and where they may work and go to school while still supported by a structured environment.

Outpatient treatment, which may follow a two- or three-day hospitalization for detoxification, also has advantages. It's less expensive; in less intensive programs, employed patients can continue working; and they receive treatment while faced with all their usual pressures and all their usual triggers of drinking, so they have a lot of support as they make changes.

Both in- and outpatient treatment usually involve alcohol education, group therapy, and training to prevent relapses. Ideally, the alcoholic's family is brought into the process; indeed, for teenagers, family therapy has emerged as the most effective treatment. Counselors also work individually with patients to address problems and develop a long-term treatment plan. Medications may be prescribed to help reduce the craving for alcohol or to treat depression and other psychiatric disorders. Some doctors offer their patients an alcohol-sensitizing medication such as Antabuse, which causes nausea, vomiting, and other unpleasant effects when combined with alcohol. Both residential and intensive outpatient treatment may be followed by extended aftercare, which involves more group therapy and individual counseling.

Today, most (but not all) treatment programs in the United States are based on the disease model of alcoholism and the twelve steps of

AA. Early treatment tends to focus on the first two steps: admitting powerlessness over alcohol (overcoming denial) and coming to believe that a higher power can "restore us to sanity." Long-term participation in AA or another recovery group is strongly recommended.

Women who live near a major city or a university may have more options, for example, cognitive behavioral therapy. This approach is based on the premise that even when genetics are a factor, alcohol abuse is a learned behavior, a bad way of dealing with problems or meeting needs. When people can identify the most powerful triggers of drinking—anger, depression, pain, seeing other people drink—they can learn to break the connection. They can also learn skills to change their behavior or avoid problems that lead them to drink. Some twelve-step-based programs have been suspicious of cognitive behavioral approaches but are now incorporating these methods into treatment, especially for preventing relapses.

"Harm reduction" and "moderation management" are highly controversial approaches, primarily because they allow the patient to set the goal, even when that goal is controlled drinking instead of abstinence. Proponents cite studies that find that a certain percentage of alcoholics do return to controlled drinking. They say controlled drinking—even if punctuated by binges—may be the best possible outcome for a determined drinker who would otherwise not make an effort. And some people who are not dependent on any substance, and have only a short history of alcohol problems, may reasonably wish for help in cutting back without becoming teetotalers. It's a pragmatic approach that suits certain people, but it has caused a lot of anger among those who have seen it seized on by women and men for whom it is not appropriate, because it feeds a fantasy that they can drink in moderation, though their history has proved otherwise.

Among women who are not severely dependent on alcohol, a brief intervention delivered by a trained physician or another health care professional—involving assessment, strategies for change, goal setting, and follow-up—may be all that is necessary. There is a growing effort to standardize and evaluate such interventions, especially as it becomes clear that they may be a powerful tool for the early treatment of alcohol problems.

WOMEN'S NEEDS

WE ARE LEARNING more about women's treatment needs, but we have a long way to go, according to Dr. Camille Barry, acting director of the Center for Substance Abuse Treatment, who told me, "Traditionally treatment has been geared for men. We know much more about what works for men than for women."

For women, the obstacles begin before treatment starts, since their families may be less supportive of treatment. The evidence for this is partly anecdotal—women in treatment who report that their husbands discouraged them from getting help and sometimes left them when they did—but it bears on the findings of a large-scale investigation of treatment referrals made by employee assistance programs. In this study of 6,400 full-time employees from eighty-four work sites, wives were often instrumental in encouraging their husbands to seek help for alcohol problems, but husbands were rarely a force in their wives' referrals.

Treatment for addictions can be costly, and women are especially hurt by cuts in federal funding. Said Camille Barry, "Women are more expensive to treat, especially if they have children. They're hesitant to go into treatment and stay if their kids can't be there with them, but this creates another unit of cost, and another barrier to treatment." As we have seen, women's addictions are often intertwined with relationship problems, they are more often victims of domestic and sexual abuse, and they frequently have mood or eating disorders. All these issues need attention if treatment is to work. "The level of awareness has been raised considerably," said Barry, "but we still have a great need for wraparound care, which is more important to women."

Today, women are still more likely to be underemployed and underinsured than men. Young women are often in low-paid jobs without benefits. In a study of men and women between ages forty-five and sixty-one, 72 percent of the men had health insurance provided by their employers, compared with 55 percent of the women; 13 percent of the women and 7 percent of the men lacked any sort of coverage at all. Even among women who work full-time, insurance coverage may be less adequate than men's. In the work site study mentioned previously, administrators of employee assistance programs indicated that among the women they referred for alcohol treatment, 22 percent did not receive the most appropriate recommendation because of inadequate insurance. This partly explains why 14 percent of these women were referred to inpatient care, compared with 30 percent of men. Minorities are even more severely affected. A study in California showed that white women entering treatment are ten times more likely than African-American women to have insurance. While women and minorities are affected most, money is a problem for most people seeking treatment. As we have noted, insurance companies often cover only hospital detoxification or outpatient services, and case management systems usually limit inpatient coverage to two or three days even when a clinician recommends a longer stay. The number of outpatient sessions may also be sharply limited. Publicly funded programs often cannot provide the range of services women need, and in particular, there is very little follow-up case management. Under these circumstances, the women who need help most are least likely to receive it.

Many clinicians in this country believe that women fare best when treatment is delivered in a setting that takes into account their interactional styles (women talk less in mixed groups); that addresses their roles in their family and society in ways that empower them; that does not allow sexual harassment; and that makes other services available, such as child care and job and relationship counseling. One well-designed study compared women-only and standard mixed-gender treatment. The two groups received comparable levels of care, but the women-only program focused specifically on women's problems. Women in the specialized program were more likely to complete treatment and had better outcomes than the women in the mixed-gender group.

Among the women I interviewed, the aspect of treatment most

consistently neglected had to do with the link between sexuality and problem drinking. As we have seen, we now have good evidence that sexual dysfunction is a powerful predictor of continuing alcohol problems in women. Sometimes alcohol itself has damaged a woman's sexuality, but more typically, the dysfunction precedes drinking problems. We know that many women and girls begin their sexual life under the influence of alcohol and are frightened by the prospect of having sex without it. Recovering women consistently report feelings of sexual shame. For example, Daphne cringed because of humiliating sex she'd had with her husband while drunk; Stephie couldn't bear the thought of sex for months after she became sober; Tamara castigated herself for having slept with men for drugs. All these women went to treatment that was excellent in other ways, but none got help with the sexual problems that plagued them well into sobriety.

Ronald Kadden, a professor in the department of psychiatry at the University of Connecticut School of Medicine, told me, "Treatment providers feel awkward with the topic, so they don't bring it up, and if they're uncomfortable, when they're trained, imagine how the woman feels. Ultimately, it is the provider's responsibility to raise issues of sexuality." Indeed, women in treatment are already feeling vulnerable, ashamed, and unwell, with limited emotional resources. Some, like Stephie, may worry that they will have to choose between sobriety and marriage. It does not have to be this way. "The tools are there to help women," said Kadden. "Women can be advised to take it slow and lower their expectations. They should know that if they've had a problem with sexuality, it might get bigger for a while. Couple sessions and sexual counseling can also make a big difference. There is help out there, but treatment programs may not be vigilant." The reality is that if women don't ask for help with their sexual anxieties, they're not likely to get it, and they'll have to deal with a continued source of stress. Stephie finally got support by forming a Women for Sobriety group where, to this day, she told me, sexuality is the number one topic. Women are enormously relieved to have an opportunity to work through their feelings with others who understand and have had similar experiences.

Finally, women who have another disorder along with their alcoholism are not getting adequate care. The situation is better than it used to be. Now, at least, many substance abuse treatment providers recognize that psychiatric problems do need immediate attention. They are less likely to recommend that a patient wait for a year or two of stable sobriety. But an alcoholic woman who, for example, suffers from depression related to a history of childhood abuse may find that she is assigned three different modes of treatment: group therapy and alcohol counseling for her addiction, visits with a psychiatrist to dispense medication, and individual therapy to deal with her personal history. This approach can work, especially if the therapist is well trained and can assist the patient in integrating all the treatment. But too often, the woman feels fragmented. Different treatments seem aimed at different problems, and she is expected to pull it all together and not just feel like a bundle of pathologies, needing pills and a whole array of doctors.

Between 30 and 60 percent of drug and alcohol abusers—women more often than men—have a concurrent mental health diagnosis. In the past ten to fifteen years, the inadequacy of treatment for this population has become apparent. The Substance Abuse and Mental Health Services Administration has piloted a multisite study developing new forms of integrated treatment. The National Institute on Drug Abuse is now emphasizing research into developing treatments to work effectively with people who have particular constellations of problems. One of these, called "Seeking Safety," was developed by Dr. Lisa Najavits at Harvard Medical School. She has had initial success using twenty-four sessions of cognitive-behavioral therapy with addicted women who also suffer from PTSD. "Safety" is the unifying theme, embracing the goals of discontinuing substance abuse, getting out of dangerous relationships, managing symptoms such as panic, and minimizing exposure to HIV.

Women with financial resources and good insurance coverage will have a range of treatment options, including private, residential programs across the country. Otherwise, what a woman finds when she goes for treatment depends largely on where she lives. In Illinois, for instance, programs based on the family unification model, with children living in residential programs with their mothers, have been in place since 1985, whereas the neighboring state of Michigan is only now developing their first such program.

Unfortunately, many of the recent gains in understanding women's needs cannot be implemented, due to budget cutbacks and managed care restrictions. "We were in a better situation in 1990 than we are now," said Nancy Paull, executive director of Stanley Street Treatment and Resources (STARR) in Fall River, Massachusetts. For example, said Paull, for about six years, STARR had same-sex units for detoxification. At first, the men fell apart. "They stopped showering and caring for themselves," said Paull, "and the nurses joked about bringing up women for visits so the men could clean up their act." Once the change was established, and men knew they were entering an all-male program, they began to do better, becoming "less macho" and more open. The women thrived from the beginning. "Women are coming in with histories of domestic violence and sexual abuse," said Paull, "and when men are around, they won't deal with these issues. When we started an all-female detox unit, they opened up. They were more receptive to treatment and more focused on what they were doing and where they were going." A few years ago, STARR was obliged to combine the units to save money, and immediately the staff saw negative results. The week I spoke with Paull, a woman had left treatment against recommendations because she "fell in love with a wonderful guy" who was also in detox. "She thought he was going to rescue her," said Paull. "They went off into the sunset. Within four hours he had dumped her." The woman wanted to be readmitted to the program, but she was turned away, because she had left against medical advice.

When possible, a woman or her family looking for treatment should consider her particular needs and look for a comfortable match. But it's worth remembering that a motivated person can take advantage of any well-run program. A study that matched patients to the most appropriate treatment—considering such factors as drinking behavior, social functioning, and personality—found, surprisingly, that a variety of people did equally well in all three forms of treatment studied: motivational enhancement therapy (which aims to strengthen patients' commitment to change), cognitive-behavioral coping skills therapy (training in self-management skills), and twelve-step facilitation (prompting active participation in AA, and discussing the first two steps). A woman may wish to find a program that has a female staff, all-women's groups, and individual counseling. Certainly she should feel confident that any such problems as eating disorders will be given attention. On the other hand, there is no need to feel she is settling for less if she simply finds a well-run program in a given community.

As for continuing support, AA, once a men's club, now counts women as more than a third of its membership, and many all-women meetings have formed. It has come a long way from the days described by Sue, whose story follows, when the only women at AA sat in the back and claimed to be doing research for a dissertation. Many women—especially those who live near a city—also have other options: Women for Sobriety, Secular Organization for Sobriety, SMART, and Rational Recovery. As we have seen, culturally specific treatment and support groups are also available. In some areas of the country, these and other holistic approaches to treatment are proliferating—everything from "intuitive healing" within Christianity to traditional aboriginal spirituality. It's noteworthy that at a time when the medical model of alcoholism is more and more dominant, there is a growing interest in spiritual approaches to the problem of substance abuse.

The rest of this chapter will look at some ways that women's paths in recovery challenge prevailing models of alcoholism and recovery, and show how some women have found their way out of the dark woods of addiction.

POWER AND POWERLESSNESS

THE LANGUAGE OF powerlessness is at the heart of AA and of treatment programs based on the twelve steps. The first step reads, *We admitted that we were powerless over alcohol—that our lives had become unmanageable.*

There is a paradox here that, when understood in its complexity, can be empowering. If we give up the struggle to control the things that are truly beyond us—for example, the effects of alcohol, and our ability to control our drinking once we start—we are freed to discover the power we do possess. A woman who knows that she loses and alcohol wins every time she takes a drink can stop spending her energy on that particular struggle. Admitting defeat on that front, she may find that the rest of the world opens up to her.

The first step of AA relates to the paradoxical dynamics of any kind of compulsive behavior, not just drinking. The harder one tries to control it, the more powerful the impulse becomes. Compulsion cannot be conquered in a head-on battle. It has to be given up, let go. You have to walk around it, not through it. When women and men have tried everything to control their behavior and found that no amount of willpower has done any good, and when they hear at AA that it is time to admit defeat, they sometimes experience overwhelming relief. They are asked to step outside the cycle of mastery and rebellion represented by their drinking and their efforts to control it. In doing so, they enter a new territory, where they can recover their freedom to make choices.

This kind of letting go is hard to do alone. You need support—someone to talk to, to hold your hand, to remind you that when you give this one thing up, a world rushes in to fill its place. For many women, AA meetings have provided that kind of support and encouragement. When AA works, women are empowered to take up their lives and make changes. They begin to feel their personal authority as they share their stories at meetings, coming to terms with their personal histories and recognizing the power they have to shape their individual future.

Accepting powerlessness is considered the essential first step in a path toward sobriety. In my interviews, however, I noticed that the stories women told me often had a different emphasis. In several cases, when a clear voice inside them said they had to stop drinking, the crucial revelation was about wanting power.

Marcia, for instance, had been in and out of detox and treatment a dozen times, and had a string of romances with abusive men. Once she lost all her money when her boyfriend persuaded her to put it in his hands. More than once, she woke up with two black eyes, unable to see.

She felt, she said, like "a broken doll." When she showed me a picture of herself from those days, I saw that she looked like a Barbie doll: a blond ponytail on top of her head, a tight midriff, and bobby socks. She described one nightmare scenario after another, including a year in an insane asylum, where she was committed against her will.

Eight years later, she was a favorite speaker at recovery programs across the country. I spoke with a man at an AA meeting in her city, who told me that he heard Marcia speak when he was in treatment and went back to his room and cried. Marcia showed him how bad life could get when drinking took over. She was also living proof that there was hope for everyone.

I asked Marcia what finally did it, what finally motivated her to be sober, and she told me that, one evening, when she and her boyfriend were walking by a lake, he told her he wanted her to forge some checks for a moneymaking scheme he had going. She'd done this before, and gotten caught. This time, she said no. "You'll do it," he said, and again she told him no. "You'll do it," he repeated.

"What are you talking about?" she said, and her boyfriend replied, "You'll do it, or I'll tell them you're going to kill yourself. They'll lock you up again."

At that moment, said Marcia, a fire lit inside her. She looked at her boyfriend with all the fury of a thunderstorm, and these words rang out in her head: *People like you will never have power over me again.* That evening, she quit drinking.

Samantha, the Ojibwa woman who counsels other alcoholics, told of two critical moments in her recovery. The first, described in Chapter 9, was a mystical moment when she lay on her husband's bed just after his death and heard the words of his favorite song coming faintly from the radio, words that spoke to her. The second came in circumstances very much like Marcia's: she got angry about other people's power over her, and she determined to make a change.

Samantha was out drinking and doing drugs. She and her boyfriend went back to her sister's to find Samantha's twelve-year-old

son, who often went there to drink. "My sister lived in this filthy, dirty
house," she said. "Dirty, dirty, dirty, the kind the city would condemn." Her sister told her the boy was in the bathroom. Samantha
went in, and there, beside a bathtub plugged and filled to the top with
cruddy black water, beside a pile of filthy clothes, her son lay on the
floor, passed out from drunkenness, in a pool of his own vomit.

"Twelve years old," said Samantha, "and he had just lost his dad.
And he was . . . Oh, man, that broke my heart. That broke my heart
like nothing."

Samantha and her boyfriend picked the boy up, washed him, and
made a bed for him. When he woke up, she fed him. And then, because
he was already under the care of child protection services, and they
were looking for him, she picked up the phone and called them to say
that he was there.

"They came and got him," she said. Furious that she had no say in
what would happen next, she decided, "I'm going to *do* something. I'm
going to put myself in a situation where I will have a say about my
kids. So I decided no matter what, come hell or high water, I'm going
to treatment. I'm going to stay there, and I'm going to get straight."
Samantha got sober so that she could be the one to make decisions
about her own and her children's lives.

You could say that recognizing powerlessness was implicit in
both Marcia's and Samantha's experiences. They quit drinking to gain
personal power because they saw that drinking was what gave other
people power over them. Yet the emphasis here is crucial. Marcia and
Samantha have a family history of abuse so severe it does not sound
real. Both were accustomed to feeling powerless. That they were controlled by alcohol, drugs, men, and the state was a depressing fact they
lived with every day. What struck them with the force of revelation was
the possibility of taking power for themselves.

Many women with histories less traumatic than Marcia's and Samantha's respond with a sinking feeling to the statement of powerlessness
in the first step. It confirms the helplessness they have felt all along; it

makes them feel sluggish, tired, and defeated. One woman told me that whenever she heard the first step at an AA meeting, she pictured herself on the floor with an array of glasses filled with bourbon, unable to stop herself from downing them one by one. Such women never imagine they can control their behavior or their destiny; they never entertain fantasies of grandeur; they always believe that the world is outside their control. They're powerless: what's new? The words of the first step heighten their anxiety, their anger, or their passivity.

The second and third steps of AA—in which alcoholics in recovery accept that a power higher than themselves can restore them to sanity, and give themselves up to that power—may have a similar effect. Some women, raised in a Christian faith, are familiar with the paradoxical language of AA, because they have grown up hearing about that central religious mystery of losing one's life to find it, of becoming a slave to Christ in order to be free. As noted in the introduction, AA grew out of a religious movement in the early twentieth century, and it draws on this tradition. Though this language can indeed be empowering—if interpreted in a positive way—it has not always been so for women. In fact, it is tied up with a very long history in which women have been exhorted to submit to male authorities, their husbands and their priests. I have spoken with religious women alcoholics—still drinking—who pray every night for God to "restore them to sanity," whose notion of turning their lives over to a higher power reinforces their idea of themselves as essentially passive, whether victims or recipients of mercy.

Though the first step asks for recognition that an alcoholic is powerlessness specifically over alcohol, women often say that in practice, at their AA meetings, there is a lot of talk about giving up power on many fronts—including relationships. The assumption is that alcoholics are self-centered, self-aggrandizing, and controlling, and that once the AA principles are applied to their lives, they will start to be more humble, more open, less demanding.

To understand the AA approach, it is helpful to know a little bit about its history. Bill Wilson, the cofounder of AA, was from a privi-

leged New England family. He was an experienced stockbrocker; he
had a law degree and a devoted wife. He based his program on the
experiences of one hundred men and one woman. These men tended to
be something like himself. All were white, and most were middle- or
upper-middle-class, privileged people. Bill Wilson noted that many of
these men had common personality traits. They tended to be arrogant,
controlling, and egocentric, unable to see their own faults and blind to
the effects of their behavior on other people. The steps of AA—including the emphasis on powerlessness—were designed to deflate the egos
of these middle-class white men who imagined they had the world by
the tail. For them it was a major—and healthy—challenge to confront
their own limitations, take seriously the damage their drinking had
done, and try to make amends.

Ironically, while AA promotes the disease concept of alcoholism
and defines it as "an allergy of mind and body," the literature of AA
betrays its roots in the moral model of alcoholism, which is precisely
what the disease model was designed to refute. In the moral model, the
alcoholic is a sinner and his drinking is a sign of his defective character.
Echoing this language, AA refers to the alcoholic's crippling "shortcomings" and "defects of character" which "made alcoholics of us in the
first place." It describes alcoholics as "grandiose and immature in the
extreme," and "an example of self-will run riot." As part of the cure, it
prescribes a "moral inventory" and a humble request to God to remove
all faults. Alcoholics who do not recover are "usually men and women
who are constitutionally incapable of being honest with themselves."

This is a story that AA members across the country tell about
themselves. I want to stress that it is clearly, for thousands of people, a
tremendously useful story. When these "defects of character" are looked
at with humor and compassion, in the presence of an accepting, supportive community, recovering women and men can learn to let go of
habits of mind that have imprisoned them.

But many people—especially women and minorities—come to
AA in a frame of mind quite different from the successful, grandiose,
white middle-class man who was Bill Wilson's archetypal alcoholic.

Many of these people never thought they had the world by the tail. They may have suffered from exploitation, trauma, or abuse. Having internalized their pain, they may have a habit of berating and attacking themselves. It's no revelation to hear that their shortcomings made them alcoholics. They always thought they were inferior to other people. For them, the ego-deflating language of AA can be damaging.

I sometimes ran into this kind of self-denigration in my interviews, as when, in a preliminary conversation by e-mail, I mentioned to a young woman in recovery that I was working on a chapter about women who began drinking after a major loss. Alarmed that I might be offering an "excuse" for drinking, she wrote back to me, "Poor me, poor me, pour me another drink. Upset by a life event? Sure, like flunking a test, falling in love with the wrong person, or murdering someone by accident. The scope matters not. My life event, whatever it is, is the center of the universe. I make it bigger than it ever is, either good or bad, and drink to mitigate the feelings of thrill or angst. We are the world's best liars. We will give up our children, our jobs, our precious selves for another drink. I drank because I was a spoiled brat. I thank Alcoholics Anonymous for keeping me sober another day, today."

Her point, that life events cannot be "blamed" for anybody's drinking, is important, but her aggression—toward me and toward herself—was also striking. She may have a long history of denigrating herself, but the language of AA has given her another way to do it.

Because of this, one therapist told me that when women she sees have problems with alcohol, she recommends AA because it's the only recovery group readily available in her small city, but "I always hold my breath when I do it, because these women usually have very little ego strength, and sometimes in AA they get worse." At AA meetings, you'll occasionally hear someone introduce herself—let's say her name is Jean—by saying, "I'm an alcoholic and my *problem* is Jean"—objectifying herself, treating herself in a manner that would be roundly disapproved of if Jean were someone other than herself. The woman from Las Vegas who felt bad when a man introduced himself by saying, "I'm

Mike, and I'm a degenerate drunk," told me, "At those meetings I learned that I had a disease called alcoholism, which meant I would always be defective, and not like other people."

Charlotte Davis Kasl, in *Many Roads, One Journey*—a book that has been tremendously useful to many who find the twelve-step program inappropriate for their needs—says that many women and minorities start off with a "crushed, nonexistent ego . . . which is not functional." They need a recovery program that shores up their sense of self, helps them recognize their negative thinking, and replaces it with modes of affirmation. She notes that a healthy ego is essential to any task. When the ego is inflated, the response should not be to "beat on it, crush it, and demolish it" but rather to infuse it with "compassion, awareness, and wisdom." A healthy ego is "porous, flowing, and flexible"; it serves the self and the society and a greater good.

Kasl developed her own sixteen steps as an alternative to AA, with the goal of promoting a balanced ego, and affirming the inner resources—sources of strength and power—of people in recovery. Her emphasis on educating people about how they have internalized society's negative views of women has been helpful to people like Margaret, who grew up walking on eggshells around a stepfather who commanded the household and called Margaret "garbage" and "a stupid Polack." "My idea of a woman's life was fear and service," Margaret told me. "The sixteen-step program opened my eyes. It helped me give my shame right back to the people who placed it on me, throw it back where it belongs. It helped me understand that I had the power to make my own decisions."

Other women discouraged by AA's emphasis on the alcoholic's "character defects" have found that Women for Sobriety, with its emphasis on positive thinking and empowerment, appeals to them. Many African-American women, in particular, turn to their churches in place of a recovery group, and groups such as Secular Organization for Sobriety, SMART, and Rational Recovery suit some women who prefer a secular approach.

For women who attend AA, there is excellent advice available, which counters the typical ego deflation. Stephanie Covington's book

A Woman's Way Through the Twelve Steps offers positive ways of adapting the steps to women's needs and reminds women of the AA adage: take what you need and leave the rest. Other women may be helped by David Berenson's reformulations, for example, for the first step: "We saw that trying to control and manipulate our feelings and relationships only led to a sense of feeling out of control and powerless." All-women AA meetings can solve a lot of problems—the language and approach naturally shift. It's good to remember, too, that the tone of AA meetings can vary enormously. Though no one is ever excluded, except in same-sex groups, like-minded people often cluster at one particular meeting. There are days and times where you'll find mostly professional women, or members of motorcycle gangs, or gays and lesbians, or twenty-somethings, or African Americans. Meetings will also vary among regions of the country (and the world). Women can try a number of meetings, if they live in a large enough area, to find one that suits.

Writing in *Tricycle* magazine, a Buddhist in recovery says he attends AA because "that's where the healing began and where it continues," but he wrestles with its polarizing judgments, believing that "wrong/right, sick/well, bad/good as they apply to my self are injurious." He writes:

> *Chicken and egg are one. No cause, no effect. No inside, no outside. No me, separate from my illness.*
>
> *So what about the "sick alcoholic," willful in the extreme, plagued by insecurity and fear, grandiose and self-loathing—"the asshole at the center of the universe" or Jung's King Baby? All of those negative traits are mine. I am grandiose, naive, and quick to anger. So are most of the people I know, alcoholic or not. I am also able to see my place in the scheme of things, to be aggressive and hard-minded, to act out of compassion and understanding. Siegfried Sassoon said, "in me the tiger sniffs the rose."*
>
> *So, rather than being either defective because of genes or gin, or perfect because of Buddhism and recovery programs, I discover that I am merely human.*

Our judgments about being well or sick, good or morally defective, powerful or powerless, reflect a culture that thinks in terms of masters and servants and sees our nature as a problem to be conquered. Ultimately, inner peace may involve transcending these dichotomies and settling for what is "merely human."

ONLY CONNECT

ONE OF the thorniest problems for people who love someone who drinks too much is how to keep close, if this is even possible. Can it be done without harming anyone?

In my own case, I have come to terms—though imperfectly—with the fact that I can do nothing to help my sister. I have set my own limits. I won't give her money; I won't ask her to visit and expose my children to her drinking. I'd be lying if I said I have come to terms completely with Carri's drinking, or that I have learned to deal with it. Still, I have picked up a thing or two. I no longer sermonize on the phone or analyze her problems like a therapist. On the other hand, I have given up on the idea that I will talk to her only when she is sober—that would be like signing off forever. Instead, I call her every week. I let her in on what is happening in my own life. I try to accept her as she is—not a problem to be solved, but my sister, whom I love. I have a little rule about telling the truth as I see it, whenever staying silent might encourage her denial, which means that our conversations are sometimes painful and sometimes make her angry. She knows I will say, on occasion, "Carri, what you're saying sounds crazy to me." I also tell her that I miss the sister hidden behind the booze, and that it hurts me to see her dying a slow death. I hope she will choose to get sober soon.

One night, after Carri called from a detox center—this time her blood alcohol level was 0.41—it dawned on me that several emergency room visits and four trips to detox in as many months meant that Carri might die sooner rather than later. I panicked. I wasn't ready to lose her. My fear threw me into doubt, and I wondered if there wasn't something I could do. It was eleven P.M. I went to the yellow pages, and I called an AA alcohol abuse hotline. A man called Joe answered, and I told him about Carri.

He asked me, "Have you ever considered cutting off contact with your sister?"

"What would that accomplish?" I asked him. "I really don't think I am enabling her. I don't think our phone calls encourage her to drink."

"I'm an alcoholic," he said. "My own mother said she never wanted to see me again. I hit bottom after that. That's why I got sober."

I argued with Joe for a while and hung up very shaken. I knew that alcoholism is insidious and can draw in an alcoholic's loved ones. I knew that, in the matter of helping an alcoholic, intuition isn't always a reliable guide. I thought of a friend whose wife is alcoholic, who had not drawn personal limits, and whose helping behavior created a context in which his wife could drink with few immediate consequences. He had to learn to stop reaching out to her when she was in pain, to allow her to experience the consequences of her drinking. He believed (as I believe) that this was the right thing to do—and something he needed to do, to preserve his sanity—but "It's completely counterintuitive," he told me. "You're in a boat, your wife is drowning in the water next to you, your impulse is to reach out your hand!"

I also thought of George McGovern, who described in his book *Terry: My Daughter's Life-and-Death Struggle with Alcoholism* how he and his wife, on the advice of an alcohol counselor, distanced themselves from their alcoholic daughter during what turned out to be the last six months of her life. He says he has always regretted this. I don't think he believes that his contact with Terry would have been the thing that saved her, but he wishes he had been close to her in the last days of her life.

If I believed that my contact with Carri were harming her, I would cut myself off, and cope willingly with my guilt if she died in the meantime. I believed Joe when he said that his mother's cutting him off was the thing that persuaded him to get sober. I appreciate the efforts of other loved ones of alcoholics who struggle to set their own

limits, and who are brave enough—often with the help of Al-Anon—
to recognize that their help is actually doing harm. I even believe that
some women might respond like Joe, and be motivated to seek treatment if a loved one cut them off.

From my own experience with Carri, however, and my interviews
with women in recovery, I have come to believe that maintaining a
connection is optimum for the alcoholic and the relative whenever this
can be accomplished without anyone's bearing inordinate pain. In all
my interviews, not one woman told me that being cut off had
prompted her recovery, but many told me about the love of some person who gave them enough faith in themselves to choose health.

Since my sample is limited, I called two therapists who are known
for their writing on women and addiction and asked them about their
experiences in this matter. Diane Byington, who practices in Denver
and has written on women and relational theory, said that she had seen
two kinds of results from being cut off by an important person. "In
some cases, it motivates a woman to get sober, but other times, it
pushes her deeper into her relationship with alcohol and drugs."

Stephanie Covington also emphasized that no one way is right for
everyone. "I'm an advocate of twelve-step programs, but many people
in recovery give advice as if there is only one way to do it. Being cut off
may have worked for Joe, but you have to think in terms of individual
cases. With women, maintaining a connection is often important. I'm
not sure it isn't just as important for men. In working with a woman to
motivate her into recovery, I would be inclined to set appropriate limits, but not disconnections.

"We all have huge individual differences. You have to ask, what's
my role, and what's my capability?

"One person might need to say, 'I can't talk to you when you're
under the influence,' or 'You can't be in this house while you're drinking.' Or a therapist might say to a client, 'I feel I am colluding in your
addiction if you come to see me when you're drinking. You're believing
we're in therapy whereas in fact we're not accomplishing anything
because you have mood-altering substances in your system.'

"Someone else might be able to take an alcoholic home and keep her safe and tolerate whatever goes on without ever trying to control her. But not everybody could do this."

Following are some stories women told me about connections that sustained their faith in themselves and allowed them to get sober. I hope that these stories will not be misinterpreted in harmful ways, encouraging families to try to "save" their alcoholic. I myself have to guard against my impulse to save my sister. To be honest, there's something in it for me: it makes me feel as if my life is in control, and it reinforces a good girl–bad girl dichotomy with which Carri and I grew up. The variety of experience offered here suggests that no one solution is right for everyone.

Benevolent Presences

Meredith is six feet tall and has an attentive, intelligent manner, and eyes that look right into you. I met her at one of the first AA meetings I attended, at a women's prison outside Burlington, Vermont. She set me at ease, taking me through the entrance rigamarole, and introducing me to the others, assuring me that my presence was okay. (I attended only open meetings of AA, where nonalcoholics are welcome.) Later, we met for an interview at a coffeehouse in Burlington, where she sipped herbal tea. I asked her what she thought about this matter of staying close to a friend or loved one who is actively alcoholic.

"I think it's optimum, if you can do it," said Meredith, "but I understand completely when people can't."

For her own part, Meredith believes that her grandmother's "benevolent presence" saved her life.

Meredith's initial problem was anorexia nervosa. She started counting calories as a college freshman; then her desire to lose a few pounds became an obsession. She soon found that she couldn't loosen up enough to eat, but a glass of wine solved the problem. "That's when I began to look forward to drinking," said Meredith. "I don't know if at that point I craved the alcohol for its own sake, because I was on the road to addiction, or if, unconsciously, I was craving food—and I knew I wouldn't get it till I drank."

When, after several stiff drinks, Meredith drove her car into a ditch, nobody checked her blood alcohol level, but the accident and her plummeting grades frightened her. She used her engagement to a boyfriend back home as an excuse to drop out of college. She didn't admit that she had a problem with alcohol, but her anorexia was obvious—she weighed only 110 pounds. Her parents were terrified, particularly her father, who had been eleven years old when his own father killed himself. "That trauma was the defining event of his life," said Meredith. "He was always afraid that I would die too. When I stopped eating, he saw his worst fears being confirmed."

Meredith's parents loved her fiancé, and they hoped that marriage would solve her eating problem. They saw that she was drinking heavily, but this didn't worry them. When she got "terribly drunk" the night of her wedding, nobody minded. As Meredith said, "My family was into partying."

Meredith wasn't the only one who had thought of alcohol as a cure for her anorexia. When, sick and hung over, she got in the car to set off on her honeymoon with her new husband, she found a bottle of rum from her father tucked between the seats. He'd gotten up early and put it there, thinking, "If she drinks, she'll eat."

Meredith's drinking escalated to a point where she could no longer ignore the problem. She entered an inpatient alcohol treatment program, but while she was there, she took laxatives to lose weight and stopped eating altogether. A gym teacher at the center saw that Meredith was too weak to do jumping jacks and took her to the hospital.

"At the hospital they fed me through the nose," Meredith remembered. "I was so afraid of getting fat from it that at night I tried to stay awake and hold the tube closed. It didn't work. If I hadn't fallen asleep, I would have died. I didn't want to die, but I was more frightened of being fat than dying. I am six feet tall. At the time I weighed eighty-eight pounds." The only calories she would accept were those she could get from beer. When her friends visited her in the hospital, she got them to sneak her several cans.

"Throughout this terrible time," said Meredith, "I lived so that I could see my grandmother again." She described her grandmother as a "tall, generous person." She had been poor as a child, but she married a wealthy man and had a beautiful house and servants, whose children she put through school. "I loved the graciousness of the world she created, but my love for her wasn't about this," said Meredith. "Her name was Serena, and I felt at peace around her. Before I went into treatment, I visited her in Florida. I was drinking, and I knew she didn't approve, but she kept on loving me. I would sit on the floor by her chair, and she would read Shakespeare's sonnets to me. She would do needlepoint, laugh, make jokes, and read to me.

"My parents loved me too, but my problems and their worrying got in the way of our relationship. My grandmother's love for me was calm and detached. It was the love of pure acceptance. When I was in treatment, I remembered what that felt like: pure acceptance. My dream was to live with her. I lived so I could see her again."

After another two years, after blackouts and drunken fights, worsening anorexia, a divorce, more alcohol-related accidents, several rounds of treatment, AA meetings, and many relapses, Meredith— "sick and tired of being sick and tired," in the words of the AA slogan—finally had her last drink. She did this by taking AA to heart and attending four or five meetings every week. Once she achieved a stable sobriety, she gradually—over the next five years—gained control over her eating. It became clear that she would never live with her grandmother—her grandmother drew a line there—but the contact she had given Meredith even when Meredith was drunk was what she needed to maintain enough faith in herself to persist in recovery, and repair her relationships with other people.

Limits to Love

Meredith was able to accept her grandmother's love in part because it came from outside her immediate family. Her relationship with her parents was complicated by personal needs and feelings of responsibility. Spouses are also in an awkward position—"unconditional love" may not be possible in a mutual relationship in which both people have needs. It may not even be desirable. AA takes a hard line about the kind of contact that can be enabling because people have a very strong tendency to get wrapped up in the lives of alcoholics, to a point where everyone is dysfunctional. Meredith's grandmother, however, was able to give love without harming herself, without losing her own sense of purpose.

When parents set limits, an alcoholic child may be too angry to accept their emotional support. Dale and her new husband have an addicted adult son, and they have found the Al-Anon principle of loving detachment quite helpful. "We are available with unconditional love," said Dale, "but we offer no resources—no loans, no house to use. He decided to go away, and we have not gone running after him. If he's going to do his addiction, he'll do it." This is painful for Dale, but mostly she can keep her equanimity, because she trusts that what she's doing is right. "I have children having problems with money, and I'm doing the same thing: I'm not going to lend you money to buy shoes if you have just bought a Jeep! I want you to learn about that." For her own part, she is ready to reestablish a connection with her son as soon as he is ready. As Covington suggests, she is setting limits but not cutting anyone off.

When the alcoholic chooses a cutoff, there may be little one can do. Sometimes, painfully, an alcoholic daughter needs not to see her parents in order to recover, and her wishes should be respected. Generally—especially for teenagers—reconnecting girls to their family and social networks is critical to recovery. This may be why family therapy is gaining ascendancy as the treatment of choice for young people.

Disconnection is appropriate whenever a relationship is doing harm to either party. Families who wish desperately to help an alcoholic can be most effective if they tend their own needs and remember the Al-Anon slogans: "You didn't cause it, you can't control it, you can't cure it." "Stop trying to make her stop." "There's nothing you can do."

A Father Who Came Through

In Amber's case, a parent did get through to her, in an unexpected way. A privileged child in a wealthy suburb of New York, Amber always had a smile on her face: "I was 'happy,' but dying inside. I felt absolutely worthless," she told me, "and I never, ever fit in in my entire life." She had a strong relationship with her parents when she was very young; later her father became alcoholic and emotionally remote, and her mother was preoccupied with his drinking.

Amber turned to alcohol when she was fifteen, because it helped her talk to boys, helped her "feel funny and cool and fit in." She had started off with "zero self-respect," but now she discovered that boys liked her—"I was an athlete, and I had a little rocket ship body." She felt better when they paid attention to her. She drank to get smashed, and, she told me, "I would let pretty much anyone fuck me."

Her drinking led to a quick downward spiral. After high school, she got a job as a hostess in a restaurant. She started drinking gin. "I would keep it in my freezer so it got nice and syrupy, and pour it over ice with a little bit of lime. Fabulous—or so I thought." She blacked out quite often and felt sick. Like Nell and Tamara and many others, she discovered that cocaine allowed her to "drink and drink and drink, and never be falling-down drunk. I loved it, because it allowed me to keep drinking, and I *loved* drinking. If you were young and cute, cocaine was also very easy to get."

Looking back, Amber believes that she knew she was doing something wrong, and that she was hurting herself, but says a part of her seemed to be enjoying her self-destruction. The highs and lows of cocaine were extreme and dramatic, and she deteriorated fast. She turned a corner one morning when, strung out, she got up early and went to the window of her apartment. "I looked out at all the stores and the railroad station, and I watched the businessmen walking down to the train to go to work in New York like normal, regular people, and it was like I was seeing myself for the first time. I'd slept with a slimy-looking guy because I'd seen his half-bag of cocaine, and he was long gone. I felt filthy. I felt like I had really hit it."

Amber called someone she knew in AA, and he referred her to a counselor at a hospital. It turned out this counselor worked at an alcohol rehabilitation center within the hospital, and Amber's first thought was, "My God, just a second here, what are we getting into, let's not blow this out of proportion." The counselor was "an absolute sweet-heart" and persuaded her to come back for a group meeting that evening. An hour before she was supposed to go, this counselor called her and said, "You're Amber Wickham, right? I have another Wickham in this program, I believe it's your father. You might want to see your dad before the meeting starts."

"Apparently," said Amber, "my dad had been told to go to these meetings or he'd lose his job, and he'd been going for a couple of months. He was fed up, though, and just about to say to hell with it, and then in walks his eldest daughter. The meeting hadn't started. I walked in completely coked up and drunk on a bottle of wine. Imagine the impact of your firstborn walking into a room and seeing her so completely wrecked, almost destroyed, a shadow of what you knew her to be. It was very emotional. I said to him, yeah, I think I've got a big problem here."

Amber will never forget the counselor introducing them as father and daughter. Her mouth dropped—she wasn't used to sharing problems with other people, particularly in her father's presence. After the meeting, her dad came back to her apartment with her, and they dumped all her cocaine down the toilet, and all her beer and wine. The next morning Amber thought: I could have sold that cocaine; how could I have done that? "It's one thing to be emotional the night before," said Amber. "I would have brushed it off the next day, but I had no opportunity to do that because my father was right there. He picked me up for a noon AA meeting. Thank God. I went to my first AA meeting, and I've been sober ever since.

"My father thinks that it's a miracle, and that if I hadn't walked into the room that night, he would not have gotten sober. If he hadn't been there, I wouldn't be either. I was his eldest daughter. . . . It meant sobriety for each of us. We have the same sobriety date.

"It was such a shock and such a slap in the face for him to see me in that condition. It made both of us realize how devastating and dangerous this disease is. When it's just yourself, you can make excuses and slough it off. But we were a mirror for each other.

"It's brought us so close together, and we have such a bond as a result. He always was a funny, gentle man, with a good sense of humor. He still is. In my earliest memory he's coming home from work, and I'm running down the stairs with my younger sister, and jumping into his arms. I loved my father, and I feel such closeness today that I think we must go back several lifetimes. And actually, I am adopted—all four of us are! It's almost as if we were brother and sister in a past life. I don't know if there's anything to that, but I feel it strongly. I have always felt connected to him."

Help Me, Help My Sister

Among the women I talked to, the inspiring presence who encouraged their sobriety was more often a sibling than a parent. For example, Ruth's brother named her and cared for her as a baby, and continued to express his faith. Louise, the African-American woman who was raped three times before the age of fourteen, is full of gratitude to her sister, who, while working full-time herself, moved in with Louise to help her with her babies at a time when Louise was driving a bus and drinking two pints of Canadian Mist a day. Louise lived in a town in Mississippi, in a whole community of women who helped her out. Her sister-in-law lived next door and baby-sat while Louise worked, and her brother's girlfriend moved in to help as well. "I don't know," said Louise, "It's just—I wanted people to be there with my kids. Deep down inside, I knew I couldn't deal with them the way I wanted to, but I always saw to it that they were taken care of."

Some years later, Louise discovered that her husband was seeing another woman. Humiliated, she decided to leave with her three children. At the bank, she discovered that her husband had withdrawn all the money from their joint account. She got a gun, intending to blow her brains out. Instead, it occurred to her that her husband ought to die. She made a plan, but first she picked up the phone and called her sister Gloria. Within minutes, Gloria was on a bus; she arrived so quickly—from several states away—that when she walked in the door

Louise looked up and said, "Where did you come from?" Her sister said, "C'mon, let's go," and held Louise sobbing in her arms all the way back on the bus from Mississippi to Saint Paul.

For a year, Louise and her children stayed with Gloria, and, said Louise, "I was like a zombie. I was just depressed, and Gloria let me sit there. I think I cried every day for about six months. When Gloria left for work I was in my nightgown, and when she came back I was still wearing it. She had to bathe me; she had to do everything. She did everything but feed me. I was just that far gone." Louise drank beer every day, and her sister—if she knew—ignored it.

Louise suspects it was her sister's prayers that pulled her out of her deepest misery. "She was a true believer of God, I'm telling you. I could hear her every day, every night, praying, *Help me, please help me, help my sister, help my sister*. I guess that helped because finally one day I just"—she snapped her fingers—"I looked around and saw my kids . . . and I started asking how I could get myself together. My sister came home that day, and I was dressed. She just looked at me and started crying and hugging. I'm looking at her, and I said, 'I want to go get me an apartment.' She couldn't believe it. It was like nothing had happened, like I hadn't gone through what I went through. All of a sudden I want to go look for an apartment. She said, 'Okay, can you make it?' I said, 'Yeah, I can make it.' So we went all day long looking for apartments."

Alcohol counselors often warn against the kind of self-sacrifice Louise's sister made, and such buffering from the consequences of drinking sometimes does turn out to be a way of killing with kindness. "If you hold your hand out to alcoholics," Dale told me, "they might catch it on their way down, and cling to you for a while, and then when they slip off they fall harder." I did not interview Louise's sister: I don't know how high a price she paid, or if her time and care were given so freely that she reaped the benefits of her compassion. Yet it looks as if Louise's sister was one of the few who could take care of an alcoholic without resentment and without trying to control her. It seems clear that Louise's children benefited from the arrangement, and that Louise, though it looked as if she was wallowing in depression and drinking herself to death, was also gathering courage to make a change. Getting her own apartment was only the first step, of course, in a process of moving toward sobriety. Even later, seven months after her last drink, Louise's sobriety remained frighteningly tentative, a matter of one day at a time.

A Stranger Among Trash Cans

Sometimes a stranger manages to get through to an alcoholic when nobody else can. Sue is now a successful real estate agent in California, managing several properties and winning awards for her work, but at the age of thirty-five she was a typical down-and-out alcoholic. "I don't always tell people at AA all of my story," she said, "because they can't relate. They'll say, 'Now, that's a real drunk, *I'm* not a real drunk.'" Sue was a bar drinker, a lover of the happy hour, in and out of jail, drunk in public, drunk at the wheel. In her twenties, she socialized with well-dressed people at country clubs, but by the age of thirty-six she resorted to the cheapest bars, unable to get men to buy her drinks "because I stank," she said. "It was coming through my pores. I'd sit in a bathtub trying to get rid of the smell, drinking a bottle of wine. With alcohol, I went so far down that I was on my knees in the gutter. God thought I was praying—my recovery was that miraculous."

Each day Sue arrived early at her favorite bar. Behind the building, there was a high wall hiding a row of trash cans, and Sue hid behind it, so that no one would see her with the shakes, waiting for the bar to open. One day a bizarre-looking woman appeared. "I thought maybe she was a palm reader," said Sue. "She was a white soul sister in a purple shirt and a green skirt with bangles up her arms. Lots of jewelry. She was six feet tall in her socks, and she was wearing heels and a turban—she was a sight to behold. When she saw me, she started laughing and laughing, and it scared the hell out of me. She said, 'I've been looking for you for nine years.'"

The woman blocked Sue's exit, and she was too big to get around. Her name was Nancy, and she took Sue back to her motel on the beach—

her husband was in town working on a nuclear plant, and Nancy was staying with him. She told Sue the story of her life. "She dropped her first kid at eleven," said Sue, "because her mom was selling her to grown men from the age of nine." Nancy had been as alcohol-dependent as Sue and had also landed in the gutter. She too had spent months hiding by the trash cans—the same place where she found Sue—until she finally got sober. For nine years she'd searched the area whenever she was in town, to try to find someone like herself whom she could help. "She told me, 'Come with me, try AA for thirty days, and I'll be your sponsor. If you don't like it, we'll gladly refund your misery.'"

At that point, said Sue, "I thought I was schizophrenic and booze was my god-given medicine to keep the demons away." She supported herself by making and selling concrete seagulls for people's yards, "squatting in someone's backyard, hooked into their electricity, sloshing cement around—people don't expect an artist to look like anything." Yet she decided to go with Nancy for the thirty-day tryout, because her hangover wouldn't clear up. "It would move around but it wouldn't go away. I knew I was in real trouble. At least I'd have this friend for a while, and I could taper back to the drinking."

The AA meetings "were kind of like brainwashing," said Sue. "I thought the people were idiots because they said the stupidest things I'd ever heard in my life. 'The name of the game is don't drink.' 'It isn't the caboose that gets you, it's the engine.' 'Don't take the first drink.' 'God could and would if he were sought.' I must have heard that last one a million times. I thought my sponsor had wet brain, because she said the same thing so often. I told her I'd pray and do *anything* to shut her up!"

A few weeks later, Sue woke up doubled over, wanting a drink. If she could have walked, she would have gone to get one. Then she remembered another AA slogan: "Put it off until tomorrow." She did, and the impulse lifted. When she got up, she went to a meeting. From then on, whenever she doubled over, she said a prayer "like I was writing a letter: *Dear God, How are you today, I'm just fine, except for the shits and the shakes.*'" The next thing she knew, said Sue, she was at a meeting, and someone asked her how she was doing. She streaked over to the calendar and saw that six weeks had passed since her first meeting. "I was so stunned that I had to run outside, because no one had ever seen me cry. I had no intention of doing more than the thirty-day trial . . . but the first thing that hit me was, I didn't want to drink."

Early in sobriety, said Sue, she was still tremendously egocentric. "The third step says to turn your life and will to God," she told me, "but instead I made a space for God to turn his will over to me. I would give God orders, like '*If you want me to do your work, get me a car.*' It worked! For a while, anyway. He must have wanted me."

When a woman at AA told Sue she loved her, Sue said, "This place is full of lesbians!" To her, at that time, love was synonymous with sex. "My sponsor had to talk me down all the time. She would always laugh her head off. It took me years to see what was so damn funny."

Things changed for Sue when her former boyfriend, "whom I'd thrown away," left for Las Vegas with a redhead. Torn up, jealous, violently distressed, Sue expressed her rage by picking up a pencil and writing "thirteen pages of garbage." When she read it later, she was horrified. "I couldn't own it. I never knew that part of me existed. It was a stranger on those pages, and it upset me." Ashamed, Sue quit going to meetings. "I went from thinking that there was nothing wrong with me to thinking that I was the worst person in the world. I thought I should have been hung on the cross with Jesus." Desperate for a drink, she called Nancy instead and told her she was living on candy bars and was never going to another meeting.

"You've got to do your fifth," said Nancy, referring to the step that requires you to admit your wrongs and your shortcomings "to God and another person." She added, "I'll be down."

Sue told Nancy everything that was in the thirteen pages and confessed the awful things she had done, which now humiliated her. "When I couldn't hold my head up, she'd tell me something horrible that she had done to survive when her mom put her out. Whatever story I told her, she laughed and told me something worse."

Afterward, Sue burned the thirteen pages.

Since that time, Sue has taken to writing out a "moral inventory" every year in November, her "AA birthday." Sometimes it's a long process, but she has reduced her shortcomings to less than a page. "All seven deadly sins are still there, but I don't always operate on them." Twenty years later, said Sue, "I don't know that my character has changed much, but what I do sure has. Alcoholism is so boring. I used to wish somebody would come into the bar and kill somebody, just for the excitement. It's boring when you have to do what booze wants you to do, and you have no choice. Being sober has been the most exciting adventure of my life."

From time to time, Sue, like Nancy, goes looking for women hiding among the trash cans. There are not many. She did find one woman who then got sober, but later she relapsed, drank, got hit by a car, and died. Sue refuses to become discouraged. In her job as a realtor, she often comes upon troubled people, and she wonders, "Did God put me here to sell this house or heal these people?" Her very first sale was a liquor store owned by a Jordanian family. "Every one of them was alcoholic, and every one of them sobered up. I like to think I influenced them."

A Link to the Larger World

The alcoholic whose world has closed down, who is imprisoned in herself, needs—when she is ready—someone else to reach out to penetrate her isolation, and to help her sense her connection to the larger world. That "someone else" may not always be a person. Michelle, the recovering alcoholic from rural Louisiana who resented having "the typical female role" in her lesbian relationship, said she was embarrassed to tell me the story of her darkest moment, and how she pulled out of it. She had been through treatment several times. Her partner Hannah had left her, she'd lost custody of her child, and she had been fired. Her utilities had been cut off, because she hadn't paid her bill. She had no lights, no air conditioning, no water, no screens on her open windows.

Holed up in her house, full of hatred for herself, she sat in the dark one sweltering night, shaking because she hadn't had a drink, making plans to kill herself. When a dog, "a big old boxer," suddenly jumped through her open window, she thought she was hallucinating. But the dog was real and stayed by her side all night. It seemed to want to be her friend. It occurred to Michelle that if this dog thought she was okay, she shouldn't give up on herself quite yet. She would go for treatment one more time.

Motivating Women

Knowing that women respond well to different modes of well-run treatment, we can see more clearly that what ultimately makes the difference is each woman's motivation and commitment to recovery.

The traditional way to think of this has been to say that each alcoholic has to hit bottom, and each alcoholic has a different bottom, high or low. When you hit your personal bottom, that's when you decide to get better. More recently, we are understanding that this hands-off attitude is not always acceptable—a person's bottom can be too low; it can devastate a family; it can mean death or a permanent loss of health. Now professional interventionists help families try to "raise the bottom." The drinker's family, loved ones, boss—all those close to her—gather with a counselor to confront her, establishing their own limits and clarifying the consequences of continued drinking. Given the telescoped progress of alcoholism in women, early intervention can be essential, whether accomplished this way or less formally. A lover's or a friend's serious concern, a doctor's early warning, a therapist's questions, all these are forms of intervention that may be most effective early on.

Of late, there is heightened interest in motivational interviewing, which starts on the premise that most people already have the tools they need to recover, that they just need help finding their own support networks and tapping into their inner resources. The research on motivational interviewing at first seemed disappointing—people treated only by this method didn't fare as well—but a follow-up found results equivalent to those obtained by two other forms of treatment that were being studied. Motivational interviewing may be especially helpful for people who are angry and independent-minded, unlikely to submit to someone else's program but perhaps more amenable when they have developed their own goals and their own reasons for sobriety. Research is ongoing.

What motivates women to get sober may not always be what we imagine—as in the case of the alcoholic mother who has lost custody of her children and wants them back. Diane Byington commented, "Some people say to a woman, 'You can't see your kids until you're sober,' hoping to motivate her, but the woman sees her kids as lost to her, and she dives deeper. But if she knows she has the possibility of getting her kids back, if she has support, and if she doesn't think she has to be perfect, it's a much stronger motivator. Her children's welfare must come first, but the mother will try harder if she doesn't think she'll lose her kids if she has one relapse."

Furthermore, our traditional ideas of motivation may be entirely irrelevant to a woman who is homeless, mentally ill, impoverished, and abused. "Among chronic relapsing alcoholics there is usually a serious breakdown in some aspect of their lives," said Ronald Kadden. "They may have housing needs, financial needs, medical or psychiatric problems. They can't be treated with just a little more of what everybody else gets. Their life issues need to be dealt with in an intensive way. This won't make the drinking go away, but my belief is that without taking care of those issues, you will never make a dent in their drinking."

Sometimes it helps to flip a question around. Instead of asking, "What motivates a woman to get sober?" the question becomes, "What motivates her to stay drunk? What does she like about it?" Women throughout this book have addressed this issue in various ways— speaking not only of physical craving but also of temporary relief from depression and anxiety, the heady pleasure of rebellion, escape from trauma, less inhibited sex, feelings of warmth and connection. These can surely be good things, but women can discover ways to get what they want that aren't so punishing.

For many chronic alcoholics, both women and men, the "bottom" they have feared all their lives is a few months of sobriety. Their relapses may be less about a physical craving—which passes over time—and more about a desperate need to return to a life that is known and understood, a life in which they can rest in what's familiar, even if that is nausea or pain or an empty park bench. Once they drink, they have no more decisions to make, since drinking carries them through the day. There is something to treasure in this: simply in knowing the contours of one's life, what one is, and what one feels.

We should not underestimate this. Even if we are sober, well-adjusted, and adaptable, our sense of well-being may depend on a clear identity. When our story about ourselves is challenged, we are likely to feel anxious. When that challenge persists, anxiety can lead to despair. When a woman has been a victim of trauma—as is so often the case with chronic alcoholics—and she has held on to this victimization as the truth about her life, then to give up that identity, to take a step toward wellness, is to revolutionize her sense of self. Any revolution involves enormous upheaval and rearrangement. It might sound paradoxical to say that someone would have a hard time giving up pain— why not hand it over? Why not choose freedom and space and possibility? But to do so requires faith—and faith, the religious will say, is a gift. Perhaps this is why many alcoholics in recovery give credit to a higher power.

Some of the women in this book describe a familiar path. They got sick and tired of being sick and tired, and they realized they didn't want to die. Some were dragged by the hand into treatment, over and over, until something clicked. Many got sober for their children. Some felt a sudden determination to get control of their lives. Others were granted a moment of understanding their connection to the human family, and this restored their hope. All of the women are sober by virtue of important choices they have made—to accept help, and to let go of life as they have known it.

Afterword

MY SISTER HAS BEEN SOBER FOR FIVE MONTHS.

When I call her, before she has finished saying "Hello," I can hear that she's all right.

It has been ten years since she has been sober this long. It's been twenty-four years since she was in school, but she's enrolled at a community college. She's not sure yet how she's doing in English, but in algebra and psychology, so far she's getting A's.

When I was starting research for this book, I went to an alcohol counselor. I told him about Carri, and he looked me in the eye and said, "What are you doing to prepare yourself for your sister's death?" That scared me, but not as much as Carri did when she called later that week. Her voice was slow and dull. When she woke up that morning, she said, the angel of death was sitting on her shoulder. She would die soon if she didn't stop drinking. She didn't know if she could.

The angel of death did not put an end to her drinking, either through death or through fear of death. Carri went on as she always did, although tests showed that her liver was affected. She had severe abdominal cramps, most likely gastritis, but possibly pancreatitis, which can be fatal. Her eyesight was deteriorating.

She found a psychiatrist who was willing to work with her on medication for her depression and anxiety, even though she was still drinking. Always, before this, antidepressants had given her panic attacks. This time, she was given one new to the market, and another new drug to counter anxiety. I was alarmed. What if Carri drank twenty beers along with her medication?

Carri continued to drink, but now, she said, she didn't have to drink. She could, when she chose to, go all day without a beer. The medication kept her from panicking and from feeling ill. To me, this sounded ridiculous. It sounded like a license to drink and a way of easing the path to death.

She did cut down on her drinking. She began reading inspirational books. She watched Gary Zukav, author of *The Seat of the Soul,* on *Oprah Winfrey* talking about addiction. He said that when a craving for alcohol overwhelms you, that craving is real, but underneath it there is pain. He said that one trick is to challenge the pain. Another trick is to look carefully at your choices. Give in to the craving, go down that path, and where does it lead you? Or challenge the pain, and stay sober, and what options open up? The message was clear and simple, said Carri, and she could use it. She taped the *Oprah* show. She planned to quit one day, and she would need tools.

When her boyfriend moved away for a while, to take a temporary job, her resolve to get sober grew. Before, whenever she stopped drinking, he had been there to tempt her with a beer. Drinking played a major role in the drama of their relationship. With him gone, she had only her own demons to battle.

She began by staying sober for four weeks. When she drank again, it was different. She didn't drink to oblivion, because she no longer needed alcohol to medicate her anxiety. She had pills to do that. Now, she said, she was drinking out of habit. Now she had the option of stopping.

Oddly enough, this relapse gave Carri the courage to start over. "Before, when I was sober, no matter how long, I always felt like I was going to fall," she told me. "I lived in fear of drinking again and how that would devastate me. Now I'm not so frightened. I had a relapse and it didn't kill me. I feel like there's more room for me to move in. I don't have to be perfect, and that gives me confidence."

This fascinates me. Many people find AA helpful specifically because it keeps reminding them how bad life was when they were drinking, and that memory stops them from taking another drink. For Carri, such memories led to a sense of doom. They were part of the fear she lived with every day, the fear she still needs to medicate. When she gets a craving, she does remind herself both of the misery alcohol would bring her and of the fruits of sobriety. But not until she stopped being terrified by the thought of a relapse could she gather her energy and make a deliberate choice to let go of her craving and the life she had known.

I am still frightened. The road ahead is a long one, and there will be obstacles. Carri hasn't taken to AA and has not established herself in another recovery group. I fear she is too isolated. What will she do when she is really challenged, when she is in one of those stretches all of us experience, in which everything seems to go wrong? Though it's been many years, she has had long periods of sobriety before. What if she has gotten sober in order to feel better so that she can taper back to drinking?

I am also full of hope. I know from the interviews in this book that women with the cards stacked against them have started brand-new lives, free of addiction. Carri is speaking and behaving in ways I've never seen before. She's preparing for a self-supporting future, and she has summoned the courage to break up with her boyfriend. She has a helpful counselor and is working well with her. This counselor urges her to start a Women for Sobriety group. Maybe she will, says Carri. Maybe, when she gets a driver's license, she'll go back to church and participate in that community.

We talk about her options for work—she's interested in nutrition—and we gossip about fashion and the family. She and I have a store of common memories dating back to a room with twin canopy beds and canary-yellow wallpaper. When she was drinking, I did not trust her with my feelings or my personal concerns. Now I am starting to open up. Because sisters are always competitors on some level, and because of the good things in my own life and her years of suffering, I would expect her to resent me, at least somewhat. Instead, I always have an advocate in Carri. I am moved by her careful listening, her enthusiasm, and her loving wishes. She has a deep fund of generosity, and it has deepened over the years. I believe what I have learned and written here about how emotional development stalls when addiction takes hold, yet my experience with Carri makes me feel that this is not quite the whole story.

Lately, I've been thinking of a boat ride I took last summer with friends. The wife brought her sister along, and the two of them sat together in one seat, chatting with each other, the Vermont hills in the distance. It was a lovely sight. It filled me with nostalgia and regret.

I am blessed to have my sister back. I give thanks for her sobriety, one day at a time.

Do You Have a Drinking Problem?

This screening tool, called TWEAK, is particularly appropriate for women. The following questions may help you determine whether or not you have a drinking problem.

1. How many drinks does it take before you begin to feel the first effects of the alcohol? (**T**olerance) (*A drink is a 12-ounce beer, a 5-ounce glass of wine, or a drink containing 1½ ounces of liquor.*)

    (If three or more, give yourself two points.)

2. Have close friends or relatives **W**orried or complained about your drinking in the past year?

    (If yes, give yourself two points.)

3. Do you sometimes take a drink in the morning when you first get up? (**E**ye-opener)

    (If yes, give yourself one point.)

4. Are there times when you drink and afterward you can't remember what you said or did? (Amnesia or blackouts)

   (*If yes, give yourself one point.*)

5. Do you sometimes feel the need to Cut down on your drinking?

   (*If yes, give yourself one point.*)

If you score a total of two or more points, or if you can hold six or more drinks without falling asleep or passing out, you may have a drinking problem. You should do something about it. It does not matter whether or not you are physically addicted to alcohol; it does not matter whether or not you can, to some extent, curtail your drinking now. If you have developed a degree of dependence on alcohol, your drinking may become worse over time. Help is available, and it is best to seek help early.

SUPPORT GROUPS, TREATMENT INFORMATION, AND BASIC INFORMATION ON ALCOHOL AND DRUGS

ALCOHOLICS ANONYMOUS
P.O. BOX 459, GRAND CENTRAL STATION, NEW YORK, NY 10163
www.alcoholics-anonymous.org

Check your phone book for local listings. A worldwide fellowship for anyone who wants to achieve and maintain sobriety. The staff—themselves recovering alcoholics—can direct you to meetings near you. They can also tell you whether there are all-women's meetings in your area.

AL-ANON FAMILY GROUP/ALATEEN
1600 CORPORATE LANDING PARKWAY, VIRGINIA BEACH, VA 23454
(800) 356-9996

www.al-anon.alateen.org
Al-Anon, whose program is adapted from the twelve steps of Alcoholics Anonymous, is a fellowship for relatives and friends of people with an alcohol problem. Alateen is primarily for teenagers.

CHILDREN OF ALCOHOLICS FOUNDATION, INC.
33 WEST 60TH STREET, 5TH FLOOR, NEW YORK, NY 10023
Information and meeting referrals: (800) 359-2623; (212) 757-2100,
extension 6370
www.coaf.org

This organization is devoted to helping young and adult children of
alcoholics, informing and educating the public and professionals about
this group, and disseminating research and new data on the effects of
family alcoholism on children.

DRUG AND ALCOHOL TREATMENT REFERRALS
(800) DRUG-HELP
www.DRUGHELP.org

This service provides advice and referrals to individuals about drug and
alcohol treatment services, including referrals to programs in the
caller's area. Run by the federal Substance Abuse and Mental Health
Services Administration, it operates twenty-four hours a day.

JACs: JEWISH ALCOHOLICS, CHEMICALLY DEPENDENT PERSONS,
AND SIGNIFICANT OTHERS
850 SEVENTH AVENUE, NEW YORK, NY 10019
212-397-4197
www.jacsweb.org

JACS meetings around the country are generally used as supplements
to twelve-step work. They provide connections among Jews in recovery
so that they will not feel alone, and they discuss ways that Judaism can
enhance their recovery. They also provide education to the Jewish community and act as advocates for Jews with treatment facilities and other
services.

LATINO COUNCIL ON ALCOHOL AND TOBACCO
1015 15TH STREET, NW, SUITE 409, WASHINGTON, DC 20005
(202) 371-1186
http://www.incacorp.com/lcat

A national organization dedicated to reducing the enormous harm caused by alcohol and tobacco in the Latino community. Advocates prevention measures ranging from education to legislation to promote better health among children and adults.

NATIONAL ASIAN PACIFIC AMERICAN FAMILIES AGAINST
SUBSTANCE ABUSE, INC.
300 WEST CESAR CHAVEZ AVENUE, #B,
LOS ANGELES, CA 90012-2818
(213) 625-5795
http://www.igc.apc.org/apiahf/napafasa.html

A private, nonprofit membership organization dedicated to strengthening families and promoting culturally competent substance abuse and related services for Asians and Pacific Islanders. Also focuses on issues and problems related to substance abuse such as health care, gang and domestic violence, mental health, and poverty.

NATIONAL BLACK ALCOHOLISM AND ADDICTIONS COUNCIL, INC.
1101 14TH STREET, NW, SUITE 630, WASHINGTON, DC 20005-5601
(202) 296-2696

An organization through which blacks concerned with alcoholism or involved in the field can exchange ideas, offer services, and coordinate and facilitate alcoholism programs that operate in the interest of black Americans.

NATIONAL CLEARINGHOUSE FOR ALCOHOL AND
DRUG INFORMATION (NCADI)
P.O. BOX 2345, ROCKVILLE, MD 20847
(800) 729-6686
www.health.org

A comprehensive resource for free informational material on alcohol and drug abuse. Offers materials from the Center for Substance Abuse Prevention, the National Institute on Drug Abuse, the National Institute of Alcohol Abuse and Addiction, and more.

NATIONAL COUNCIL ON ALCOHOLISM AND
DRUG DEPENDENCE, INC. (NCADD)
12 WEST 21ST STREET, 7TH FLOOR, NEW YORK, NY 10010
(800) NCA-CALL
(212) 206-6770
www.ncadd.org

NCADD advocates prevention, intervention, and treatment; it is committed to fighting the stigma, denial, and shame of alcoholism and drug addiction. Through the automated service at the national number, callers may be connected to their local NCADD affiliate for referrals to treatment services in their area.

NATIONAL INSTITUTE ON ALCOHOL ABUSE AND
ALCOHOLISM (NIAAA)
6000 EXECUTIVE BOULEVARD, SUITE 400,
BETHESDA, MD 20892-7003
(301) 443-3860
http://www.niaaa.nih.gov

The primary purpose of this federal government agency is to fund research on alcohol abuse and alcoholism. Available information on alcoholism includes accessible "Most Frequently Asked Questions" and "Alcohol Alert" bulletins to professional research publications. Several publications are available on the web in full text. Publications are also available from NCADI (see above).

RATIONAL RECOVERY SELF-HELP NETWORK
Box 8100, LOTUS, CA 95651
(530) 621-4374 or (530) 621-2667
http://www.rational.org/recovery

An abstinence-based, non-twelve-step recovery program with no religious, spiritual, or psychological content. Based on Addictive Voice Recognition Technique, a tutorial which can be found on the organization's website.

SECULAR ORGANIZATIONS FOR SOBRIETY (SOS)
CENTER FOR INQUIRY—WEST, 5521 GROSVENOR BOULEVARD, LOS ANGELES, CA 90066
(310) 821-8430
http://www.secularhumanism.org/sos/

A non–spiritually based recovery fellowship.

S.M.A.R.T. Recovery
24000 Mercantile Road, Suite #11, Beachwood, OH 44122
(216) 292-0220
http://www.smartrecovery.org

An abstinence-based, non-twelve-step self-help program for people having problems with drinking and drugs. Based on the principles of rational emotive behavior therapy.

WOMEN FOR SOBRIETY
P.O. Box 618, QUAKERTOWN, PA 18951-0618
(800) 333-1606
http://www.womenforsobriety.org

A national membership organization that aims to help all women with a drinking problem find a way to sobriety and a fulfilling way of life. Small, local groups of women meet to discuss their shared problems and needs.

INTERNET RECOVERY RESOURCES

In addition to the sites listed above:

ADDICTION RESOURCE GUIDE: <www.hubplace.com/addictions/>   A comprehensive set of links to addiction treatment facilities online.

CENTER FOR SUBSTANCE ABUSE TREATMENT (CSAT): <www.samsha.gov/csat/csat.htm/>   This site allows you to search for treatment and prevention programs nationwide. Gives information on location, services, and payment.

CESAR BOARD: General Information on Alcohol: <www.bsos.umd.edu/cesar/alcohol.html>   Provides basic information about alcohol, including direct and indirect effects of alcohol on the brain and the liver.

CHRISTIANS IN RECOVERY, INC.: <www.christians-in-recovery.com> Resources for Christians in recovery, including online meetings and e-mail fellowships.

CLOSE TO HOME: MOYERS ON ADDICTION: <www.wnet.org/closetohome/>   This is a companion site to Bill Moyers's television series on addiction. It includes such links as self-help and treatment, general information about addiction, and information for health professionals.

CSAP WORKPLACE HELPLINE: <www.health.org/pubs/workcap.htm> Or call 1-800-WORKPLACE. Center for Substance Abuse Prevention offers a consulting service for business, labor, and community alcohol and drug abuse prevention organizations.

HAZELDEN FOUNDATION: <www.hazelden.org/index.htm> Hazelden, a twelve-step-based substance abuse treatment center, offers educational materials on chemical dependency and related areas. This site includes an index of publications, and meditations for recovery.

ONLINE AA RECOVERY RESOURCES: <www.recovery.org>   This site contains a wealth of information, including online AA meetings, worldwide Intergroup phone numbers, convention information, and an online version of the Big Book.

RECOVERY NETWORK: <www.recoverynetwork.com>   This commercial site contains links to hundreds of recovery-oriented websites, including twelve-step groups, secular groups, and religious groups such as Christians in Recovery and JACS (see above). There are also links to information on addiction and recovery.

Notes

FOREWORD

xiv. public policy initiatives: S. B. Blume, "Women and Alcohol: Issues in Social
Policy," in Gender and Alcohol: Individual and Social Perspectives, eds.
R. W. Wilsnack and S. C. Wilsnack (New Brunswick, N.J.: Rutgers Center
of Alcohol Studies, 1997), 462–489.

INTRODUCTION

2. Reviving Ophelia: M. Pipher, Reviving Ophelia: Saving the Selves of Adolescent
Girls (New York: Ballantine, 1994), 19.

6. tale of addiction: For an analysis of the limitations of the AA model, see Jeffer-
son Singer, Message in a Bottle: Stories of Men and Addiction (New York: Free
Press, 1997).

6. evangelical Oxford Group: Alcoholics Anonymous World Services, Inc., Dr. Bob
and the Good Oldtimers (New York: Author, 1980).

6. particular story: In Many Roads, One Journey: Moving Beyond the Twelve Steps
(New York: HarperCollins, 1992), Charlotte Davis Kasl gives a sympathetic
account of the origins of AA, and why it works better for some people than
for others.

7. "thirteenth stepping": For discussions of women and AA, see Margaret Coker,
"Overcoming Sexism in AA: How Women Cope," in Gender and Addictions:
Men and Women in Treatment, eds. S. L. A. Straussner and E. Zelvin (Northvale,
N.J.: Jason Aronson, 1997), 264–281; S. S. Covington, "Sororities of Help-
ing and Healing: Women and Mutual Help Groups," in Alcohol and Drugs
Are Women's Issues, ed. P. Roth (Metuchen, N.J.: Women's Action Alliance
and Scarecrow, 1991); S. S. Covington, A Woman's Way Through the Twelve
Steps (Center City, Minn.: Hazelden, 1994). See also Kasl, Many Roads, One
Journey.

9. process is circular: Systems theory emphasizes the need to remove the frame of
causality from our thinking about human behavior. See C. Bepko with

J. Krestan, *The Responsibility Trap: A Blueprint for Treating the Alcoholic Family* (New York: Free Press, 1985).

9. *dopamine functioning*: For a review of research on neurotransmitters as mediators of alcohol-related behavior, see the *Ninth Special Report to Congress on Alcohol and Health* (U.S. Department of Health and Human Services, 1997), 99–130.

9. *manageable range*: This paragraph draws on "Moyers on Addiction: Close to Home," a production of Public Affairs Television, Princeton, N.J., Films for the Humanities and Sciences (FFH 7681).

10. *study of alcoholic women*: K.S. Kendler, A.S. Heath, R.C. Kessler, and L.J. Euves, "A Twin-Family Study of Alcoholism in Women," *American Journal of Psychiatry* 151 (5): 707–715, 1994. Cited in *Ninth Special Report,* 36.

10. *Asian-American woman*: M.R. Gillmore et al., "Racial Differences in Acceptability and Availability of Drugs and Early Initiation of Substance Abuse," *American Journal of Drug and Alcohol Abuse* 16, no. 3–4 (1990): 185–206.

10. *familial level*: G.M. Barnes, M.P. Farrell, and S. Banerjee, "Family Influences on Alcohol Abuse and Other Problem Behaviors Among Black and White Adolescents in a General Population Sample," in *Alcohol Problems Among Adolescents: Current Directions in Prevention Research,* eds. G.M. Boyd, J. Howard, and R.A. Zucker (Hillsdale, N.J.: Lawrence Erlbaum Associates, 1995), 13–31.

10. *George Vaillant*: G.E. Vaillant, "Prospective Evidence for the Effects of Environment upon Alcoholism," in *Alcoholism and the Family*, eds. S. Saitoh, P. Steinglass, and M.A. Schuckit (New York: Brunner/Mazel, 1992), 71–83. John Searles cites this example in an unpublished paper, "The Genetics of Alcoholism: Implications for Prevention and Treatment."

10. *certain personality scores*: *Ninth Special Report*, 48–49.

11. *study published in 1973*: G.A. Marlatt, B. Demming, and J.B. Reid, "Loss of Control Drinking in Alcoholics: An Experimental Analogue," *Journal of Abnormal Psychology* 81, no. 3 (1973): 233–241.

11. *Biochemical expressions*: Except for the example of cortisol, I am drawing on R.J. Degrandpré, "Just Cause?" *The Sciences* (March/April 1999): 14–18.

12. *clarifies certain points*: H. Begleiter and B. Porjesz, "What Is Inherited in the Predisposition to Alcoholism," *Alcoholism: Clinical and Experimental Research* 23, no. 7 (July 1999); also, Henri Begleiter, personal conversation with the author, July 13, 1999.

13. *"No gene exists"*: *Ninth Special Report*, 43.

13. *the clearest association*: M.A. Schuckit, "Genetics of the Risk for Alcoholism," *American Journal on Addictions,* in press.

13. *study of 450 sons*: Ibid.

14. *Andrew Heath*: A.C. Heath, P.A.F. Madden, et al., "Genetic Differences in Alcohol Sensitivity and the Inheritance of Alcoholism Risk," *Psychological Medicine* 29, no. 5 (1999): 1069–1981. Heath's findings present an interesting vari-

ation of emphasis from Schuckit's: among the men in his study, the protective effect of being highly sensitive to alcohol was significant, while having a low sensitivity to alcohol was only somewhat associated with alcohol dependence.

14. *Another (somewhat contradictory)*: *Ninth Special Report*, 44.

14. *study of Japanese-Americans*: T. V. Nakawatase et al., "The Association Between Fast-Flushing Response and Alcohol Use Among Japanese Americans, *Journal of Studies on Alcohol* 54, no. 1 (1993): 48–53.

14. *Dr. Henri Begleiter's group*: Begleiter and Porjesz, "What Is Inherited in the Predisposition to Alcoholism," 1125–1135; also, Henri Begleiter, personal conversation with the author, July 13, 1999.

15. *multidimensional research agenda*: National Institute on Drug Abuse, "Research on the Origins of and Pathways to Drug Abuse," *NIH Guide* 26, no. 8 (March 14, 1997), PA 97–043.

16. *redefine it as a biological illness*: Interestingly, even many of the staunchest proponents of the disease concept acknowledge that it is a simplification. For instance, George Vaillant, in his influential book *The Natural History of Alcoholism Revisited* (Cambridge: Harvard University Press, 1995), argues that "to treat alcoholics effectively we need to invoke the model of the medical practitioner," but he concedes that "alcohol dependence lies on a continuum and . . . in scientific terms *behavior disorder* will often be a happier choice than *disease*," 22.

CHAPTER 1: WHY MEN CAN OUTDRINK WOMEN

23. *Harvard Nurses' Health Study*: C. S. Fuchs, M. J. Stampfer, G. A. Colditz, et al. "Alcohol Consumption and Mortality Among Women," *New England Journal of Medicine* 332, no. 19 (1995): 1245–1250.

23. *moderate and acceptable alcohol intake*: U.S. Department of Agriculture, Agricultural Research Service, Advisory Guidelines Committee, *Report of the Dietary Guidelines Advisory Committee on the Dietary Guidelines for Americans to the Secretary of Health and Human Services and the Secretary of Agriculture* (Washington, D.C.: U.S. Department of Agriculture, 1995).

24. *Women metabolize alcohol differently*: S. B. Blume, "Women and Addictive Disorders," in *Principles of Addiction Medicine*, ed. N. S. Miller (Chevy Chase, Md.: American Society of Addiction Medicine, 1994), 1–16. Current research is also investigating size of the liver as a factor in women's alcohol metabolism.

24. *risk of cirrhosis*: B. F. Grant et al., "Epidemiology of Alcoholic Liver Disease," *Seminars in Liver Disease* 8, no. 1 (1988): 12–25. Other estimates range from 20 to 40 grams of pure alcohol for women and from 40 to 80 grams for men. See *Eighth Special Report to the U.S. Congress on Alcohol and Health* (Alexandria, Va.: National Institute on Alcohol Abuse and Alcoholism, 1993).

24. *developing high blood pressure*: J.C.M. Witteman et al., "Relation of Moderate Alcohol Consumption and Risk of Systemic Hypertension in Women," *American Journal of Cardiology* 65 (1990): 633–637. Cited in Blume, "Women and Addictive Disorders."

24–25. *counteract osteoporosis*: See S. Hill, "Mental and Physical Health Consequences of Alcohol Use in Women," in *Recent Developments in Alcoholism*, Vol. 12: *Alcoholism and Women*, ed. Marc Galanter (New York: Plenum Press, 1995), 186; and L.J. Tivis and J. Gavaler, "Alcohol, Hormones, and Health in Post-Menopausal Women," *Alcohol Health and Research World* 18, no. 3: 185–188.

25. *menstrual irregularities: Ninth Special Report*, 160.

25. *spontaneous abortion*: S. Harlap and P.H. Shiono, "Alcohol, Smoking and Incidence of Spontaneous Abortions in the First and Second Trimesters," *Lancet* 2, no. 8187 (July 1980): 173–176. Cited in National Center on Addiction and Substance Abuse at Columbia University (CASA), *Substance Abuse and the American Woman* (New York: Author, 1996), 80. This study found that women who had more than three drinks daily had 3.5 times greater risk of spontaneous abortion than nondrinkers.

25. *fetal alcohol effects*: K.A. Tolo Passaro and R.E. Little, "Childbearing and Alcohol Use," in *Gender and Alcohol: Individual and Social Perspectives*, eds. R.W. Wilsnack and S.C. Wilsnack (New Brunswick, N.J.: Rutgers Center of Alcohol Studies, 1997), 90–113.

25. *infant death rate*: Center for Disease Control and Prevention, National Center for Health Statistics, Linked Birth/Infant Death Data Set, 1991.

25. *Framingham Heart Study*: Y. Zhang et al., "Alcohol Consumption and Risk of Breast Cancer: The Framingham Study Revisited," *American Journal of Epidemiology* 149, no. 2 (January 1999): 93–101.

25. *Earlier studies suggest*: Hill, "Mental and Physical Health Consequences of Alcohol Use in Women," 186; M.P. Longnecker, "Alcoholic Beverage Consumption in Relation to Risk of Breast Cancer: Meta-analysis and Review," *Cancer Causes and Control* 5, no. 1 (1994): 73–82.

25. *a study conducted by the American Cancer Society*: M.J. Thun, A.D. Lopez, et al., "Alcohol Consumption and Mortality Among Middle-Aged and Elderly U.S. Adults," *New England Journal of Medicine* 337, no. 24 (1997): 1705–1714.

26. *When a woman's production of estrogen*: Tivis and Gavaler, "Alcohol, Hormones, and Health in Post-Menopausal Women," 185–188; Fuchs, Stampfer, Colditz, et al.): 1245–1250; CASA, *Substance Abuse and the American Woman*, 47–48.

26. *consumed six or more drinks*: A.L. Klatsky, "Blood Pressure and Alcohol Intake," in *Hypertension, Pathophysiology, Diagnosis and Management*, eds. J.H. Laragh and B.M. Brenner (New York: Raven Press, 1990), 277–294.

26. *8,000 cardiovascular deaths*: E. Hanna et al., "Dying to Be Equal: Women, Alcohol, and Cardiovascular Disease," *British Journal of Addiction* 87 (1992): 1593–1597.

26. *depresses the immune system*: B. A. Miller and W. R. Downs, "The Impact of Family Violence on the Use of Alcohol by Women," *Alcohol Health and Research World* 17, no. 2 (1993): 176.

26. *esophageal cancer*: *Ninth Special Report*, 139.

26. *both suffer damage to the liver*: For reviews of the literature on gender differences in susceptibility to alcohol, see Hill, "Mental and Physical Health Consequences of Alcohol Use in Women," 181–197; C. S. Lieber, "Gender Differences in Alcohol Metabolism and Susceptibility," in *Gender and Alcohol: Individual and Social Perspectives*, eds. R. W. Wilsnack and S. C. Wilsnack (New Brunswick, N.J.: Rutgers Center of Alcohol Studies, 1997), 77–113; M. Schuckit, J. Daeppen, J. Tipp, M. Hesselbrock, and K. Bucholz, "The Clinical Course of Alcohol-Related Problems in Alcohol Dependent and Nonalcohol Dependent Drinking Women and Men," *Journal of Studies on Alcohol* (September 1998): 581–590.

27. *women's rate of completed suicide*: Hill, "Mental and Physical Health Consequences of Alcohol Use in Women," 181–197.

27. *five times more likely to commit suicide*: E. M. Smith et al., "Predictors of Mortality in Alcoholic Women: Prospective Follow-Up Study," *Alcohol and Clinical Experimental Research* 7 (1983): 237–243; S. B. Blume, "Gender Differences in Alcohol-Related Disorders," *Harvard Review of Psychiatry* 2, no. 1 (1994): 7–14.

27. *criteria defined by the American Psychiatric Association*: American Psychiatric Association, *Diagnostic and Statistical Manual of Mental Disorders* (4th ed.). Washington, D.C.: Author, 1994.

27. *In short, says one doctor*: J. W. West, *The Betty Ford Center Book of Answers* (New York: Pocket Books, 1997), 17.

27. *An individual's pattern of drinking*: Hill, "Mental and Physical Health Consequences of Alcohol Use in Women," 183.

28. *highest rates of problem drinking*: Blume, "Women and Addictive Disorders," 2.

28. *leading single drug of abuse*: N. D. Volgeltanz and S. C. Wilsnack, "Alcohol Problems in Women: Risk Factors, Consequences, and Treatment Strategies," in *Health Care for Women: Psychological, Social, and Behavioral Influences*, eds. S. J. Gallant, G. Puryear Keita, and R. Royak-Schaler (Washington, D.C.: American Psychological Association, 1997), 75.

28. *Institute of Medicine*: Institute of Medicine, *Broadening the Base of Treatment for Alcohol Problems* (Washington, D.C.: National Academy Press, 1990).

28. *In a follow-up analysis*: R. W. Wilsnack, S. C. Wilsnack, A. F. Kristjanson, and T. R. Harris, "Ten-Year Prediction of Women's Drinking Behavior in a Nationally Representative Sample," *Women's Health: Research on Gender, Behavior, and Policy* 4, no. 3 (1998): 199–230.

28. *Typically, both young women and young men*: E. L. Gomberg, "Alcohol Abuse: Age and Gender Differences," in *Gender and Alcohol: Individual and Social Per-*

spectives, eds. R. W. Wilsnack and S. C. Wilsnack (New Brunswick, N.J.: Rutgers Center of Alcohol Studies, 1997), 225.

29. *The alcoholic beverage industry*: Blume, "Women and Addictive Disorders," 13.

29. *Women in treatment*: Miller and Downs, "The Impact of Family Violence on the Use of Alcohol by Women"; B. A. Miller et al., "Spousal Violence Among Alcoholic Women as Compared to a Random Household Sample of Women," *Journal of Studies on Alcohol* 50, no. 6 (1989): 533–540.

29. *particular barriers*: Blume, "Women and Alcohol," 462–489.

29. *wind up with a cross-addiction*: National Center on Addiction and Substance Abuse at Columbia University (CASA), *Under the Rug: Substance Abuse and the Mature Woman* (New York: Author, 1998).

30. *Oral contraceptives reduce*: Blume, "Women and Addictive Disorders."

30. *high rates of sexual problems*: S. C. Wilsnack, J. J. Plaud, R. W. Wilsnack, and A. D. Klassen, "Sexuality, Gender, and Alcohol Use," in *Gender and Alcohol: Individual and Social Perspectives*, eds. R. W. Wilsnack and S. C. Wilsnack (New Brunswick, N.J.: Rutgers Center of Alcohol Studies, 1997), 250–288.

30. *form of self-treatment*: E. S. L. Gomberg summarizes this research in "Women's Drinking Practices and Problems from a Lifespan Perspective," in *Women and Alcohol: Issues for Prevention Research*, NIAAA *Research Monograph* 32, eds. J. M. Howard, S. E. Martin, P. D. Mail, M. E. Hilton, E. D. Taylor (Bethesda, Md.: National Institutes of Health, 1996): 188–189. Gomberg notes the ambiguity of some of the early studies emphasizing traumatic events as precipitating women's abusive drinking. She suggests that a woman's coping style may be a more important factor in alcohol problems than the number of traumatic events in her life but also notes the growing evidence linking childhood trauma with alcohol and drug abuse.

30. *the number of male drivers*: National Institute on Alcohol Abuse and Alcoholism (NIAAA), "Trends in Alcohol-Related Fatal Traffic Crashes, United States, 1977–1994 (December 1996): 1.

30. *responding to visual cues*: NIAAA, Alcohol Alert, no. 46, December 1999: "Are Women More Vulnerable to Alcohol's Effects?"

30. *more likely than alcoholic men to have a mental health disorder*: M. N. Hesselbrock and V. M. Hesselbrock, "Gender, Alcoholism, and Psychiatric Comorbidity," in *Gender and Alcohol: Individual and Social Perspectives*, eds. R. W. Wilsnack and S. C. Wilsnack (New Brunswick, N.J.: Rutgers Center of Alcohol Studies, 1997), 49–71.

30. *childhood sexual abuse twice as often*: Miller and Downs, "Impact of Family Violence."

31. *Girls who are sexually or physically abused*: C. S. Widom, "Alcohol Abuse in Abused and Neglected Children Followed Up: Are They at Increased Risk?" *Journal of Studies on Alcohol* 56 (1995): 207–217.

31. *Lesbian and bisexual women*: For a review of the research on drinking in lesbian populations, see Wilsnack, Plaud, Wilsnack, and Klassen, "Sexuality, Gender, and Alcohol Use," 258–260.

31. *number of women who drink has increased sharply*: CASA, *Substance Abuse and the American Woman*, 42–43.

31. *572 women in treatment*: P. A. Harrison, "Women in Treatment: Changing Over Time," *International Journal of the Addictions* 24, no. 7 (1989): 655–673.

31. *men leave their alcoholic wives*: See CASA, *Substance Abuse and the American Woman*, 113, for citations of literature on family responses to alcohol problems in women.

31. *Women who are not married*: Vogeltanz and Wilsnack, "Alcohol Problems in Women," 80.

31. *threats of prosecution*: CASA, *Substance Abuse and the American Woman*, 112–130.

32. *African-American women who drink heavily*: R. J. Sokol et al., "Significant Determinants of Susceptibility to Alcohol Teratogenicity," *Annals of the New York Academy of Sciences* 477 (1986): 87–102. *Ninth Special Report* refers to a study which concludes, "Although FAS occurs in all racial groups, its incidence is greater in populations with low socioeconomic status, regardless of race." Genetic influences may also play a role in different levels of vulnerability to FAS. See *Ninth Special Report*, 210.

32. *dependence is lower for African-American women*: CASA, *Substance Abuse and the American Woman*, 46.

32. *Statistically, a woman is somewhat more at risk*: Vogeltanz and Wilsnack, "Alcohol Problems in Women," 75–96.

CHAPTER 2: WOMEN AND DRINKING: A LONG STORY IN BRIEF

35. *Dr. Marc Schuckit*: M. A. Schuckit, "The Alcoholic Woman: A Literature Review," *Psychiatry in Medicine* 3, no. 1 (1972): 44.

35. *In a survey*: Wilsnack, Plaud, Wilsnack, and Klassen, "Sexuality, Gender, and Alcohol Use," 250–288.

36. *rape scenarios*: See S. B. Blume, "Alcoholism in Women," *Harvard Mental Health Letter* (March 1998): 5–7; and Wilsnack, Plaud, Wilsnack, and Klassen, "Sexuality, Gender, and Alcohol Use," 250–288.

36. *worse anxiety*: S. Hill, "Vulnerability to the Biomedical Consequences of Alcoholism and Alcohol-Related Problems Among Women," in *Alcohol Problems in Women*, eds. S. C. Wilsnack and L. J. Beckman (New York: Guilford Press, 1984), 121–154.

37. *alcohol-related accident*: K. M. Fillmore et al., "Patterns and Trends in Women's and Men's Drinking," in *Gender and Alcohol: Individual and Social*

Perspectives, eds. R. W. Wilsnack and S. C. Wilsnack (New Brunswick, N. J.: Rutgers Center of Alcohol Studies, 1997), 21–48.

37. *Kaye Middleton Fillmore*: Kaye Middleton Fillmore, personal interview with the author, December 10, 1998.

37. *Barry Carr*: Barry Carr, personal conversation with the author, December 10, 1998.

37. *"When she is drunk"*: Quoted in N. Purcell, "Women and Wine in Ancient Rome," in *Gender, Drink and Drugs*, ed. M. McDonald (Oxford: Berg, 1994), 191–208.

38. *"The real issue"*: M. Sandmaier, *The Invisible Alcoholics: Women and Alcohol Abuse in America* (New York: McGraw-Hill, 1980), 24.

39. *biological factors*: Fillmore et al., "Patterns and Trends in Women's and Men's Drinking," 21–48.

39. *cross-cultural study*: Richard W. Wilsnack, Nancy D. Vogeltanz, Sharon C. Wilsnack, and T. Robert Harris, et al., "Gender Differences in Alcohol Consumption and Adverse Drinking Consequences: Cross-Cultural Patterns," *Addiction* 95, No. 2 (2000): 251–265.

40. *"Olympian height"*: B. A. Ikuesan, "Drinking Problems and the Position of Women in Nigeria," *Addiction* 89 (1994): 941–944.

40. *native Korean*: S. Hill, "Vulnerability to Alcoholism in Women: Genetic and Cultural Factors," in *Recent Developments in Alcoholism*, Vol. 12: *Women and Alcoholism*, ed. Marc Galanter (New York: Plenum Press, 1995), 23.

41. *monastic rules*: Quoted in E. Amt, *Women's Lives in Medieval Europe: A Sourcebook* (London: Routledge, 1993), 226.

41. *noble women*: M. Plant, *Women and Alcohol: Contemporary & Historical Perspectives* (London: Free Association Books, 1997), 35.

42. *inappropriate medication*: See S. R. Kandall, *Substance and Shadow: Women and Addiction in the United States* (Cambridge, Mass.: Harvard University Press, 1996).

42. *drink alone*: Harrison, "Women in Treatment: Changing Over Time."

42. *Seventy-five percent*: M. D. George, *London Life in the Eighteenth Century* (New York: Capricorn, 1965), 26. Cited in M. Plant, *Women and Alcohol: Contemporary and Historical Perspectives* (London: Free Association Books, 1997), 35.

43. *Sandmaier writes*: Sandmaier, *Invisible Alcoholics*, 33. I draw on Sandmaier for much of this history.

43. *"necessary weapon"*: A. Sinclair, *The Better Half: The Emancipation of the American Woman* (New York: Harper and Row, 1965), 224. Quoted in Sandmaier, *Invisible Alcoholics*.

44. *40 percent of American women*: S. C. Wilsnack, R. W. Wilsnack, and S. Hiller-Sturmhöfel, "How Women Drink: Epidemiology of Women's Drinking and Problem Drinking," *Alcohol Health and Research World* 18, no. 3 (1994): 173–184.

44. *Britain and Australia*: Plant, *Women and Alcohol*, 1997, 13.

45. *according to Richard and Sharon Wilsnack*: R. W. Wilsnack and S. C. Wilsnack, "Introduction" in *Gender and Alcohol: Individual and Social Perspectives*, eds. R. W. Wilsnack and S. C. Wilsnack (New Brunswick, N.J.: Rutgers Center of Alcohol Studies, 1997), 9. See also S. B. Blume, "Sexuality and Stigma: The Alcoholic Woman," *Alcohol Health and Research World* 15, no. 2 (1991): 139–146.

CHAPTER 3: MARRIAGE AND PARTNERSHIPS

49. *It has been known*: S. C. Wilsnack and R. W. Wilsnack, "Drinking and Problem Drinking in U.S. Women: Patterns and Recent Trends," in *Recent Developments in Alcoholism,* Vol. 12: *Alcoholism and Women,* ed. Marc Galanter (New York: Plenum Press, 1995), 30–60.

49. *Heavy drinkers get together*: L. J. Roberts and K. E. Leonard, "Gender Differences and Similarities in the Alcohol and Marriage Relationship," in *Gender and Alcohol: Individual and Social Perspectives,* eds. R. W. Wilsnack and S. C. Wilsnack (New Brunswick, N.J.: Rutgers Center of Alcohol Studies, 1997), 289–311.

58. *Dr. Josette Mondanaro*: J. Mondanaro, *Chemically Dependent Women: Assessment and Treatment* (Lexington, Mass.: Lexington Books, 1989), 24.

58. *Elizabeth Zelvin*: Elizabeth Zelvin, personal conversation with the author, April 9, 1999. See also E. Zelvin, "Codependency Issues of Substance-Abusing Women," in *Gender and Addictions: Men and Women in Treatment,* eds. S. L. A. Straussner and E. Zelvin (Northvale, N.J.: Jason Aronson, 1997), 47–70.

61. *Charlotte Davis Kasl*: Kasl, *Many Roads, One Journey,* 279.

61. *Claudia Bepko and Jo-Ann Krestan*: Bepko and Krestan, *Responsibility Trap.*

62. *"It's tempting to assume"*: Claudia Bepko, personal conversation with the author, April 8, 1999.

62. *"disorders of power"*: C. Bepko, "Disorders of Power: Women and Addiction in the Family," in *Women in Families,* eds. M. McGoldrick, C. Anderson, and F. Walsh (New York: W. W. Norton, 1989), 406–426.

64. *conflict has been framed*: Ibid., 57.

64. *"males are pitted against females"*: Ibid., 69.

CHAPTER 4: MOTHERS: A MESSAGE FROM THE OWL

70. *"Woman needs to give"*: Quoted in P. J. Caplan, *Don't Blame Mother: Mending the Mother-Daughter Relationship* (New York: Harper and Row, 1989), 77. Caplan lists myths about the perfect mother. Myth 2 is, "Mothers are endless founts of nurturance."

70. *"lost their maternal instinct"*: See Kandall, *Substance and Shadow,* 285.

71. *"When a woman's shame gets intense"*: Sandy Kleven, coordinator of the Women and Children's Program, Hazelden Women and Children's Recovery Community, personal conversation with the author, February 22, 1999.

71. *Claudia Bepko*: Claudia Bepko, personal conversation with the author, April 8, 1999. All quotations from Claudia Bepko are taken from this conversation.

74. *Jean Kirkpatrick*: J. Kirkpatrick, *Turnabout: New Help for the Woman Alcoholic* (New York: Bantam Books, 1990), 69.

74. *"not caused by weakness:"* Alcoholics Anonymous pamphlet.

76. *early loss of her mother*: See Chapter 8 for a discussion of early separation from a parent as a predictor of continuing alcohol problems in women.

76. *"role deprivation"*: Wilsnack and Wilsnack, "Drinking and Problem Drinking in U.S. Women," 30–60.

77. *Naomi Lowinsky*: N. R. Lowinsky, *The Motherline* (Los Angeles: Tarcher, 1993).

79. *Judith Viorst*: J. Viorst, *Necessary Losses: The Loves, Illusions, Dependencies, and Impossible Expectations That All of Us Have to Give Up in Order to Grow* (New York: Fireside, 1998): 249.

81. *Fetal alcohol syndrome:* I am drawing on a summary of the research in Passaro and Little, "Childbearing and Alcohol Use," 90–113.

82. *U.S. Department of Health*: U.S. Department of Health and Human Services, National Clearinghouse for Alcohol and Drug Information, "Making the Link: Alcohol, Tobacco, and Other Drugs and Pregnancy and Parenthood," Spring 1995.

82. *uncritical focus on the effects of light drinking*: Maura Plant makes this argument in *Women and Alcohol: Contemporary and Historical Perspectives,* 140–173.

82. *Native American populations*: Drinking rates vary among tribes, and FAS statistics also vary.

82. *it appears in populations*: *Ninth Special Report,* 210.

82. *Since 1985, prosecutors*: CASA, *Substance Abuse and the American Woman,* 119–130.

83. *$88.2 million*: Kandall, *Substance and Shadow,* 286.

83. *moving away from treatment*: For a thorough discussion of this issue, see ibid.

85. *mothers who currently abuse*: I am drawing on N. J. Smyth and B. A. Miller, "Parenting Issues for Substance-Abusing Women," in *Gender and Addictions: Men and Women in Treatment,* eds. S. L. A. Straussner and E. Zelvin (Northvale, N. J.: Jason Aronson, 1997), 125–150.

85. *"They create another unit of cost"*: Dr. Camille Barry, personal conversation with the author, July 8, 1998.

85. *she may be overwhelmed*: Smyth and Miller, "Parenting Issues for Substance-Abusing Women."

86. *Shirley Coletti*: Shirley Coletti, personal conversation with the author, February 3, 1999. Quotations from Shirley Coletti are all from this conversation.

86. *Women's Alcoholism Center*: K. Bishop, "Alcoholic Women: New Approach in San Francisco," *New York Times,* May 17, 1997.

87. *Sandy Klevens*: Sandy Klevens, personal conversation with the author, February 22, 1999. For information about the Hazelden Women and Children's Recovery Community, call 1-800-257-7800.

87. *loss of their mothering role*: C. N. Williams and L. V. Klerman, "Female Alcohol Abuse: Its Effects on the Family," in *Alcohol Problems in Women,* eds. S. C. Wilsnack and L. J. Beckman (New York: Guilford Press, 1984), 302.

CHAPTER 5: TEENAGE GIRLS AND COLLEGE WOMEN

94. *American Association of University Women*: American Association of University Women, *Shortchanging Girls, Shortchanging America* (Washington, D.C.: Greenberg-Lake, 1991).

95. *"girls' true selves"*: Pipher, *Reviving Ophelia,* 22.

95. *Relational theory suggests*: I am drawing on J. P. Salzman, "Save the World, Save Myself," in *Making Connections: The Relational Worlds of Adolescent Girls at Emma Willard School,* eds. N. P. Lyons and T. J. Hanmer (New York: Troy, 1989), 113.

96. *regular drinking begins*: CASA, *Substance Abuse and the American Woman,* 43.

96. *some of this drinking is "normal"*: Pipher, *Reviving Ophelia,* 190.

96. *research has linked drinking in adolescence*: Chassin and DeLucia, "Drinking During Adolescence," 177.

97. *drinking habits of adolescents*: R. W. Edwards, P. J. Thurman, and F. Beauvais, "Patterns of Alcohol Use Among Ethnic Minority Adolescent Women," in *Recent Developments in Alcoholism,* Vol. 12, ed. Marc Galanter (New York: Plenum Press, 1995), 369–386.

97. *Among Hispanic students*: M. Windle, "Alcohol Use and Abuse," *Alcohol Health and Research World* 15, no. 1 (1991): 5–10.

97. *among ethnic minority communities, family values*: Edwards, Thurman, and Beauvais, "Patterns of Alcohol Use Among Ethnic Minority Adolescent Women."

97. *religiosity in teenagers*: K. M. Thompson and R. W. Wilsnack, "Drinking and Drinking Problems Among Female Adolescents: Patterns and Influences," in *Alcohol Problems in Women,* eds. S. C. Wilsnack and L. J. Beckman (New York: Guilford Press, 1984), 37–65.

98. *dramatic increase in the use of illicit drugs*: National Institute on Drug Abuse Media Advisory, December 17, 1999.

99. *spend more on alcohol*: L. Eigen, *Alcohol Practices, Policies, and Potentials of American Colleges and Universities: An OSAP White Paper* (Rockville, MD: U.S. Department of Health and Human Services, Office of Substance Abuse Prevention, 1991).

99. *Henry Wechsler*: H. Wechsler, G. W. Dowdall, G. Maenner, J. Gledhill-Hoyt, and H. Lee, "Changes in Binge Drinking and Related Problems Among American College Students Between 1993 and 1997," *Journal of American College Health* 47, no. 2 (1998): 57–68.

100. *one northeastern university*: Cited in H. Wechsler and S. Bryn Austin, "Binge Drinking: The Five/Four Measure," *Journal of Studies on Alcohol* Correspondence 59, no. 1 (January 1998).

101. *As many as 360,000*: Eigen, *Alcohol Practices, Policies, and Potentials*.

101. *Studies of college students suggest*: J. S. Baer, A. Stacy, and M. Larimer, "Biases in the Perception of Drinking Norms Among College Students," *Journal of Studies on Alcohol* 52, no. 6 (1991): 580–586.

101. *Prospective students and their parents*: Yonna McShane, prevention specialist at Middlebury College, personal conversation with the author, February 19, 2000.

101. *a single motivational session*: G. A. Marlatt, J. S. Baer, and M. Larimer, "Preventing Alcohol Abuse in College Students: A Harm-Reduction Approach," in G. M. Boyd, J. Howard, and R. A. Zucker, eds., *Alcohol Problems Among Adolescents: Current Directions in Prevention Research* (Hillsdale, N.J.: Lawrence Erlbaum Associates, 1995), 147–172; D. R. Kivlahan, G. A. Marlatt, K. Fromme, D. B. Coppel, and E. Williams, "Secondary Prevention with College Drinkers: Evaluation of an Alcohol Skills Training Program," *Journal of Consulting and Clinical Psychology* 61, no. 2 (1990): 344–353.

101. *"Alcohol Alert" bulletin*: D. Shalala, NIAAA, Alcohol Alert, no. 29PH 357, July 1995.

102. *Studies of teenagers in treatment*: L. Chassin and C. DeLucia, "Drinking During Adolescence," *Alcohol, Health, and Research World* 20, no. 3 (1996): 175–180; A. Arria, R. Tarter, and D. Van Thiel, "The Effects of Alcohol Abuse on the Health of Adolescents," *Alcohol, Health, and Research World* 15, no. 1 (1991): 52–57; L. Acoca, "Profile of a Chemically Dependent Adolescent and Whole Child Assessment," *Juvenile and Family Court Journal* (1995): 11–18; U.S. Department of Health and Human Services, National Institute of Drug Abuse Capsule 36: "Facts Supporting NIDA's Drug Abuse and AIDS Prevention Campaign for Teens," revised March 1996.

102. *Dr. Sandra Brown*: D. Shalala, NIAAA, NIH News Release, February 14, 2000. The study cited is by S. B. Brown and colleagues and is published in *Alcoholism: Clinical and Experimental Research* 24, No. 2.

103. *complications of eating disorders*: A. Kaplan and P. E. Garfinkel, *Medical Issues and the Eating Disorders: An Interface* (New York: Brunner/Mazel, 1993).

103. *teenage girls who drink more than five times a month*: D. B. Clark, N. Pollack, O. G. Bukstein, A. C. Mezzich, J. T. Bromberger, and J. E. Donovan, "Gender and Comorbid Psychopathology in Adolescents with Alcohol Dependence," *Journal of the American Academy of Child and Adolescent Psychiatry* 36, no. 9 (September 1997): 1195–1204.

104. *early sexual activity puts them at risk*: B. C. Coleman, "Researchers: All Sexually Active Girls Need Pap-Smear Screenings," *Naples Daily News*, March 2, 1999, 10A.

104. *girls' coexisting disorders*: M. Lynne Cooper, M. R. Frone, M. Russell, and R. S. Peirce, "Gender, Stress, Coping, and Alcohol Use," in *Gender and Alcohol: Individual and Social Perspectives*, eds. R. W. Wilsnack and S. C. Wilsnack (New Brunswick, N.J.: Rutgers Center of Alcohol Studies, 1997), 199–224.

104. *In a study of adolescents*: D. B. Clark, L. Lesnick, and A. M. Hegedus, "Traumas and Other Adverse Life Events in Adolescents with Alcohol Abuse and Dependence," *Journal of the American Academy of Child and Adolescent Psychiatry* 36, no. 12 (1997): 1744–1751.

104. *coping styles*: See, for example, D. B. Levit, "Gender Differences in Ego Defenses in Adolescence: Sex Roles as One Way to Understand the Differences," *Journal of Personality and Social Psychology* 61, no. 6 (December 1991): 992–1000.

104. *Patrice Selmari*: Patrice Selmari, personal conversation with the author, January 13, 1999.

105. *Shirley Coletti*: Shirley Coletti, personal conversation with the author, February 3, 1999.

106. *convergence of drinking patterns*: P. W. Mercer and K. A. Khavari, "Are Women Drinking More Like Men? An Empirical Examination of the Convergence Hypothesis," *Alcohol: Clinical and Experimental Research* 14, no. 3 (1990): 461–466. Cited in Blume, "Women and Addictive Disorders," 2.

106. *Daughters are fifteen times*: CASA, *Substance Abuse and the American Woman*, 5.

106. *early start with alcohol*: B. F. Grant and D. A. Dawson, "Age of Onset of Drug Use and Its Association with DSM-IV Drug Abuse and Dependence: Results from the National Longitudinal Alcohol Epidemiologic Survey," *Journal of Substance Abuse* 10, no. 2 (1998): 163–173.

106. *Dr. Camille Barry*: Dr. Camille Barry, personal conversation with the author, July 8, 1998.

108. *David Elkind*: D. Elkind, *The Hurried Child: Growing Up Too Fast Too Soon* (Reading, Mass.: Addison-Wesley, 1981), 111.

111. *David Elkind*: Ibid.

113. *Today, the vast majority*: Acoca, "Profile of a Chemically Dependent Adolescent and Whole Child Assessment"; C. S. Martin, A. M. Arria, A. C. Mezzich, and O. G. Bukstein, "Patterns of Polydrug Use in Adolescent Alcohol Abusers," *American Journal of Alcohol Abuse* 19 (1993): 511–521.

114. *unquestioning adherence*: See Kasl, *Many Roads, One Journey*, 21–23.

116. *Sharon Wilsnack and Richard Wilsnack*: Wilsnack, Plaud, Wilsnack, and Klassen, "Sexuality, Gender, and Alcohol Use." In their national longitudinal study of women's drinking, the Wilsnacks have collected data at five-year intervals, beginning in 1981. New questions and procedures, and a larger

pool of respondents, were introduced at various points in the survey. When I refer to the Wilsnacks' work in subsequent chapters, the data may not seem consistent at first glance, because I will be drawing on results that have been measured and analyzed in different contexts and at different times. In each case, I cite the specific article on which I draw.

116. *Pipher*: Pipher, *Reviving Ophelia,* 207–208.

117. *most likely to drink*: See H. Raskin White and R. Farmer Huselid, "Gender Differences in Alcohol Use During Adolescence," *Gender and Alcohol: Individual and Social Perspectives,* eds. R. W. Wilsnack and S. C. Wilsnack (New Brunswick, N.J.: Rutgers Center of Alcohol Studies, 1997), 187.

118. *Current estimates*: Wilsnack, Plaud, Wilsnack, and Klassen, "Sexuality, Gender, and Alcohol Use," 262.

118. *one university*: NIAAA, Alcohol Alert, no. 29PH 357, July 1995.

118. *Yonna McShane*: Yonna McShane, personal conversation with the author, February 19, 2000.

122. *Seventy-two percent*: L. R. Lilenfeld and W. H. Kaye, "The Link Between Alcoholism and Eating Disorders," *Alcohol Health and Research World* 20, no. 2 (Spring 1996): 94–100. For a discussion of the etiology of alcoholism and eating disorders, see also Hesselbrock and Hesselbrock, "Gender, Alcoholism, and Psychiatric Comorbidity," 49–71.

123. *Charlotte Davis Kasl*: C. D. Kasl, *Women, Sex, and Addiction: A Search for Love and Power* (New York: Ticknor & Fields, 1989).

124. *Evelyn Basoff*: E. Basoff, *Mothers and Daughters: Loving and Letting Go* (New York: Plume, 1989), 45.

CHAPTER 6: ON THE JOB

126. *newspaper headlines*: Cited in B. McConville, *Women Under the Influence: Alcohol and Its Impact* (London: Pandora, 1995), 63.

126. *social roles*: S. C. Wilsnack, "Patterns and Trends in Women's Drinking: Recent Findings and Some Implications for Prevention," in *Women and Alcohol: Issues for Prevention Research,* eds. J. M. Howard, S. E. Martin, P. D. Mail, M. E. Hilton, and E. D. Taylor. NIAAA Research Monograph No. 32, *Women and Alcohol: Issues for Prevention Research* (Bethesda, Md.: National Institutes of Health, 1996): 19–63.

127. *job stress*: T. C. Blum and P. M. Roman, "Employment and Drinking," in *Gender and Alcohol: Individual and Social Perspectives,* eds. R. W. Wilsnack and S. C. Wilsnack (New Brunswick, N.J.: Rutgers Center of Alcohol Studies, 1997), 379–394.

127. *study of middle-aged*: F. C. Breslin, M. K. O'Keeffe, L. Burrell, J. Ratliff-Crain, and A. Baum, "The Effects of Stress and Coping on Daily Alcohol Use in Women," *Addictive Behavior* 20, no. 2 (1995): 141–147.

127. *National Household Survey*: Cited in CASA, *Substance Abuse and the American Woman*, 31.

127. *the great increase*: M. Lundy and B. Younger, "Forward Women: The Invisible Majority," *Empowering Women in the Workplace* (New York: Haworth Press, 1994), xv–xxvi.

128. *National Employment Survey*: Blum and Roman, "Employment and Drinking," 379–394.

128. *Work and Occupations*: J. K. Martin and P. M. Roman, "Job Satisfaction, Job Reward Characteristics, and Employees' Problem Drinking Behaviors," *Work and Occupations* 23, no. 1 (1996): 4–25.

128. *Mexican-American women*: G. M. Ames and L. A. Rebhun, "Occupational Culture, Drinking, and Women: An Incomplete Research Picture," in *Women and Alcohol: Issues for Prevention Research*, eds. S. M. Howard et al., NIAAA Research Monograph No. 32 (Bethesda, Md.: National Institutes of Health, 1996): 261–290.

128. *unwanted status*: Wilsnack, Wilsnack, and Hiller-Sturmhöfel, "How Women Drink," 173–181.

129. *male-dominated occupations*: Wilsnack, "Patterns and Trends in Women's Drinking," 30.

131. *Women lawyers are increasing*: American Bar Association, *The Report of "At the Breaking Point: A National Conference on the Emerging Crisis in the Quality of Lawyers' Health and Lives—Its Impact on Law Firms and Client Services"* (Chicago: Author, 1991), 6.

131. *New Jersey Lawyer*: W. J. Kane and C. Blaisden, "Use and Abuse: Are You Controlling the Substance, or Is the Substance Controlling You?" *New Jersey Lawyer*, December 1996, 12–14.

132. *railroad workers*: Ames and Rebhun, "Occupational Culture, Drinking, and Women," 269.

132. *G. Andrew Benjamin*: Quoted in H. V. Samborn, "Plays Well with Others," *ABA Journal: The Lawyer's Magazine* 85 (April 1999): 78–79.

132. *commonly cited study*: G. A. H. Benjamin, E. J. Darling, and B. D. Sales, "The Prevalance of Depression, Alcohol Abuse, and Cocaine Abuse Among United States Lawyers," 13 *International Journal of Law and Psychiatry* 233 (1990): 233–246.

133. *18 percent of lawyers*: Kane and Blaisden, "Use and Abuse: Are You Controlling the Substance, or Is the Substance Controlling You?"

133. *William John Kane*: William John Kane, personal conversation with the author, April 17, 2000.

135. *physicians and airline pilots*: R. B. Allan, "Alcoholism, Drug Abuse and Lawyers: Are We Ready to Address the Denial?" *Creighton Law Review* 31 (1997): 265–277.

135. *Historically, women*: B. R. Spiegel and D. D. Friedman, "High-Achieving Women: Issues in Addiction and Recovery," in *Gender and Addictions: Men*

and Women in Treatment, eds. S. L. A. Straussner and E. Zelvin (Northvale, N.J.: Jason Aronson, 1997), 151–166.

136. *female-dominated occupations:* Ames and Rebhun, "Occupational Culture, Drinking, and Women," 271–276.

136. *England and Wales:* Plant, *Women and Alcohol,* 30.

136. *Edith Gomberg:* Gomberg, "Alcohol Abuse," 235.

137. *employee assistance programs:* Blum and Roman, "Employment and Drinking," 390.

137. *professional or graduate degree:* J. H. LaRosa, "Executive Women and Health: Perceptions and Practices," *American Journal of Public Health* 80 (1990): 1450–1454.

137. *higher prevalence of drinking:* Blum and Roman, "Employment and Drinking."

137. *explosive situations:* See Spiegel and Friedman, "High-Achieving Women."

140. *Walter Brownsword:* Walter Brownsword, personal conversation with the author, March 24, 2000.

CHAPTER 7: LOVE HUNGER

149. *"Alcohol was my true love":* Cited in S. S. Covington and J. L. Surrey, "The Relational Model of Women's Psychological Development: Implications for Substance Abuse," in *Gender and Alcohol: Individual and Social Perspectives,* eds. R. W. Wilsnack and S. C. Wilsnack (New Brunswick, N.J.: Rutgers Center of Alcohol Studies, 1997), 335–351.

149. *Caroline Knapp:* C. Knapp, *Drinking: A Love Story* (New York: Dell, 1997), 6.

150. *Diane Byington:* Diane Byington, personal conversation with the author, April 15, 1999.

151. *696 American women:* R. W. Wilsnack, S. C. Wilsnack, A. F. Kristjanson, and T. R. Harris, "Ten-Year Prediction of Women's Drinking Behavior in a Nationally Representative Sample," *Women's Health: Research on Gender, Behavior, and Policy* 4, no. 3 (1998): 199–230.

151. *Sharon Wilsnack:* Sharon Wilsnack, personal conversation with the author, June 16, 1999.

153. *Linda Beckman:* S. M. Harvey and L. J. Beckman, "Alcohol Consumption, Female Sexual Behavior and Contraceptive Use," *Journal of Studies on Alcohol* 47(1986): 327–332.

153. *This should not surprise:* Sheila Blume, personal correspondence with the author, March 5, 2000.

153. *Researchers suspect:* Wilsnack, Plaud, Wilsnack, and Klassen, "Sexuality, Gender, and Alcohol Use," 250–288.

164. *Judith Viorst:* Viorst, *Necessary Losses,* 35.

165. *male drinker's psyche:* For a discussion of the early work on alcoholism, dependency, and power, see Sandmaier, *Invisible Alcoholics,* 82–105.

166. *article on high-achieving women*: Spiegel and Friedman, "High-Achieving Women," 151–166.

169. *Caroline Knapp*: Knapp, *Drinking*, 137.

171. *In our secular society*: See R.J. Lifton, *The Broken Connection: On Death and the Continuity of Life* (New York: Simon & Schuster, 1979).

171. *As connections strengthen*: For a discussion of expanding relationships as part of recovery, see Covington and Surrey, "The Relational Model of Women's Psychological Development"; and Covington, *A Woman's Way Through the Twelve Steps*.

CHAPTER 8: SPRINGS OF SORROW: DRINKING AT TIMES OF LOSS

174. *primal renunciation*: For a discussion of the losses at each stage of life, see Viorst, *Necessary Losses*.

174. *Daniel Levinson*: D.J. Levinson, *The Seasons of a Woman's Life* (New York: Alfred A. Knopf, 1996).

175. *Judith Viorst*: Viorst, *Necessary Losses*, 272.

176. *More often than men*: CASA, *Substance Abuse and the American Woman*, 33.

176. *early-onset and late-onset*: See Gomberg, "Alcohol Abuse," 225–244.

177. *mean age of onset*: Ibid., 228.

177. *Shirley Hill*: Hill, "Vulnerability to Alcoholism in Women," 9–28.

177. *scientists dispute*: See Gomberg, "Alcohol Abuse," 228.

177. *number of negative events*: E.S.L. Gomberg, "Alcoholic Women in Treatment: Early Histories and Early Problem Behaviors," *Advances in Alcohol and Substance Abuse* 8, no. 2 (1989): 133–147.

178. *What protects*: *Ninth Special Report*, 35.

179. *DSM IV*: American Psychiatric Association, *Diagnostic and Statistical Manual of Mental Disorders*, 4th ed. Washington, D.C.: Author (1994), 684.

179. *Assessing an alcoholic's depression*: A study of 2,945 alcoholics published in 1997, as part of the Collaborative Study on the Genetics of Alcoholism, used a time-line method to determine whether depressive episodes were independent or substance-induced; it found that 15.2 percent of the alcoholics experienced independent depressions, whereas 26.4 percent experienced substance-induced episodes. Those who experienced independent major depressive episodes were more likely to be married, Caucasian, and female; to have had less experience with drugs and less treatment for alcoholism; to have attempted suicide; and to have a close relative with a major mood disorder. M.A. Schuckit, J.E. Tipp, M. Bergman, W. Reich, V.M. Hesselbrock, and T.L. Smith, "Comparison of Induced and Independent Major Depressive Disorders in 2,945 Alcoholics," in *American Journal of Psychiatry* 154, no. 7 (July 1997): 948–958.

179. *Until 1994*: D. Samuels, "Saying Yes to Drugs," *New Yorker*, March 23, 1998.

180. *synergistic effect*: E. Z. Hanna and B. F. Grant, "Gender Differences in DSM-IV Alcohol Use Disorders and Major Depression as Distributed in the General Population: Clinical Implications," in *Comprehensive Psychiatry* (D09) 38, no. 4 (July/August 1997): 202–212. Note also a study that collected self-reports from more than 42,000 U.S. adults from the general population, supporting prior research that showed that there is more alcoholism in the families of both male and female alcoholics who are also diagnosed with depression than there is among alcoholics without depression. D. A. Dawson and B. F. Grant, "Family History of Alcoholism and Gender: Their Combined Effects on DSM-IV Alcohol Dependence and Major Depression," *Journal of Studies on Alcohol* 59, no. 1 (January 1998): 97–107.

180. *Estimates of the prevalence*: Hesselbrock and Hesselbrock, "Gender, Alcoholism, and Psychiatric Comorbidity," 49–71.

180. *higher rates of depression among women*: Terrence Real, in *I Don't Want to Talk About It: Overcoming the Secret Legacy of Male Depression* (Scribner: New York, 1997), argues that men's depression is often hidden or covert, making it difficult to diagnose according to the usual symptoms. It may be that depression in male alcoholics is underdiagnosed, just as alcoholism is underdiagnosed in depressed women.

180. *exceeds men's by two to one*: C. Brown and H. C. Schulberg, "Depression and Anxiety Disorders: Diagnosis and Treatment in Primary Care Practice," in *Health Care for Women: Psychological, Social, and Behavioral Influences*, eds. S. J. Gallant, G. Puryear Keita, and R. Royak-Schaler (Washington, D.C.: American Psychological Association, 1997), 237–256.

180. *more reactive*: E. S. L. Gomberg, "Older Women and Alcohol Use and Abuse," in *Recent Developments in Alcoholism*, Vol. 12: *Alcoholism and Women*, ed. M. Galanter (New York: Plenum Press, 1995), 61–79.

180. *Daniel Levinson*: Levinson, *Seasons of a Woman's Life*.

183. *typical pattern*: Gomberg, "Older Women and Alcohol Use and Abuse."

183. *a national survey*: S. C. Wilsnack, N. D. Vogeltanz, L. E. Diers, and R. W. Wilsnack, "Drinking and Problem Drinking in Older Women," in *Alcohol and Aging*, eds. T. P. Beresford and E. S. L. Gomberg (London: Oxford University Press, 1995), 263–292.

184. *Released in June 1998*: CASA, *Under the Rug*, iii.

185. *Dr. Sylvia Staub*: Sylvia Staub, personal conversation with the author, October 11, 1999.

186. *physiological response*: A. Breier, J. R. Kelsoe, P. D. Kirwin, S. A. Beller, O. M. Wolkowitz, and D. Pickar, "Early Parental Loss and Development of Adult Psychopathology," *Archives of General Psychiatry* 45 (1988): 987–993.

186. *Sharon and Richard Wilsnack*: Wilsnack, Wilsnack, Kristjanson, and Harris, "Ten-Year Prediction of Women's Drinking Behavior"; and Sharon

Wilsnack, personal conversation with the author, June 6, 1999. Sharon Wilsnack noted that early separation from parents predicted a range of problems. Sharon and Richard Wilsnack's survey was of women in the general population, and those who were experiencing symptoms from alcohol abuse were not necessarily clinically diagnosed alcoholics. Sharon Wilsnack points out that among these women, there is a good deal of shifting in and out of problems over time, and that the longitudinal study—which allows them to make predictions about whose problems will continue to get worse—is a much stronger statement than a snapshot in time. Richard and Sharon Wilsnack were recently granted continued funding for their research; in 2001 they will be able to collect data from over a twenty-year period.

CHAPTER 9: STEALING COURAGE FROM A TURTLE'S HEART: SEXUALLY ABUSED WOMEN FIGHTING ALCOHOL

192. *disrupted early family life*: E.S.L. Gomberg, "Antecedents of Alcohol Problems in Women," in *Alcohol Problems in Women*, eds. S.C. Wilsnack and L.J. Beckman (New York: Guilford Press, 1984), 243; B.A. Miller, W.R. Downs, D.M. Gondoli, and A. Keil, "The Role of Childhood Sexual Abuse in the Development of Alcoholism in Women," *Violence and Victims* 2 (1987): 157–172; Wilsnack, Wilsnack, Kristjanson, and Harris,"Ten-Year Prediction of Women's Drinking Behavior."

192. *Edith Gomberg*: Gomberg, "Alcoholic Women in Treatment," 133–147.

192. *long-term consequences*: W. Langeland and C. Hartgers, "Child Sexual and Physical Abuse and Alcoholism: A Review," *Journal of Studies on Alcohol* 59 (1998): 336; F.W. Putman and P.K. Trickett, "Child Sexual Abuse: A Model of Chronic Trauma," *Psychiatry* 56, no. 1 (February 1993): 85–86.

192. *Primarily, girls*: Putnam and Trickett, "Child Sexual Abuse," 83.

192. *numbers were startling*: K. Bollerud, "A Model for the Treatment of Trauma-Related Syndromes Among Chemically Dependent Inpatient Women," *Journal of Substance Abuse Treatment* 7 (1990): 83–87; J.L. Forth-Finegan, "Sugar and Spice and Everything Nice: Gender Socialization and Women's Addiction—A Literature Review," in *Feminism and Addiction*, ed. C. Bepko (New York: Haworth Press, 1991), 19–48; D.J. Rohsenow, R. Corbett, and D. Devine, "Molested as Children: A Hidden Contribution to Substance Abuse?" *Journal of Substance Abuse Treatment* 5 (1988): 13–15; V. Yandow, "Alcoholism in Women," *Psychiatric Annals* 19 (1989): 243–247.

192. *a study reported in 1993*: B.A. Miller, W.R. Downs, and M. Testa, "Interrelationships Between Victimization Experience and Women's Alcohol Use," *Journal of Studies on Alcohol,* supplement no. 11 (1993): 107–117.

193. *compared with female psychiatric patients*: Putnam and Trickett, "Child Sexual Abuse," 85.

193. *vaginal penetration*: J. H. Beitchman, K. J. Zucker, J. E. Hood, G. A. daCosta, D. Akman, and E. Cassavia, "A Review of the Long-Term Effects of Child Sexual Abuse," *Child Abuse and Neglect* 16, no. 1 (1992): 101–118.

193. *Childhood rape*: J. N. Epstein, B. E. Saunders, D. G. Kilpatrick, and H. S. Resnick, "PTSD as a Mediator Between Childhood Rape and Alcohol Use in Adult Women," *Child Abuse and Neglect* 22, no. 3 (March 1998): 223–234.

193. *Some of these studies have been criticized*: In my summary of methodological problems I am drawing largely on Langeland and Hartgers, "Child Sexual and Physical Abuse and Alcoholism."

194. *In Norway*: W. Pedersen and A. Skrondal, "Alcohol and Sexual Victimization: A Longitudinal Study of Norwegian Girls," *Addiction* (BM3) 91, no. 4 (April 1996): 565–581.

194. *a landmark study*: S. C. Wilsnack, N. D. Vogeltanz, A. D. Klassen, and T. R. Harris, "Childhood Sexual Abuse and Women's Substance Abuse: National Survey Findings," *Journal of Studies on Alcohol* 58, no. 3 (May 1997): 264–271.

195. *"single strongest predictor"*: Sharon Wilsnack, personal conversation with the author, October 1, 1998. In 1996, questions about physical abuse and other childhood traumas were added to Wilsnack's study. Analysis of this material will be completed in the next few years.

196. *Judith Viorst*: Viorst, *Necessary Losses*, 48.

196. *"Instead of parts"*: Ibid., 49.

197. *Rita Teusch*: Rita Teusch, personal conversation with the author, September 12, 1998. All quotations from Rita Teusch are from this conversation.

197. *has written on the connection*: R. Teusch, "Substance-Abusing Women and Sexual Abuse," in *Gender and Addictions: Men and Women in Treatment*, eds. S. L. A. Straussner and E. Zelvin (Northvale, N.J.: Jason Aronson, 1997), 97–122.

197. *Dissociation is commonly used*: Putman and Trickett, "Child Sexual Abuse," 86–87.

199. *David Elkind*: D. Elkind, *The Child's Reality* (Hillsdale, N.J.: Lawrence Erlbaum Associates, 1978), 119.

203. *Monitoring the Future*: NIAAA, Alcohol Alert, no. 37, July 1997.

203. *consensual sexual intercourse*: Wilsnack, Vogeltanz, Klassen, and Harris, "Childhood Sexual Abuse and Women's Substance Abuse," 264–271.

205. *Jennifer Egan*: J. Egan, "The Thin Red Line," *New York Times Magazine*, July 27, 1997, 25.

208. *In the Wilsnacks' survey*: Wilsnack, Wilsnack, Kristjanson, and Harris, "Ten-Year Prediction of Women's Drinking Behavior."

209. *Dr. Bessel van der Kolk*: Quoted in Egan, "Thin Red Line," 34.

210. *Corinna Stewart*: Corinna Stewart, personal conversation with the author, September 10, 1998.

212. *Joan Ellen Zweben*: J.E. Zweben, H.W. Clark, and D.E. Smith, "Traumatic Experiences and Substance Abuse: Mapping the Territory," *Journal of Psychoactive Drugs 26*, no. 4 (October–December 1994): 334.

218. *Some researchers point out*: Langeland and Hartgers, "Child Sexual and Physical Abuse and Alcoholism," 337.

CHAPTER 10: DOCTORS STILL DON'T GET IT

225. *apt to visit physicians*: CASA, *Substance Abuse and the American Woman*, 108.

226. *hypothetical patients*: This example is given by Marc Schuckit in *Educating Yourself About Alcohol and Drugs: A People's Primer* (New York: Plenum Press, 1995), 322.

227. *particularly blind*: For example, N.V. Dawson, G. Dadheech, T. Speroff, R.L. Smith, and D.S. Schubert, "The Effect of Patient Gender on the Prevalence and Recognition of Alcoholism on a General, Medicine Inpatient Service," *Journal of General Internal Medicine* 7 (1992): 38–45; D.G. Buschbaum, R.G. Buchanan, R.M. Pses, S.H. Schnoll, and M.J. Lawton, "Physician Detection of Drinking Problems in Patients Attending a General Medicine Practice," *Journal of General Internal Medicine* 7 (1992): 517–521; E.R. Brown, R. Wyn, W.G. Cumberland, H. Yu, E. Abel, L. Gelberg, and L. Ngu, *Women's Health-Related Behaviors and Use of Clinical Preventive Services: A Report to the Commonwealth Fund* (Los Angeles: UCLA Center for Health Policy Research, 1995). All cited in CASA, *Substance Abuse and the American Woman*.

227. *three times more likely*: Dawson, Dadheech, Speroff, Smith, and Schubert, "The Effect of Patient Gender on the Prevalence and Recognition of Alcoholism on a General Medicine Inpatient Service."

227. *only 24 percent*: B. Bush, S. Shaw, P. Cleary, T.L. Delbanco, and M.D. Aronson, "Screening for Alcohol Abuse Using the CAGE Questionnaire," *American Journal of Medicine* 82, no. 2 (1987): 231–235, cited in CASA, *Substance Abuse and the Mature Woman*, 63.

227. *A range of studies*: M.F. Fleming, K.L. Barry, L.B. Manwell, K. Johnson, and R. London, "Brief Physician Advice for Problem Alcohol Drinkers: A Randomized Controlled Trial in Community-Based Primary Care Practices," *Journal of the American Medical Association* 27, no. 5 (1997): 1039–1045; D.C. Parish, "Another Indication for Screening and Early Intervention: Problem Drinking," *Journal of the American Medical Association* 277 (1997): 1079–1080. See also CASA, *Under the Rug*, 63.

227. *Among men who consumed*: Fleming, Barry, Manwell, Johnson, and London, "Brief Physician Advice for Problem Alcohol Drinkers."

227. *single motivational session*: Marlatt, Baer, and Larimer, "Preventing Alcohol Abuse in College Students," 147–172; Kivlahan, Marlatt, Fromme, Coppel, and Williams, "Secondary Prevention with College Drinkers," 344–353.

228. *American Medical Association*: American Medical Association, Council on Scientific Affairs Report, *Alcoholism and Alcohol Abuse Among Women* (Chicago: Author, 1997).

228. *survey of 400 physicians*: CASA, *Under the Rug*, 45–56.

228. *CAGE*: If a woman answers yes at least once, or has at least eight drinks per week or at least four drinks per occasion, her doctor should ask her more about her patterns of use, her reasons for drinking, any alcohol-related medical problems, and her family history of alcoholism. NIAAA, *The Physician's Guide to Helping Patients with Alcohol Problems* (Rockville, Md.: Author, 1995). Cited in CASA, *Substance Abuse and the American Woman*, 111.

229. *82 percent of these physicians*: CASA, *Under the Rug,* 47.

229. *alcohol and prescription drugs*: E.S.L. Gomberg, "Women and Alcohol: Use and Abuse," *Journal of Nervous and Mental Disease* 181, no. 4 (1993): 211–219.

229. *doctors confuse the signs*: CASA, *Substance Abuse and the American Woman*.

229. *400 physicians*: CASA, *Under the Rug*, 56.

230. *Stephen R. Kandall*: Kandall, *Substance and Shadow*, 8.

230. *Victorian era*: Ibid., 3.

230. *A national panel*: S. Gilbert, "Doctors Found to Fail in Diagnosing Addictions," *New York Times,* February 14, 1996, C8.

230. *Doctors may not know*: Schuckit, *Educating Yourself About Alcohol and Drugs,* 321–326. Schuckit notes that his medical colleagues often misdiagnose patients with alcohol problems, and he suggests that the situation might be improved if doctors change erroneous stereotypes of what alcoholics look like, pay attention to less obvious alcohol-related medical disorders, and note which blood tests can be important clues to identifying the "hidden" alcoholic.

231. *more common markers*: D. Wilke, "Women and Alcoholism: How a Male-as-Norm Bias Affects Research, Assessment, and Treatment," *Health and Social Work* 19, no. 1 (1994): 29–35; T.L. Hughes, "Evaluating Research on Chemical Dependency Among Women: A Women's Health Perspective," *Family and Community Health* 13, no. 3 (1990): 35–46, cited in CASA, *Substance Abuse and the American Woman*, 110.

232. *"We must pay physicians"*: CASA, *Under the Rug*, 54.

232. *Indirect measures*: Schuckit, *Educating Yourself About Alcohol and Drugs,* 315–321.

233. *Charlotte Davis Kasl*: Kasl, *Many Roads, One Journey*, 115–116.

235. *Recently, addiction specialists*: M. Freimuth, "Psychotherapists' Beliefs About the Benefits of 12-Step Groups," *Alcoholism Treatment Quarterly* 14, no. 3 (1996): 95–102.

235. *Evaluations of alcohol treatment*: K. M. Schneider, F. J. Kviz, M. L. Isola, and W. J. Filstead, "Evaluating Multiple Outcomes and Gender Differences in Alcoholism Treatment," *Addictive Behaviors* 20, no. 1 (1995): 1–21.

235. *guide to substance abuse services*: E. Sullivan and M. Fleming, *A Guide to Substance Abuse Services for Primary Care Clinicians: Treatment Protocol (TIP) Series 24* (Rockville, Md.: U.S. Department of Health and Human Services, Center for Substance Abuse Treatment, 1997).

236. *Vogeltanz and Wilsnack*: Vogeltanz and Wilsnack, "Alcohol Problems in Women," 75–96.

236. *effective prevention strategies*: Kandall's book *Substance and Shadow* also offers a range of treatment and prevention strategies for addicted women in chap. 11, 280–299.

CHAPTER 11: WORKING WITH DIFFERENCE: MINNESOTA INDIAN WOMEN'S RESOURCE CENTER AND AFRICAN-AMERICAN FAMILY SERVICES

243. *Maya Hennessey*: Maya Hennessey, personal conversation with the author, April 25, 2000.

244. *one counselor commented*: "Moyers on Addiction: Close to Home," a production of Public Affairs Television, Princeton, N.J., Films for the Humanities and Sciences (FFH 7681).

245. *treatment record charts*: "Evaluating the Effectiveness of Alcohol and Substance Abuse Services for American Indian and Alaska Native Women," Evaluation Phase 2, Final Report, Executive Summary (San Francisco: Institute for Health Policy Studies, 1995).

245. *When treatment providers*: C. H. Woll, "What Difference Does Culture Make? Providing Treatment to Women Different from You," in *Chemical Dependency: Women at Risk*, eds. B. L. Underhill and D. G. Finnegan (New York: Haworth Press, 1996), 70–71.

245. *imply that minority women*: R. Rhodes and A. Johnson, "A Feminist Approach to Treating Alcohol and Drug-Addicted African-American Women," *Women and Therapy* 20, no. 3 (1997): 34.

247. *"cultural pain"*: P. Bell, with assistance from D. Peterson, *Cultural Pain and African Americans: Unspoken Issues in Early Recovery* (Center City, Minn.: Hazelden Educational Materials, 1992), 36.

248. *"insecure, embarrassed"*: Ibid., 8–9.

249. *"As African Americans in treatment"*: Ibid., 9.

263. *Audre Lorde*: A. Lorde, in *Sister Outsider* (Trumansberg, N.Y.: Crossing Press, 1984), 53.

263. *Patricia Hill Collins*: P.H. Collins, *Black Feminist Thought: Knowledge, Consciousness, and the Politics of Empowerment* (Cambridge, Mass.: Unwin Hyman, 1990), 166.

264. Cool Pose: R. Majors and J.M. Billson, *Cool Pose: The Dilemmas of Black Manhood in America* (New York: Simon & Schuster, 1992).

265. *Ice T*: Ice T, *The Ice Opinion* (New York: St. Martin's Press, 1994), 10.

266. *In a culture where addicted*: A study of 582 women (200 Anglo-American and 382 African-American) recruited from substance abuse treatment centers showed that Anglo-American female drug users were more likely than African-American women to deal drugs. R. Moise, J. Kovach, B. Reed, and N. Bellows, "A Comparison of Black and White Women Entering Drug Abuse Treatment Programs," *International Journal on Addiction* 17, no. 1 (1982): 35–49.

273. *a new study has found*: cited in A. Zuger, "Many Prostitutes Suffer Combat Disorder, Study Finds," *New York Times*, August 18, 1998, C8.

274. *Angela Davis*: A. Davis, "Rape, Racism and the Capitalist Setting," *Black Scholar* 9, no. 7 (1978): 24–30.

274. *Alice Walker*: A. Walker, *In Search of Our Mothers' Gardens* (San Diego: Harcourt Brace Jovanovich, 1983).

274. *either-or options*: If Walker's analysis is accurate, it follows that the descendants of white slave owners would also be particularly subject to violence. This inference turns out to be supported by the prevalence of murder in the South. Statistics tell part of the story: in cities with a population between 50,000 and 20,000, white males in the South commit murder at twice the rate of white men in the rest of the country; in smaller cities, the ratio is three to one; in rural areas, it is four to one. Louisiana—where conditions under slavery were most brutal—has the highest homicide rate in the country. The *New York Times* reports that "the high Southern murder rate is a key factor behind America's disproportionately high homicide rate compared with other democratic, industrialized nations." F. Butterfield, "Why America's Murder Rate Is So High," *New York Times*, July 26, 1998, section 4, 1.

275. *Patricia Hill Collins*: P.H. Collins, "The Sexual Politics of Black Womanhood," in *Black Feminist Thought*, 163–180.

275. *No matter that they*: Ibid.

275. *popular conservative critics*: For example, D. D'Souza, *The End of Racism* (New York: Simon & Schuster, 1995).

276. *study of African-American college students*: M.J. Gilbert and R.L. Collins, "Ethnic Variation in Women's and Men's Drinking," in *Gender and Alcohol: Individual and Social Perspectives*, eds. R.W. Wilsnack and S.C. Wilsnack (New Brunswick, N.J.: Rutgers Center of Alcohol Studies, 1997), 369.

276. *less accepting than men*: R. Caetano and D. Herd, "Black Drinking Practices in Northern California," *American Journal of Drug and Alcohol Abuse* 10 (1984): 571–587.

276. *more tolerance*: M. B. Bailey, P. W. Haberman, and H. Alksne, "The Epidemiology of Alcoholism in an Urban Residential Area," *Quarterly Journal of Studies on Alcohol* 26 (1965): 19–40.

277. *more likely than whites to abstain*: M. Lillie-Blanton, E. MacKenzie, and J. C. Anthony, "Black-White Differences in Alcohol Use by Women: Baltimore Survey Findings," *Public Health Reports* 106, no. 2 (March-April 1991): 124–134.

277. *Trying to make sense*: I am drawing on Gilbert and Collins, "Ethnic Variation in Women's and Men's Drinking," 357–378.

277. *national survey*: D. Herd, "Sex Ratios of Drinking Patterns and Problems Among Blacks and Whites: Results from a National Survey," *Journal of Studies on Alcohol* (January 1997): 75–82.

277. *Death from cirrhosis*: CASA, *Substance Abuse and the American Woman*, 46.

277. *fetal alcohol syndrome*: NIAAA, *Alcohol Alert*, no. 23 PH 347, January 1994.

278. *sixty-three women*: N. H. Turner et al., "Community's Role in the Promotion of Recovery from Addiction and Prevention of Relapse Among Women: An Exploratory Study," *Ethnicity and Disease* 8 (Winter 1998): 26–35.

278. *AIDS*: G. M. Wingood and R. J. DiClemente, "Pattern Influences and Gender-Related Factors Associated with Noncondom Use Among Young Adult African American Women," *American Journal of Community Psychology* 26, no. 1 (February 1998): 29.

278. *Survey on Drug Abuse*: B. A. Rouse, J. Carter, and S. Rodriguez-Andrew, "Race/Ethnicity and Other Sociocultural Influences on Alcoholism Treatment for Women," in *Recent Developments in Alcoholism*, Vol. 12: *Alcoholism and Women*, ed. Marc Galanter (New York: Plenum Press, 1995), 348.

278. *2.2 million white women*: CASA, *Substance Abuse and the American Woman*, 39.

278. *criminalized*: A. H. Tana-Cisse, "Issues for African American Women." In *Alcohol and Drugs Are Women's Issues*, Vol. 1: *A Review of the Issues*, ed. P. Roth (Metuchen, N.J.: Women's Action Alliance and Scarecrow Press, 1991), 54–60.

278. *criminally charged*: CASA, *Substance Abuse and the American Woman*, 119–122.

CHAPTER 12: RECOVERY: ONLY CONNECT

285. *designed for men*: Covington and Surrey, "The Relational Model of Women's Psychological Development," 348.

285. *About 10 percent of alcohol-dependent patients*: M. E. McCaul and J. Furst, "Alcoholism Treatment in the United States," *Alcohol Health and Research World* 18, no. 4 (1994): 253–260. My overview of treatment draws on this article and on R. M. Kadden, "Cognitive-Behavioral Approaches to Alcoholism Treatment," *Alcohol Health and Research World* 18, no. 4 (1994): 279–286.

286. *Outpatient treatment*: See M. Schuckit's chapter "How Do I Find the Right Program?" in Schuckit, *Educating Yourself About Alcohol and Drugs*, 155–170.

287. *based on the premise*: Kadden, "Cognitive-Behavioral Approaches to Alcoholism Treatment."

287. *"Harm reduction"*: For information on the "harm reduction" approach, see the Harm Reduction Coalition's website, at *http://www.harmreduction.org.*

288. *Dr. Camille Barry*: Camille Barry, personal conversation with the author, July 8, 1998. Further quotes from Barry are from this conversation.

288. *a large-scale investigation*: T. Blume, P. Roman, and E. Harwood, "Employed Women with Alcohol Problems Who Seek Help from Employee Assistance Programs," in *Recent Developments in Alcoholism,* Vol. 12: *Alcoholism and Women*, ed. Marc Galanter (New York: Plenum Press, 1995), 125–156.

288. *underemployed and underinsured*: Blume, "Women and Alcohol," 462–489.

289. *the work site study*: Blum, Roman, and Harwood, "Employed Women with Alcohol Problems."

289. *well-designed study*: L. Dahlgren and A. Willander, "Are Special Treatment Facilities for Female Alcoholics Needed?" *Alcoholism: Clinical and Experimental Research* 13, no. 4 (1989): 499–504.

290. *Ronald Kadden*: Ronald Kadden, personal conversation with the author, September 24, 1999. Further quotes from Kadden are from this conversation.

291. *Between 30 and 60 percent*: A. I. Leshner, "Drug Abuse and Mental Disorders: Comorbidity is Reality," *NIDA Notes: Director's Column* 14, no. 4, 2000.

291. *Dr. Lisa Najavits*: Lisa Najavits, personal conversation with the author, May 10, 2000.

291. *family unification model*: See chapter 4, 84–87.

292. *Nancy Paull*: Nancy Paull, personal conversation with the author, July 18, 2000.

292. *A study that matched patients*: See M. E. Mattson, "Finding the Right Approach," in *Treating Addictive Behaviors*, 2nd edition, eds. W. R. Miller and N. Heather (New York: Plenum Press, 1998): 163–172.

297. *To understand the AA approach*: See Kasl's *Many Roads, One Journey.*

300. *Charlotte Davis Kasl*: Ibid., 18.

300. *sixteen steps*: Ibid., and C. D. Kasl, *Yes, You Can! A Guide to Empowerment Groups* (Lolo, MT: Many Roads, One Journey, 1994), which can be ordered from Many Roads, One Journey, P.O. Box 1302, Lolo, MT 59847; 406-273-6080.

300. *Stephanie Covington's book*: Covington, *A Woman's Way Through the Twelve Steps.*

301. *Berenson's reformulations*: D. Berenson, "Powerlessness—Liberating or Enslaving? Responding to the Feminist Critique of the Twelve Steps," in *Feminism and Addiction*, ed. C. Bepko (New York: Haworth Press, 1991), 67–84.

301. *"Chicken and egg"*: W. Alexander, "From A to Z," *Tricycle: The Buddhist Review* (Fall 1998): 61–65.

303. *George McGovern*: G. McGovern, *Terry: My Daughter's Life-and-Death Struggle with Alcoholism* (New York: Villard, 1996).

304. *Diane Byington*: D. Byington, personal conversation with the author, July 26, 1999.

304. *Stephanie Covington:* personal conversation with the author, July 30, 1999.

Selected Readings

Research Findings and Clinical Perspectives

Please consult endnotes for a complete list of books, studies, and articles. The following books and reports provide information about alcoholism in women and its treatment.

Bepko, Claudia, ed. *Feminism and Addiction*. New York: Haworth Press, 1991.

————, with Jo-Ann Krestan. *The Responsibility Trap: A Blueprint for Treating the Alcoholic Family*. New York: The Free Press, 1985.

Covington, Stephanie S. *Helping Women Recover: A Program for Treating Addiction*. San Francisco: Jossey-Bass, 1999.

Department of Health and Human Services. *Ninth Special Report to the U.S. Congress on Alcohol and Health*. Rockville, Md.: U.S. Department of Health and Human Services, 1997.

Ettore, Elizabeth. *Women and Substance Abuse*. New Brunswick, N.J.: Rutgers University Press, 1992.

Howard, J.M., S.E. Martin, P.D. Mail, M.E. Hilton, and E.D. Taylor, eds. *National Institute on Alcohol Abuse and Alcoholism Research Monograph No. 32, Women and Alcohol: Issues for Prevention Research*. Bethesda, Md.: National Institutes of Health, 1996.

National Center on Addiction and Substance Abuse at Columbia University (CASA). *Substance Abuse and the American Woman*. New York: CASA, 1996.

————. *Under the Rug: Substance Abuse and the Mature Woman.* New York: CASA, 1998.

Plant, Moira. *Women and Alcohol: Contemporary and Historical Perspectives.* London: Free Association Books Ltd., 1997.

Straussner, S. L. A., and Elizabeth Zelvin, eds. *Gender and Addictions: Men and Women in Treatment.* London: Jason Aronson, 1997.

Van Den Bergh, Nan, ed. *Feminist Perspectives on Addictions.* New York: Springer, 1991.

Wilsnack, Sharon C., and Richard W. Wilsnack, eds. *Gender and Alcohol: Individual and Social Perspectives.* New Brunswick, N.J.: Rutgers Center of Alcohol Studies, 1997.

Novels, Memoirs, and Stories

Allen, Chaney. *I'm Black and I'm Sober: The Timeless Story of a Woman's Journey Back to Sanity.* 2d ed. Center City, Minn.: Hazelden, 1995.

Fisher, Carrie. *Postcards from the Edge.* New York: Pocket Books, 1990.

Gilliam, Marianne. *How Alcoholics Anonymous Failed Me: My Personal Journey to Sobriety Through Self-Empowerment.* New York: Eagle Brook, 1999.

Hafner, Sarah. *Nice Girls Don't Drink.* New York: Bergin & Garvey, 1992.

Knapp, Caroline. *Drinking: A Love Story.* New York: Delta, 1997.

Lamott, Anne. *Operating Instructions: A Journal of My Son's First Year.* New York: Fawcett Books, 1994.

————. *Rosie.* New York: Penguin, 1997.

McGovern, George. *Terry: My Daughter's Life-and-Death Struggle with Alcoholism.* New York: Villard, 1996.

Self-Help for Women Alcoholics and Their Families

Agnew, Eleanor and Sharon Robideaux. *My Mama's Waltz: A Book for Daughters of Alcoholic Mothers.* New York: Pocket Books, 1998.

Alcoholics Anonymous. New York: Alcoholics Anonymous World Service, 1993.

Babbit, Nikki. *Adolescent Drug and Alcohol Abuse: How to Spot It, Stop It, and Get Help for Your Family.* O'Reilly & Associates, 2000.

Black, Claudia. *It Will Never Happen to Me.* New York: Ballantine, 1991.

Chopra, Deepak. *Overcoming Addictions: The Spiritual Solution.* New York: Three Rivers Press, 1998.

Covington, Stephanie S. *A Woman's Way Through the Twelve Steps.* Center City, Minn.: Hazelden, 1994.

———. *Awakening Your Sexuality: A Guide for Recovering Women.* Center City, Minn.: Hazelden, 2000.

Englemann, Jeanne. *Claiming My Power in Recovery: The First Step for Women.* Center City, Minn.: Hazelden Educational Materials, 1992.

———. *Women and Spirituality.* Center City, Minn.: Hazelden Educational Materials, 1992.

Kasl, Charlotte Davis. *Many Roads, One Journey: Moving Beyond the 12 Steps.* New York: HarperPerennial, 1992.

———. *Yes, You Can! A Guide to Empowerment Groups.* Lolo, Mont.: Many Roads, One Journey, 1995. (Write to P.O. Box 1302, Lolo, MT. 59847 for information about ordering.)

Kirkpatrick, Jean. *Goodbye Hangovers, Hello Life: Self-Help for Women.* New York, Atheneum, 1986.

———. *Turnabout: New Help for the Woman Alcoholic.* New York: Bantam Books, 1990.

Knigge, Barbara, Elizabeth Farrell, and Patricia Pardun. *Women's Voices: Our Process of Recovery.* Center City, Minn.: Hazelden Educational Materials, 1993.

Robertson, Nan. *Getting Better: Inside Alcoholics Anonymous.* New York: William Morrow, 1988.

Vogler, Roger, and Wayne Bartz. *Teenagers and Alcohol: When Saying No Isn't Enough.* Philadelphia: The Charles Press, 1992.

Wegscheider-Cruse, Sharon. *Another Chance: Hope and Health for the Alcoholic Family.* Science & Behavior Books, 1989.

Woititz, Janet Geringer. *Adult Children of Alcoholics.* Health Communications, 1990.

RELATED TOPICS

Bepko, Claudia, and Jo-Ann Krestan, *Too Good for Her Own Good: Searching for Self and Intimacy in Important Relationships.* New York: HarperPerennial, 1990.

Borysenko, Joan. *A Woman's Book of Life: The Biology, Psychology, and Spirituality of the Feminine Life Cycle.* New York: Riverhead Books, 1996.

Chernin, Kim. *The Hungry Self: Women, Eating, and Identity.* New York: HarperPerennial, 1994.

Covington, Stephanie, and Linda Beckett. *Leaving the Enchanted Forest: The Path from Relationship Addiction to Intimacy.* HarperSanFrancisco, 1988.

Edelman, Hope. *Motherless Daughters: The Legacy of Loss.* New York: Addison-Wesley, 1994.

Kasl, Charlotte Davis. *Women, Sex, and Addiction: A Search for Love and Power.* New York: Ticknor & Fields, 1989.

Lerner, Harriet G. *The Dance of Anger.* New York: Harper & Row, 1985.

Rapping, Elayne. *The Culture of Recovery: Making Sense of the Self-Help Movement in Women's Lives.* Boston: Beacon Press, 1997.

Scarf, Maggie. *Unfinished Business: Pressure Points in the Lives of Women.* Garden City, N.Y.: Doubleday & Company, 1980.

Viorst, Judith. *Necessary Losses: The Loves, Illusions, Dependencies, and Impossible Expectations That All of Us Have to Give Up in Order to Grow.* New York: Fireside, 1986.

Young-Eisendrath, Polly. *Women and Desire: Beyond Wanting to Be Wanted.* New York: Harmony Books, 1999.

Index

African-American Family Services
(AAFS):
 antidrug efforts of, 276, 277
 culturally specific work of, 238–39,
  240, 248–49
 founding of, 249
 holistic approach of, 245–46
 multitude of programs of, 249–50
 violence elimination programs of,
  242, 250
 women's program of, 242–43,
  250–52, 258, 271–72, 283–84
African-American women, 50
 adolescent, 97
 attitudes on alcohol use of,
  276–77
 communication styles of, 240
 cultural pain experienced by, 249,
  274–76
 drug use of, 277–79
 fetal alcohol syndrome and, 32, 82,
  277
 insurance coverage of, 289
 motherhood-related prosecutions of,
  83, 278–79
 recovery groups of, 300
 sexual pressures on, 263–65,
  274–75
 slave history of, 274–75
age, alcohol/drug tolerance decreased
 with, 30
aging, losses of, 174
AIDS, 278
Al-Anon, 59–60, 61, 308, 327
alcohol dehydrogenase (ADH), 13
Alcoholics Anonymous (AA), 327
 anonymity stressed in, 238
 apolitical stance of, 144
 confessional step of, 315–16

confrontational strategies in, 241
dependency problems transformed
 within, 158
as disciplined program for change,
 139–40
diverse attendance of, 238
on enabling relationships, 307–8
female membership of, 7, 114–15,
 293, 299–301
first female recovery in, xiv
founder of, 6, 296–97
male alcoholic model addressed in,
 5–7
power concepts of, 287–88, 293,
 298, 301
psychotherapy vs., 234–35
recovery vernacular of, 114, 314
safe emotional atmosphere of, 67
self-critical approach of, 139, 141,
 298–300
sexual-abuse survivors in, 215
for teenagers, 115
variety among meeting groups in,
 143–44, 301
women's self-help alternatives to,
 74, 141, 144–45, 162–63, 293,
 300
alcoholism:
 alcohol sensitivity vs., 13–14
 denial of, 206–7, 226
 diagnosis of, 27, 225–33, 325–26
 disease concept of, 16–17, 139–41,
  238, 286, 298
 early intervention against, 137,
  287–88, 317
 environmental influences on, 10–11,
  33, 177, 192
 genetic risk of, xii, 9–10, 11,
  12–15, 33, 176–77